CONTEMPORARY COGNITIVE THERAPY

Contemporary Cognitive Therapy

Theory, Research, and Practice

Edited by
ROBERT L. LEAHY

THE GUILFORD PRESS
New York   London

© 2004 The Guilford Press
A Division of Guilford Publications, Inc.
72 Spring Street, New York, NY 10012
www.guilford.com

Chapter 1 © 2004 Christine A. Padesky

Printed in the United States of America

This book is printed on acid-free paper.

Last digit is print number: 9   8   7   6   5   4   3   2   1

Library of Congress Cataloging-in-Publication Data

Contemporary cognitive therapy : theory, research, and practice / edited by
    Robert L. Leahy.
       p. cm.
    Includes bibliographical references and index.
    ISBN 1-59385-062-X (hardcover : alk. paper)
    1. Cognitive therapy.   I. Leahy, Robert L.
    RC489.C63C665 2004
    616.89′142—dc22   2004011772

For Aaron T. Beck, man of vision

About the Editor

Robert L. Leahy, PhD, is President of the International Association for Cognitive Psychotherapy, Founder and Director of the American Institute for Cognitive Therapy (*www.CognitiveTherapyNYC.com*), and Professor of Psychiatry at Weill–Cornell University Medical College. He is the author or editor of many publications, including *Roadblocks in Cognitive-Behavioral Therapy, Psychological Treatment of Bipolar Disorder* (with Sheri L. Johnson), *Overcoming Resistance in Cognitive Therapy, Cognitive Therapy Techniques,* and *Treatment Plans and Interventions for Depression and Anxiety Disorders* (with Stephen J. Holland).

Dr. Leahy is frequently invited to lecture nationally and internationally. He is Associate Editor of the *Journal of Cognitive Psychotherapy* (having served as Editor from 1998 to 2003) and is a Founding Fellow of the Academy of Cognitive Therapy. He serves on the Executive Committee of the International Association of Cognitive Psychotherapy, the Executive Board of the Academy of Cognitive Therapy, and the Scientific Advisory Committee of the National Alliance for the Mentally Ill, as well as on advisory committees for numerous national and international conferences on cognitive-behavioral therapy.

Contributors

Judith S. Beck, PhD, Beck Institute for Cognitive Therapy, Bala Cynwyd, Pennsylvania

Dianne L. Chambless, PhD, Department of Psychology, University of Pennsylvania, Philadelphia, Pennsylvania

David A. Clark, PhD, Department of Psychology, University of New Brunswick, Fredericton, New Brunswick, Canada

David M. Clark, PhD, Department of Psychology, Institute of Psychiatry, London, United Kingdom

Frank M. Dattilio, PhD, Department of Psychiatry, Harvard University Medical School, Boston, Massachusetts

Robert J. DeRubeis, PhD, Department of Psychology, University of Pennsylvania, Philadelphia, Pennsylvania

Anke Ehlers, PhD, Department of Psychology, Institute of Psychiatry, London, United Kingdom

Norman B. Epstein, PhD, Department of Family Studies, University of Maryland, College Park, Maryland

Arthur Freeman, EdD, Department of Clinical Psychology, Philadelphia College of Osteopathic Medicine, Philadelphia, Pennsylvania

Steven D. Hollon, PhD, Department of Psychology, Vanderbilt University, Nashville, Tennessee

Rick E. Ingram, PhD, Department of Psychology, Southern Methodist University, Dallas, Texas

Janet Klosko, PhD, private practice, Great Neck, New York

Robert L. Leahy, PhD, American Institute for Cognitive Therapy, New York, New York

Cory F. Newman, PhD, Center for Cognitive Therapy, University of Pennsylvania School of Medicine, Philadelphia, Pennsylvania

Christine A. Padesky, PhD, Center for Cognitive Therapy, Huntington Beach, California, *www.padesky.com*

Michael Peterman, PhD, Department of Psychology, University of North Carolina, Chapel Hill, North Carolina

James Pretzer, PhD, Cleveland Center for Cognitive Therapy, Beachwood, Ohio

Neil A. Rector, PhD, Centre for Addiction and Mental Health, University of Toronto, Toronto, Ontario, Canada

John H. Riskind, PhD, Department of Psychology, George Mason University, Fairfax, Virginia

Christine D. Scher, PhD, Department of Psychology, California State University, San Bernardino, California

Jan Scott, MD, Department of Psychological Medicine, Institute of Psychiatry, London, United Kingdom

Zindel V. Segal, PhD, Centre for Addiction and Mental Health, University of Toronto, Toronto, Ontario, Canada

Adrian Wells, PhD, School of Psychiatry and Behavioural Sciences, University of Manchester, Manchester, United Kingdom

Jesse H. Wright, MD, PhD, Department of Psychiatry and Behavioral Sciences, University of Louisville School of Medicine, Louisville, Kentucky

Jeffrey Young, PhD, Department of Psychiatry, Columbia University, New York, New York

Preface

The idea for this book grew from a full-day preconference meeting at the Association for Advancement of Behavior Therapy in November 2001. A number of leading cognitive therapists who had worked with Aaron T. Beck presented their work. This was to be the "Beck Festschrift." Appropriately, the conference was in Philadelphia—the Mecca of cognitive therapy—and the audience was standing room only. The speakers were Christine Padesky, Zindel Segal, John Riskind, David A. Clark, Cory Newman, Kelly Bemis Vitousek, James Pretzer, Norman Epstein, Robert DeRubeis, Steve Hollon, Jan Scott, Andy Butler, Greg Brown, Dianne Chambless, Judith Beck, Jeffrey Young, Neil Rector, Jesse Wright, and Art Freeman. The closing comments were by Aaron Beck. I was honored to be asked to participate—and even more honored when Beck asked me to organize a book based on these presentations. Since some of our British colleagues were not able to make it to the conference, we invited them to contribute to the book as well.

Who is this Aaron T. Beck, and how did he merit a Festschrift?

The contributors to this book provide an answer to this question. In our opening chapter, Christine Padesky provides an historical review of Beck's life and work. By any standards, this is a remarkable life. At the writing of this preface, Beck—who is now 82—continues to make significant contributions. But Beck had to struggle as a lone voice in psychiatry against the dominant, if not doctrinaire, psychoanalysts. Beck got the patient off the couch and into the real world to test out their "cognitions" with behavioral experiments. He was a revolutionary of the mind—literally turning psychology on its head.

As Christine Padesky notes in her chapter, Aaron T. Beck is known as "Tim" to those who have been fortunate enough to get to know him personally. I must say, it took me a few years of calling him "Dr. Beck" to finally be corrected by him: "Call me Tim." So, Tim it is.

In any case, the first time I met Tim was at my interview for a post-doctoral fellowship at the Center for Cognitive Therapy. After meeting with Art Freeman, whose charisma and energy impress me to this day, I was led to a small, windowless office where I met a rather quiet, gentle-speaking, white-haired Tim Beck. I was fortunate enough to pass the Beck interview, and the following September I began the post-doc. Beck held a weekly "anxiety seminar," an open discussion of the cognitive processes of the different anxiety disorders. To this day, my thinking about clinical issues is affected by the probing—even, at times, relentless—questioning of "Why?" and "What does that mean?" Beck was a Piagetian of the mind—"How does this make sense to this person?" "How does hopelessness make sense?"

Tim led with an inquisitive open style of curiosity about what makes someone think—whatever he or she thinks. There was a sense among all of us that we were part of something much bigger than any one person; we were at the center of a new revolution in clinical psychology. Indeed, the only books to guide us in this new cognitive therapy were Beck's books on depression and cognitive therapy and the emotional disorders.

At that time, we thought we knew that cognitive therapy worked for depression, and we were beginning to see its value in anxiety. Norm Epstein was developing ideas about a cognitive therapy for couples. But there was nothing yet for substance abuse, families, personality disorders—or even the specific anxiety disorders. Tim was cautious about making any unsubstantiated claims about cognitive therapy as an effective treatment beyond a small range of problems.

This book is a testimony to the power of ideas. The cognitive model—or, I should say, the cognitive models—have been extended to a range of problems unforeseen during the early days of cognitive therapy. In the book, we have gathered many of the leading figures in the world, covering a range of topics including every anxiety disorder, unipolar and bipolar disorder, schizophrenia, couples and families, children and adolescents, borderline personality—even the use of pharmacotherapy.

Today there are cognitive therapy centers in most major cities in the United States and cognitive-behavioral organizations in every major country in the world. The 2004 World Congress of Cognitive Psychotherapy was held in Kobe, Japan, a long way from the halls of the University of Pennsylvania.

I can only imagine what thoughts and feelings were running through Tim's mind and heart at the 2001 Festschrift. The pursuit of truth and the courage to carve out a road less traveled has led to one of the most significant contributions in the history of psychiatry and psychology. I know that the contributors to this volume feel a strong connection to—and gratitude toward—Tim for providing us with the path.

The current volume recognizes the influence of Beck's work across a wide range of issues. Moreover, as testimony to the intellectual richness of the cognitive model, the reader will recognize that the chapters in this volume develop a number of "cognitive models"—models of psychopathology and treatment that were unforeseen in the early days of cognitive therapy. This is not a collection of individuals reminiscing about the "early days" but rather a collection of the cutting edges of the new frontiers of the field.

Although the earlier model stressed the nature of depressive cognition once the depressive episode was activated, it is important to recognize that the cognitive model also implied underlying or latent schemas that differentiated individuals with varied predispositions toward depression. Moreover, cognitive therapy directly addressed both the active cognitive distortions during depression and the cognitive diathesis. In the current volume, Christine Scher, Zindel Segal, and Rick Ingram (Chapter 2) and Steven Hollon and Robert DeRubeis (Chapter 3) review the evidence that provides support to a range of cognitive vulnerabilities to depression and the efficacy of cognitive therapy for depression. There can be no reasonable question that cognitive therapy is as effective as medication in the treatment of depression—and provides an added benefit of protection against suicidal risk and future depressive episodes.

The earlier model of schematic processing, maladaptive assumptions, and automatic thoughts—which characterized Beck's theories of depression and anxiety—has been expanded and elaborated into newer models of psychopathology and treatment. In the current volume, several leading researchers and theoreticians provide these new and effective models for a range of anxiety disorders. John Riskind's looming vulnerability model (Chapter 4) suggests a cognitive vulnerability to anxiety disorders that places emphasis on the imminence and impending danger of approaching threat. Dianne Chambless and Michael Peterman (Chapter 5) review the evidence supporting the efficacy of cognitive-behavioral treatments for generalized anxiety and panic disorders.

In Chapter 6, on decision making and psychopathology, I draw on the current cognitive psychology literature on how individuals utilize heuristics or self-protective strategies in making decisions. Since depressed and anxious individuals contemplate change—and especially the risk of change—I suggest that models of anxious and pessimistic decision making may assist us in understanding how these strategies makes sense to these individuals—even when they seem to be self-defeating to the clinician.

As will become apparent to the reader in these chapters, the cognitive model of anxiety has moved beyond the schematic model of evaluating threat and one's ability to cope with it. Indeed, several of these models share a metacognitive emphasis—with a focus on how anxious individuals evaluate their thoughts and emotions. Strategies of mental control, the sense of responsibility for one's intrusive thoughts, fear of losing control of one's thinking, and the tendency to pathologize one's mental processing are the cognitive vulnerabilities for the anxiety disorders. These mental strategies—and evaluations of one's own experience—are often adapted by anxious individuals to solve the problem of anxiety. Ironically, the solution has become the problem.

David M. Clark and Anke Ehlers delineate their cognitive model of posttraumatic stress disorder in Chapter 7, indicating how these individuals evaluate their intrusions and how a specific cognitive model of intervention can be employed. David A. Clark (Chapter 8) describes a cognitive model of obsessive–compulsive disorder, again emphasizing how individuals evaluate their intrusions and strategize on how to cope with them. In Chapter 9, Adrian Wells describes his metacognitive model of intrusion and mental control, indicating its relevance to understanding and treating generalized anxiety disorder, trauma, and depression.

The cognitive model—or, again, models—are applied to specific populations, with apparently no foreseeable limit to the groups that we can address. Cory Newman (Chapter 10) describes the utility of this approach in understanding and treating individuals with substance abuse—a major problem that is comorbid with every one of the disorders that we treat. In Chapter 11, Jan Scott reviews the new and exciting work on the use of cognitive models of treatment for bipolar disorder, a group that only 10 years ago was relegated to a biological diathesis and treatment approach. Today, psychological treatments—accompanied by the use of mood-stabilizing medications—help reduce the frequency, severity, and length of mood episodes, and reduce the necessity for hospitalization. Similarly, Neil Rector's review of the application of the cognitive model to schizophrenia (Chapter 12) offers new hope for combined pharmacological and psychosocial approaches. Again, an important element here is encouraging the patient to evaluate how delusions or hallucinations are processed or acted on. We should note that this is one of Tim Beck's current areas of research and interest, as he travels worldwide to lecture on his latest research and theory in this area.

Janet Klosko and Jeffrey Young (Chapter 13), James Pretzer and Judith Beck (Chapter 14), and Arthur Freeman (Chapter 15) review the latest advances in the treatment of personality disorders. Klosko and Young provide a model that integrates various approaches other than the cognitive model, including object relations theory, transactional analysis, and Gestalt theory. Pretzer and Beck describe the development of approaches to personality disorders, which now include an integration of cognitive and interpersonal phenomena in the model the authors elaborate. Of particular interest are the various cognitions that may have an impact on the patient's utilization of cognitive therapy interventions and the specific feedback mechanisms that may "verify" dysfunctional beliefs through schema-driven interpersonal strategies. Freeman develops a cognitive model for evaluating and treating personality disorders in children and adolescents. Given the extension of the cognitive model to younger age groups—and given the plausible assumption that personality disorders do not arise at voting age—Freeman's new territory for the cognitive model holds immense promise.

In Chapter 16, Jesse Wright reviews the importance of integrating pharmacological treatments with psychosocial treatments, such as cognitive therapy. Wright avoids the dichotomous thinking that suggests that psychopathology is *either* biological or psychological. Rather, he suggests how pharmacological approaches can enhance cognitive interventions and how cognitive therapy can increase the efficacy of and compliance with biological treatments. This is a balanced and empowering approach that Wright shows has relevance for depression, anxiety, bulimia nervosa, and psychosis—and one that practicing clinicians are likely to endorse.

Finally, Norman Epstein and Frank Dattilio, who have been contributing to their respective fields for over 20 years, provide reviews of the use of the cognitive model in treating couples and families. Epstein (Chapter 17) traces the history of the cognitive approach to couples and outlines methods for assessment, cognitive-behavioral interventions, and the current empirical status of these treatments. Dattilio (Chapter 18) begins his discussion with a review of the early "resistance" to a cognitive model in the family therapy field and then develops a detailed clinical-intervention model for cognitive family therapy that incorporates systems approaches that are commonly used by family therapists. Since each family member views the family dynamic through his or her own schematic process, addressing these different individual models can facilitate change.

We hope that these contributions will reflect admirably on Beck's legacy—to which he himself continues to make contributions. Quite infrequently in the field of psychology, someone comes along with a vision that changes everything. Tim Beck has given us this vision. He has taken the road less traveled—and it has made all the difference.

ROBERT L. LEAHY

Contents

Contents

Part I

INTRODUCTION

Aaron T. Beck

Mind, Man, and Mentor

CHRISTINE A. PADESKY

Aaron T. Beck has won more than 25 prestigious special recognition awards, including 4 lifetime achievement awards. And yet even those of us who have worked closely with "Tim" (as he is known to his friends) can lose sight of how revolutionary some of his accomplishments were, and how pervasive his influence continues to be on the leaders in our field— many of whom are represented in this book as chapter authors. All the research and theories presented in this book relate to Beck's seminal ideas.

This chapter provides a frame for the remainder of the book by offering an overview of Beck's career to date in three broad areas. The first section, "Beck: Mind," provides a brief synopsis of his key conceptual, empirical, and psychotherapy contributions. Second, "Beck: Man" suggests how his personal qualities and the environmental context in which he works have fostered his wide influence. Third, to understand his sociological influence on the field, in "Beck: Mentor" I extract the values he models that mark his career and inspire all of us who follow.

Personal commentaries in this chapter are based on observations of Tim Beck since 1978. During this time, I have enjoyed a close professional relationship and friendship with him, and our interactions on various projects and at professional meetings have led to a wealth of insight-laden anecdotes. Those who are intrigued by this chapter and wish to pursue a more thorough review of Beck's life can read Weishaar's (1993) articulate biography of Beck.

The impetus for this book was a Festschrift honoring Beck in November 2001. Festschrifts are usually held in honor of people who have made great empirical or conceptual contributions to a field. Beck's conceptual and empirical contributions are considered among the greatest in the history of psychology and psychiatry. In addition, he not only introduced a new form of psychotherapy; he was a pioneer in the development of an empirically validated system of psychotherapy (Padesky & Beck, 2003).

Beck's influence on conceptualization, research, and psychotherapy in so many areas of clinical focus (e.g., depression, suicide, anxiety, schizophrenia, substance abuse, relationship anger, chronic pain) far exceeds the usual criteria for a Festschrift. Thus I propose a new term to celebrate work of such breadth and depth: a "Beckschrift." A Beckschrift would be celebrated on behalf of anyone who, in many different areas of clinical investigation, makes profound contributions in all three areas: conceptualization, empirical research, and psychotherapy. No one in the history of psychotherapy is as worthy of this recognition as Beck.

In addition to his extensive professional contributions in books and journals, Beck has spearheaded the development of an international network of researchers, clinicians, and educators. He has helped form a large, active community of those dedicated to developing and evaluating cognitive therapy. His personal effectiveness in shaping collaborative international efforts is remarkable and stands firmly with his publications as a success likely to influence the development of psychotherapy theory, practice, and research for decades to come.

BECK: MIND

An intriguing way to review Beck's publications is to recount key contributions for each decade. Since Beck was born in 1921, calendar decades roughly approximate his own personal decade shifts. In addition to indicating how old Beck was when he accomplished various career highlights, an age-related review is encouraging for younger colleagues and students, because Beck had fewer than 40 publications by the age of 50. That goal is attainable for many. For those reaching midcareer, the age tracking is more daunting: Beck published 370 articles and books between the ages of 50 and 80. At the time this volume went to press, he had already published an additional 60 articles and 2 books in the opening years of his ninth decade. He is a case study for those who argue that there is no reason why productivity needs to decline with age.

A longitudinal view also shows how Beck's ideas have evolved over time. It captures more accurately the slow pooling of innovative and substantive ideas that preceded the rapid expansion of his vision and influence. The quick expansion of cognitive therapy since 1990 is remarkable—and yet by that time cognitive therapy had already experienced nearly three decades of development, many of these years below the radar of mainstream psychology.

The 1940s

While in his 20s, Beck completed his undergraduate degree at Brown University, received a medical degree from Yale University, and completed residencies in pathology and psychiatry (Weishaar, 1993). Showing early promise as a diligent scholar, Beck won awards for scholarship and oratory at Brown and for research during his first residency.

The 1950s

During the 1950s, Beck continued his psychiatric studies—first at the Austen Riggs Center in Stockbridge, Massachusetts, and then at the Philadelphia Psychoanalytic Society, where he graduated as a psychoanalyst in 1956 (at age 35). He also began a long and fruitful career on the faculty of the University of Pennsylvania starting as an instructor in psychiatry. By the end of this decade he was an assistant professor in psychiatry. Within 40 years, the University of Pennsylvania would name him University Professor Emeritus in the Department of Psychiatry.

He published his first psychiatric articles in the 1950s. Two of these are seminal for cognitive therapy. In 1952 (at age 31) he published his first psychiatric article, a case study of treatment of schizophrenic delusion (Beck, 1952). Fifty years later, his case study was republished and discussed within the "new" framework for cognitive therapy of schizophrenia (Beck, 1952/2002a, 2002b). This was the first of many early Beck publications recognized later as a significant precursor to innovative cognitive therapy developments.

The middle of this decade comprises 3 of the 6 "missing years" of Beck's presence in psychiatry. There have been only 6 years since 1952 in which he did not publish at least one paper. These years are 1955, 1957, 1958, 1960, 1965, and 1966. It is not coincidental that Tim's children were born in 1952, 1954, 1956, and 1959. Apparently one child is compatible with publishing, but several toddlers and young children make publishing more difficult. His active role as a parent accounts for a publishing decline in his 30s. The lack of publications in 1965 and 1966 reflects years dedicated to writing his first book.

A study at the end of this decade (Beck & Hurvich, 1959) foreshadowed the end of his psychoanalytic career and the beginning of cognitive therapy, even though no one, including Beck, foresaw its significance at the time. Beck set out to empirically demonstrate the psychoanalytic theory that depression is anger turned inward. He predicted that the dreams of depressed patients would support this theory. In fact, his hypothesis was not supported. The content of dreams in depressed patients was similar to the content of their waking thoughts (self-critical, pessimistic, and negative). To his credit, Beck did not discard these unexpected data. Instead, over the next decade, his belief in the psychoanalytic theory of depression gradually eroded, and Beck set out to develop a new empirically derived theory of depression.

The 1960s

As he approached age 40, Beck began to take a new look at depression and developed a new instrument to measure it—the Beck Depression Inventory (Beck, Ward, Mendelson, Mock, & Erbaugh, 1961). Over time, this simple self-report scale became one of the most widely used measures of depression, updated in 1996 as the Beck Depression Inventory—II (Beck & Steer, 1996). The Beck Depression Inventory not only captures signature changes in mood, but also taps changes in motivation, physical functioning, and cognitive features of depression.

He began to notice characteristic "cognitive distortions" that occur in depression (Beck, 1963). His empirical observations led Beck to begin to view this "mood" disorder as primarily a thinking disorder. Beck's clinical observations and empirical findings were published in 1967 in a landmark book—*Depression: Clinical, Experimental, and Theoretical Aspects* (Beck, 1967), republished a few years later as *Depression: Causes and Treatment* (Beck, 1967/1972). In this text he reviewed the current biological and psychological theories of depression (including "manic–depression," now called "bipolar disorder") and the empirical evidence in favor of each. Then he outlined a new cognitive theory of depression, based on findings in his own research and the related research of others.

Many new and enduring concepts related to depression were introduced in this book. Beck coined the term "automatic thoughts" to describe the thoughts that occur spontaneously throughout the day. He showed how, in depression, these thoughts are characteristically negative and include many negative cognitive distortions. He demonstrated how a "negative cognitive triad" (the negative beliefs depressed people hold about themselves, the world, and the future) could lead to the emotional and motivational symptoms in depression. His book also proposed a new "schema" theory to describe systematic interactions between cognition and emotion. The final sentence of his theoretical presentation of his cognitive model quietly upended the psychoanalytic theory he had set out to support a decade earlier: "The relative absence of anger in depression is attributed to the displacement of schemas relevant to blaming others by schemas of self-blame" (Beck, 1967, p. 290).

The 1970s

Beck's contributions increased exponentially after he turned 50 in 1971. In the final 12 pages of Beck's 1967 book, he outlined some broad ideas about how cognitive therapy for depression might work, including the importance of identifying and testing the beliefs maintaining the depression. During the 1970s he worked with many colleagues, students, and residents at the University of Pennsylvania to detail and refine these ideas, published at the end of the decade in *Cognitive Therapy for Depression* (Beck, Rush, Shaw, & Emery, 1979).

Just as Beck's book on the cognitive theory of depression introduced new concepts that transformed professional dialogues about depression, the new treatment manual included ideas that were revolutionary in psychotherapy practice. Behavior therapists had introduced empirical data collection into psychotherapy, but in most cases in behavior therapy at that time, the therapist was the empiricist in treatment; the client was a source of data or a data collector. Beck introduced the concept of "collaborative empiricism" to convey that the therapist and client could form an equal working partnership. Both therapist and client devise experiments and proposed ideas about how to test key beliefs and evaluate the effectiveness of particular behavioral strategies. Therapists were urged to encourage clients' curiosity and active engagement in therapy procedures.

New therapy procedures included imagination exercises to capture automatic thoughts linked to depression; thought records to identify and test these automatic thoughts; and behavioral experiments to evaluate beliefs related to motivation and coping strategies. These procedures were intertwined with a new interviewing style that Beck called "Socratic questioning." Socratic questioning requires a therapist to ask a client questions to retrieve information relevant to depressed automatic thoughts that is out of awareness in the depressed state, but easily accessible with prompting. For example, a depressed client who thinks, "I never do anything right," is asked questions to recall prior and current accomplishments. New information, once considered, helps balance depressive conclusions about self, world, and future (the negative cognitive triad) and temporarily lifts mood. Furthermore, cognitive therapy took a bold step in asserting that clients can learn to do this process themselves, to reduce the long-term need for a therapist and to prevent relapse. The self-help nature of cognitive therapy contradicted the Zeitgeist of the time that only highly trained therapists could understand and treat psychological problems.

Cognitive Therapy for Depression was one of the first attempts to detail step-by-step therapy procedures. In addition, prior to its publication, Beck and colleagues conducted a treatment outcome study to evaluate and demonstrate its effectiveness (Rush, Beck, Kovacs, & Hollon, 1977). Other clinical research teams also empirically evaluated the treatment protocol and found it to be an effective treatment for depression (cf. Blackburn, Bishop, Glen, Whalley, & Christie, 1981)—the first psychotherapy treatment to do as well as or better than pharmacological treatments of depression.

The combination of a detailed treatment protocol manual with outcome research was an innovation in psychotherapy practice that had only previously been attempted by behavior therapists in treating discrete behavioral problems. By accomplishing the same feat with a more complex set of clinical interventions that included cognitive, emotional, and behavioral components, Beck pioneered a model for what psychologists many years later defined as an "empirically validated psychological treatment" (Task Force on Promotion and Dissemination of Psychological Procedures, 1995; Task Force on Psychological Intervention Guidelines, 1995).

Beck also developed international renown in the theory and prediction of suicide. He identified hopelessness as a key cognitive predictor of suicide (Beck, Brown, & Steer, 1989; Beck, Kovacs, & Weissman, 1975; Minkoff, Bergman, Beck, & Beck, 1973), even when suicide was studied in the context of drug abuse (Weissman, Beck, & Kovacs, 1979) or other factors previously recognized as prime correlates of suicide. He developed and validated a series of scales to help measure suicide risk, including the Beck Hopelessness Scale (Beck, Weissman, Lester, & Trexler, 1974), the Beck Suicide Intent Scale (Beck, Schuyler, & Herman, 1974), and the Beck Scale for Suicidal Ideation (Beck, Kovacs, & Weissman, 1979). Work begun in this decade continues to shape the profession's understanding of suicide and clinical interventions designed to prevent suicide (cf. Brown, Beck, Steer, & Grisham, 2000; Weishaar, 1996, 2004; Weishaar & Beck, 1992).

Simultaneously with these in-depth explorations of depression and suicide, Beck proposed wider applications of his cognitive theory and methods. In his first book written for lay readers, *Cognitive Therapy and the Emotional Disorders* (Beck, 1976), Beck eloquently described his therapy and cognitive theory of emotions. He proposed that clinical depression and anxiety are on a continuum with normal emotional experiences, and that all emotional experiences are linked to cognitions. Beck outlined his theory of cognitive specificity, in which each emotion is associated with particular cognitive themes. Depression is paired with cognitive themes of pessimism, self-criticism, and hopelessness. Anxiety is accompanied by cognitive themes of threat, danger, and vulnerability. Anger is marked by themes of violation and hurt, along with perceptions of others as malevolent.

The 1980s

Just as Beck dramatically transformed psychological views of depression and suicide in the 1970s, in the 1980s he and his colleagues created new frameworks for understanding anxiety, substance abuse, and relationship conflict. In addition, Beck devoted significant time and energy during this decade to creation of an interactive and visible international community of scholars. Beck initiated an international meeting of cognitive therapists and researchers in Philadelphia (1983) and encouraged subsequent meetings in Umeå, Sweden (1986) and Oxford, England (1989) for the increasingly well-attended World Congresses of Cognitive Therapy. Beck made it clear to colleagues that he was as committed to collaborative empiricism among researchers and therapists as between therapists and clients.

His cognitive model of anxiety (Beck & Emery with Greenberg, 1985) is his best-known contribution of this decade. Using an evolutionary model to demonstrate the adaptive nature of anxiety, Beck proposed that all anxiety results from overestimations of danger and/or underestimations of coping and resources. Based on empirical findings (Beck, Laude, & Bohnert, 1974), he also noted that anxiety is often accompanied by images. Therefore, methods for identifying and testing images were elaborated in greater detail in this anxiety text than in previous cognitive therapy texts.

Just as he had done for depression, Beck developed and validated a scale for measuring anxiety, the Beck Anxiety Inventory (Beck, Epstein, Brown & Steer, 1988; Beck & Steer, 1990). Despite the strength of Beck's general cognitive theory of anxiety, he did not develop a single protocol for treating anxiety. Due to the idiosyncratic nature of specific cognitions in various anxiety disorders, specific treatment protocols were developed for each of the anxiety disorder diagnoses. Many researchers and theorists contributed to development and empirical evaluation of these treatment models, as described in detail in Chapters 4, 5, 7, 8, and 9 of this book.

In addition to anxiety, Beck worked with colleagues to develop cognitive models of stress (Pretzer, Beck, & Newman, 1989) and anger (Beck, 1988). His cognitive model of anger was applied to couple conflict in his popular press book *Love Is Never Enough* (Beck, 1988). In this book, he demonstrates how the same principles of cognitive distortion delineated for depression and anxiety can operate within close relationships and turn love into hate. Furthermore, he shows how cognitive therapy principles can help calm the turmoil in relationships, and can restore and maintain positive relationships.

Beck also was principal investigator or coinvestigator for several large national research grants examining the utility of cognitive therapy with substance abuse, particularly heroin, cocaine, and alcohol abuse. Although his involvement in substance abuse research began as an adjunct to his studies of suicide (Beck, Steer, & Shaw, 1984; Beck, Weissman, & Kovacs, 1976; Weissman et al., 1979), Beck's work in this area gradually shifted to development of a cognitive model for understanding addiction and delineation of successful treatment methods (Beck, Wright, Newman, & Liese, 1993).

The 1990s

By the 1990s, cognitive therapy was no longer a novel therapy; it had become a mainstream choice for effective brief therapy for depression and anxiety among therapists in North America and the United Kingdom. As Beck entered his 70s, cognitive therapy for depression had been so widely studied that a new book summarizing the empirical findings relevant to cognitive theory and therapy was merited: *Scientific Foundations of Cognitive Theory and Therapy of Depression* (Clark & Beck with Alford, 1999). The publication of *Cognitive Therapy with Inpatients: Developing a Cognitive Milieu* (Wright, Thase, Beck, & Ludgate, 1993) recognized that cognitive therapy was becoming a widely disseminated model for inpatient programs. In addition, cognitive therapy was rapidly spreading throughout the world, as cognitive therapy texts were translated into many different languages.

While continuing his research and refinements of the treatments for depression, suicide, and anxiety disorders, Beck increasingly turned his attention to applications of cognitive therapy to more complex problems. To do so, he both articulated new aspects of cognitive theory and clarified how traditional cognitive concepts could explain such diverse human experiences as panic disorder and schizophrenia (Alford & Beck, 1997).

Cognitive Therapy of Personality Disorders (Beck, Freeman, et al., 1990) offered the first vision of longer-term cognitive therapy as applied to personality disorders—diagnoses usually considered treatment-resistant. In this book Beck employed his schema theory to provide a detailed developmental cognitive theory of personality. Several years later he expanded his schema theory to include the concepts of "modes," defined as "networks of cognitive, affective, motivational, and behavioral components," and "charges," which "explain the fluctuations in the intensity gradients of cognitive structures" (Beck, 1996, p. 2). Early research findings regarding cognitive therapy for personality disorders are encouraging (Pretzer & Beck, 1996; Beck, Freeman, et al., 2004). The demonstration that beliefs alone could differentially discriminate among personality disorder diagnoses lent some empirical support for his cognitive theory of personality (Beck et al., 2001). Chapter 14 of this volume reviews the current status of this still-evolving cognitive therapy application.

In the latter half of this decade, Beck wrote *Prisoners of Hate: The Cognitive Basis of Anger, Hostility, and Violence* (Beck, 1999) to show how the cognitive model for anger can explain larger conflicts as well as it describes interfamilial interpersonal conflicts. He then offers concrete ideas derived from cognitive theory and therapy for healing broad global, national, religious, and ethnic divisions.

Beck increasingly focused his attention on new cognitive models and therapies for schizophrenia as the 20th century came to a close (Alford & Beck, 1994; Beck, 1994; Beck & Rector, 1998). His first psychiatric paper as a young psychiatrist had addressed therapy for schizophrenic delusions (Beck, 1952). Preliminary research was demonstrating that his modern cognitive therapy might prove a mighty intervention for all schizophrenic symptoms (Beck, 2000).

The 2000s

Hearing Beck speak about cognitive therapy of schizophrenia, one would not think he has been thinking, writing, and practicing psychiatry for more than 50 years. He expresses the enthusiasm of someone newly discovering cognitive therapy when he describes the growing empirical evidence that cognitive therapy can effectively help persons with schizophrenia (Beck & Rector, 2002; Morrison, 2002; Rector & Beck, 2001, 2002; Warman & Beck, 2003).

In 2001, Beck celebrated his 80th birthday. This landmark is often accompanied by fond memories of a life well lived. Beck marked the start of his ninth decade with the publication of his 15th book, *Bipolar Disorder: A Cognitive Therapy Approach* (Newman, Leahy, Beck, Reilly-Harrington, & Gyulai, 2002). This was one of nearly 40 publications for him in 2001 and 2002, spanning the topics of depression, suicide, panic disorder, personality disorders, schizophrenia, obsessive–compulsive disorder, geriatric medical outpatients, and the Clark–Beck Obsessive–Compulsive Inventory (Clark & Beck, 2002).

The *Beck Youth Inventories of Emotional and Social Impairment* (J. S. Beck & Beck with Jolly, 2001) assess symptoms of depression, anxiety, anger, disruptive behavior, and self-concept in children. These measures suggest an additional emphasis for Beck and colleagues on using cognitive theory and therapy with children for purposes of prevention, early identification, and treatment of problems.

As evidenced by the publications just described, as well as his first book on cognitive therapy for chronic pain (Winterowd, Beck, & Gruener,

2003), Beck continues to expand, elaborate, refine, and conduct empirical research on the many implications and applications of his cognitive theory and therapy. The second edition of *Cognitive Therapy of Personality Disorders* (Beck et al., 2004) further articulated his theory of personality and elaborated the cognitive therapy treatment of personality disorders. Between 1952 and the time the present volume went to press, he has published 17 books and more than 450 articles and book chapters. Surely Beck is one of the most prolific thinkers and writers in the history of psychiatry.

Of course, the quality of what one publishes is more important than the quantity. Beck's career models the exponential effectiveness of working equally hard in the areas of conceptualization, empirical research, and therapy applications. His discoveries and innovations in each area are enhanced by knowledge gained in the other two areas.

For example, beginning with the 1959 paper on dream content of depressed patients (Beck & Hurvich, 1959), his *empirical* work in the area of depression preceded development of his cognitive *theory* of depression, first published in 1967. His *therapy*, so familiar to us today, developed over the next 15 years; principles of that therapy protocol were first published between 1974 and 1979. Yet, even while the psychotherapy was developing, the empirical work continued with carefully constructed outcome studies. Beck continues to this day to refine his conceptual model for depression, informed by new research and psychotherapy practices (Clark et al., 1999).

Table 1.1 summarizes the links among his contributions in the areas of conceptualization, empiricism, and development of his psychotherapy. Each date listed in Table 1.1 is generally that of the first published work in which the concept or finding was described by Beck. In some cases, a date range is cited because his ideas developed and were elaborated in print over a time span. A scan of Table 1.1 shows how empirical studies occur before and after conceptual breakthroughs. Psychotherapy developments both follow and lead research and new conceptual models. Furthermore, Beck continues to be active in all these areas today. For example, in 2003 he published works related to anxiety, depression, schizophrenia, psychosis, personality disorders, suicide, and chronic pain.

BECK: MAN

It is not only the sheer brilliance of his *mind* that has led to Beck's central role in the evolution of psychotherapy over the past 50 years. Early in his career, Beck envisioned a science of mind, emotion, behavior, and social context to stand proudly alongside the sciences of biochemistry and neuroscience that also inform psychiatry. Beck helped form this new cognitively based biopsychosocial science; he also gave birth to a movement and a

TABLE 1.1. Beck's Original Contributions on Selected Topics

Focus	Conceptual innovations	Empirical contributions	Psychotherapy
Depression	Cognitive distortions (1963) Cognitive model (1967) Automatic thoughts (1967) Cognitive triad (1970)	Dream content not masochistic (1959) Beck Depression Inventory (1961–1996) Outcome studies (1977–1982)	Cognitive therapy (CT) for depression (1974–1979): "Collaborative empiricism" Thought records Behavioral experiments Socratic questioning

Anxiety disorders	Cognitive model of anxiety (1972–1979):
	  Overestimations of danger
	  Underestimations of coping/ resources
	Cognitive specificity (1976–1994)
		Beck Anxiety Inventory (1988)
		Outcome studies (1988–1997)
		Clark–Beck Obsessive–Compulsive Inventory (2002)
			CT principles of treatment (1976–1985)
			Idiosyncratic nature of automatic thoughts
			Importance of imagery

Schizophrenia	Cognitive model of schizophrenia (1979–present)	Case study (1952) Outcome studies (1994–present)	CT of schizophrenia (1994–present)
Suicide	Hopelessness as key (1973)	Predictors of suicide (1971–2001) Beck Hopelessness Scale (1974) Suicidal Intent Scale (1974) Scale for Suicidal Ideation (1979)	CT for suicidal behavior (1990)
Personality	Schema theory (1967) Cognitive model (1990) Theory of modes (1996)	Dysfunctional Attitude Scale (1991) Sociotropy and Autonomy Scales (1991) Personality Belief Questionnaire (1995)	CT for personality disorders (1990–present)
Addictions	Links to depression (1977–present) Links to suicide (1975–present)	Links to depression (1977–present) Links to suicide (1975–present) Outcome studies (1997–1999)	CT for substance abuse (1983–2001)

community of researchers, educators, and therapists loyal to him and his vision.

How is it that he has been able to form such a vibrant and active community of scientist-practitioners? How has Beck generated such enthusiasm with his ideas, often simple, such as the link between thoughts and emotion? Others have proposed similar ideas over the years, and yet they do not stand as tall in our minds as Beck does. In this section, Beck's personal qualities and the environmental contexts in which he has lived are linked to his ability to build a robust community of cognitive therapists and researchers.

Curiosity

The fruits of his mind have already been reviewed. What qualities of mind contribute to such productive efforts? It goes without saying that Beck is highly intelligent. One of the most important features of Beck's intelligence is curiosity. Those who know him well expect every encounter to include questions and exploration of new ideas. I have enjoyed listening to Beck question servers in restaurants, graduate students at conferences, and tennis players at courtside to gather information relevant to his theories. Since his theories strive to account for all human experiences, his insatiable curiosity serves him well.

Flexibility

Equally important, his thinking is flexible. It is rare for a leader in any field to be so open to changing his own theory and models based on empirical evidence. And yet Beck has done so again and again, firmly convinced that the best ideas are shaped by data. He is a positive thinker—not in the genre of Norman Vincent Peale, but in the school of those who see every obstacle as a problem waiting to be solved.

Vision

Beck envisioned revolutions in psychiatric theory and in psychotherapy. He envisioned wide acceptance of a theory of emotion that focused on beliefs. He envisioned an empirically based psychotherapy that would be short-term, would be effective, and could actively engage the client in solving problems. These visions have been achieved with greater professional and public acceptance than most would have expected. And yet his vision seems to be ever expanding. By the time cognitive therapy achieves a vision he held 10 years earlier, Beck has already increased his visionary efforts to encompass new challenges and applications. For this reason, Beck's visionary ideas hold the respect of his colleagues, even if some seem a bit improbable. Last decade's improbable ideas are already this decade's proudest achievements.

Personal Awareness

Beck is an active participant in the world. He uses lessons and opportunities throughout his life to build better models of theory, research, and therapy. Beck is aware of his own moods and is willing to learn from them. Many principles central to cognitive theory were derived from careful observation of his own moods and those of people around him. Just as is done in cognitive therapy, Beck tries to understand his own emotional reactions and use these constructively. He observes his own thinking processes and notes which experiences are convergent with and which are divergent from his theories. Such personal observations are then compared with the self-reports of others before empirical studies are constructed.

Persistence

Beck is renowned for his stamina, maintained by regular exercise, meditation, and a moderate diet. His work pace and the demands he places on those who work with him exhaust many of his younger colleagues. Even more important than physical endurance, Beck has great emotional and cognitive persistence. During the first 20 years he taught them, his cognitive therapy lectures and workshops were attended by only a handful of people, and these colleagues often arrived with great reservations toward and vocal criticism of his ideas. Yet he continued talking about cognitive theory with anyone who would accommodate him.

Audiences grew with cognitive therapy's success, yet even in the mid-1980s Beck's presentations were attended by skeptics and challenged by antagonistic voices. His simple ideas were revolutionary in their challenge of current theories and treatments, and he evoked the ire that revolutionary voices often do. Yet Beck persisted, encouraged by data when personal support was not forthcoming.

Environmental Contexts

Despite the antagonism of some colleagues, Beck benefited from the larger social and intellectual environments in which he worked. The spirit of collaboration in cognitive therapy was influenced by and received a receptive audience, in part because of the human empowerment movements of the 1960s and 1970s—civil rights, women's rights, and gay liberation. During the evolution of cognitive therapy, empiricism was on the rise in psychol-

ogy, due at least in part to a burgeoning respect for behaviorism. Cognitive
theory and therapy emerged at the dawn of a cognitive revolution in psychology and an emerging information-processing Zeitgeist in public discourse. Cognitive therapy is one of the few health-related services to benefit
from financial constraints on the health care marketplace at the beginning
of the 21st century. With fewer dollars, leading care providers started paying greater attention to brief therapies with empirically proven
effectiveness. Most of the time, this has meant that cognitive therapy is a
preferred therapy.

Community Leadership

However advantageous the environment, the spread of enthusiasm for cognitive therapy has been greatly enhanced by Beck's own behavior. His career is marked by productive collaborations with people in many countries
around the world. His interactions with colleagues are marked by generosity, loyalty, and kindness. As such, he has helped create a community of
cognitive therapists that lives by those values to the benefit of all.

His professional generosity is legendary. Many of today's leading cognitive therapists and researchers can point to early career advancements
that came about because of Beck. He has invited young scholars to participate in prestigious research projects, offered talented clinicians the opportunity to coteach workshops with him, and written numerous letters of rec-
ommendation for professionals around the globe.

My first invitation to coteach with Beck came in 1984, when I was a
recent PhD and 31 years old—the same age Beck was when he wrote his
first psychiatric paper. He invited me to coteach with him in Washington,
D.C., at a large workshop at the annual meeting of the Association for Advancement of Behavior Therapy. This and subsequent coteaching invita-
tions literally launched my career as a cognitive therapy workshop
presenter.

He is loyal and encourages loyalty among the cognitive therapy community. He has traveled thousands of miles to support the openings of cognitive therapy clinics and research institutes. He rarely makes negative comments about colleagues and privately takes to task cognitive therapists who
do. When he does offer criticism of a position or behavior among cognitive
therapists, such comments are backed by empirical evidence and bracketed
by an effort at understanding the other therapists' position.

His kindness toward colleagues is only surpassed by his kindness toward clients and other people in the community who might benefit from
cognitive therapy. In the hundreds of hours I have spent with Beck teaching
workshops, attending conferences, discussing theory, and having casual
conversations, he has never made a negative comment about a client. His

compassionate caring for others is the engine that drives his passion to improve cognitive therapy.

One personal story best illustrates the sincerity of Tim's personal caring. He and I were featured at an evening presentation for several hundred psychiatrists. At this event, we interviewed a volunteer patient from a local cognitive therapy psychiatric inpatient program, to discuss what she had learned about her depression during her stay in the hospital. She spoke about the suicide attempt that had led to her hospitalization and about the new hope cognitive therapy offered her.

The following morning, I met Tim at his hotel, and he asked me to drive him to the hospital before we began our planned activities. At the hospital, he and I met in a private consultation room with the woman who had been on stage with us the night before. Tim talked to her with gentle concern about the issues that had brought her into the hospital. He discussed her plans following discharge. Toward the end of this private meeting, he took out a piece of paper and began writing something down. He would often do this in conversations, so I assumed some new idea had occurred to him that he did not want to forget. At the end of our meeting, he handed the woman the piece of paper. "This is my home telephone number," he told her with a smile. "I want you to call me after you have been home a few weeks, to let me know how it is going for you." As we drove away from the hospital, all he said to me was this: "She was so generous in talking about her life so others can learn. This is a small thing I can do for her in return."

Community Vision

Beck's personal attitude toward patients is mirrored in the vision he holds for the cognitive therapy community. He strives to create a community that is global, inclusive, collaborative, empowering, and benevolent.

Global

Beck's vision for cognitive therapy has always been global. He never wanted to start an American Cognitive Therapy Association. Instead, he hosted the first World Congress of Cognitive Therapy in Philadelphia. He inspired the foundation of the International Association of Cognitive Psychotherapy. He was instrumental in the establishment of a global Academy of Cognitive Therapy to credential qualified cognitive therapists. And before any of these existed, he personally linked cognitive researchers, therapists and educators around the world. He nudged us to write, travel, and meet each other, encouraging friendships as well as work collaborations.

Inclusive

His community vision for cognitive therapy is inclusive, welcoming people from diverse educational and professional backgrounds (e.g., psychiatrists, psychologists, social workers, nurses, occupational therapists, pastoral counselors, drug abuse counselors), of all ages, races, ethnic identifications, sexual orientations, and religions. His inclusive values have led to dialogue and collaboration between colleagues from quite different cultural and professional communities.

In one cognitive therapy meeting, cognitive therapists from Israel offered to collaborate with cognitive therapists from neighboring Arab countries, even though the home nations of these cognitive therapists were politically hostile. Such interchanges please Beck enormously, because he wants cognitive therapists to form a single community with diverse membership. He dreams that cognitive theory as described in *Prisoners of Hate* (Beck, 1999) might contribute to world healing of divisions.

Collaborative

Beck encourages collaboration. Furthermore, he performs a matchmaking service to bring together colleagues for projects that he thinks would be improved by collaborative efforts. He models the strength inherent in sharing ideas by freely sharing his own ideas. When Beck speaks about cognitive therapy, he acknowledges the contributions of colleagues within and outside of cognitive therapy:

> In formulating my first theory of depression, I drew on some of the early cognitive psychologists such as Allport, Piaget, and particularly George Kelly. I was also influenced by the work of Karen Horney and Alfred Adler. Up to this point, I was not aware of the work of Ellis, which had been published primarily in papers in psychology journals (which I had not subscribed to) and in books. After my 1963 and 1964 papers were published, I was introduced to Ellis's work by a letter from Ellis, himself, who noted our work was similar. (Beck, personal communication, October 15, 2002)

In formal presentations, he describes the work of other cognitive therapists with such enthusiasm that a naïve listener may not recognize Beck's own work as the origin of novel advances.

Empowering

Beck empowers cognitive therapists around the world by supporting funding for cognitive therapy research; publicly recognizing others' contributions; citing international contributions in his own publications; and offering advice and other forms of help via e-mail, telephone, and in-person conversations. Such recognition by someone of Beck's stature can boost a researcher's standing in a university department or call public attention to a clinician's special skill. He also empowers others by encouraging them to undertake research, develop psychotherapy innovations, and initiate writing projects. Once, at lunch, he urged a graduate student to develop her own questionnaire rather than continue searching fruitlessly in the literature for an existing questionnaire related to her topic. Beck wrote the student's ideas on a napkin and endorsed her ideas as being as worthy of research as those in published questionnaires.

Benevolent

Finally, his vision is that the cognitive therapy community will be benevolent. He models behavior that is benevolent toward colleagues; he respects diverse ideas and helps others advance in their work. His therapy is designed to be benevolent toward and empowering of clients. He encourages cognitive therapists in conflict to work out disagreements amicably.

BECK: MENTOR

What can we learn from Beck as a mentor? When I think over the first 25 years of my relationship with Tim, I am struck by his intensity and focus. There is ferocity in his pursuit of ideas and research. And yet his ferocity is counterbalanced by respect for divergent ideas, and his intensity is counterbalanced by a sweetness of celebration when goals are met. Although he makes great demands on colleagues and students, he also offers great encouragement and enthusiasm when tasks are overwhelming.

The lesson I draw from observing Tim is that no single personal quality is as potent alone as in combination with a counterbalancing quality. In my opinion, Tim's great success is fostered by a combination of qualities that are remarkable in their coexistence. Table 1.2 shows paired qualities that I believe exemplify Beck in his work. These qualities can offer guidance to those who want to learn from Beck as a model for their own professional lives.

TABLE 1.2. Paired Beck Qualities

Visionary	Humble
Tenacious	Flexible
Independent	Collaborative
Data-driven	Heartfelt
Theoretical	Practical applications
Individualistic	Community-minded
Proud	Appreciative

Beck is visionary, and he also is humble. Those who want to emulate him should envision the big picture of human potential in order to reinvent and go beyond current theories. Yet it is equally important to stay humble to data and to what our clients, colleagues, and personal experience teach us.

Beck has terrific tenacity, and he also is flexible. To walk in his footsteps is to prepare for a marathon. To match his contributions, one should be tenacious in research projects, theory and therapy development, and dissemination of information to others. While being a persistent champion of what has been accomplished, it is equally important to stay flexible and integrate new ideas if they are backed by empirical support.

Beck has been an independent thinker, and he also collaborates with many. Independence of thought can be difficult. For many years, Beck had only a few colleagues who took his ideas seriously. And yet it is important to be willing to work hard—alone, if necessary—if one wants to chart new territory. It is also critical to the growth of ideas to collaborate with others when possible, so that ideas gain added strength and diversity of application.

Beck has followed the data, and he also has followed his heart. In this way, Beck is a humanistic scientist. Those who imitate him will be firmly wedded to the empirical foundations of theories and practice. Yet there is no conflict between a scientific commitment and careful concern for the human implications of work. Deep caring for the people with whom we work and whom our work touches ennobles the work we do. A focus on human need also provides a wise road map to those committed to making important career contributions.

This chapter illustrates how Beck exemplifies the balance of theory and practice more fully than most. Few people will be able to make such balanced and innovative contributions to theory, clinical practice, and empirical research. Yet each professional in a mental health field can make a commitment to learn more about theory, practice, and research, and to reflect each of these in his or her work.

Finally, Tim Beck has always been proud of his contributions, and at the same time very publicly appreciative of others' help and their influence on his work. All the contributors to this book are justifiably proud of all that has been accomplished during their careers. And we are also appreciative of and indebted to Tim Beck, who is one of very few who have given so much and contributed to so many areas of inquiry and service.

I end this chapter with a challenge to readers of this book, especially students and those at the beginning of their careers. If what you read leads you to greater appreciation of Beck's contributions, demonstrate your respect for him in ways that will be very meaningful to him. Try to emulate aspects of Beck's varied and valuable career to date: (1) Maintain a more curious mind; (2) learn from your own moods; (3) work with greater stamina; (4) learn to benefit from the environment in which you live and work; (5) be more collaborative, generous, and kind; (6) empower others; and (7) practice these steps with a global vision. These are ways we can all begin to thank Aaron T. Beck for his invaluable and enduring contributions to our field.

REFERENCES

Alford, B. A., & Beck, A. T. (1994). Cognitive therapy of delusional beliefs. *Behaviour Research and Therapy, 32*(3), 369–380.

Alford, B., & Beck, A. T. (1997). *The integrative power of cognitive therapy.* New York: Guilford Press.

Beck, A. T. (1952). Successful outpatient psychotherapy of a chronic schizophrenic with a delusion based on borrowed guilt. *Psychiatry, 15,* 305–312.

Beck, A. T. (1963). Thinking and depression: Idiosyncratic content and cognitive distortions. *Archives of General Psychiatry, 9,* 324–333.

Beck, A. T. (1967). *Depression: Clinical, experimental, and theoretical aspects.* New York: Harper & Row.

Beck, A. T. (1972). *Depression: Causes and treatment.* Philadelphia: University of Pennsylvania Press. (Original work published 1967)

Beck, A. T. (1976). *Cognitive therapy and the emotional disorders.* New York: International Universities Press.

Beck, A. T. (1988). *Love is never enough.* New York: Harper & Row.

Beck, A. T. (1994). Foreword. In D. Kingdon & D. Turkington (Eds.), *Cognitive-behavioral therapy of schizophrenia* (pp. v–vii). New York: Guilford Press.

Beck, A. T. (1996). Beyond belief: a theory of modes, personality, and psychopathology. In P. Salkovskis (Ed.), *Frontiers of cognitive therapy* (pp. 1–25). New York: Guilford Press.

Beck, A. T. (1999). *Prisoners of hate: The cognitive basis of anger, hostility and violence.* New York: HarperCollins.

Beck, A. T. (2000). Member's corner: Cognitive approaches to schizophrenia: A paradigm shift? Based on the 1999 Joseph Zubin Award Address. *Psychopathology Research, 10*(2), 3–10.

Beck, A. T. (2002a). Successful outpatient psychotherapy of a chronic schizophrenic with a delusion based on borrowed guilt: A 1952 case study (reprinted). In A. Morrison (Ed.), *A casebook of cognitive therapy for psychosis* (pp. 3–14). Hove, UK: Brunner-Routledge. (Original work published 1952)

Beck, A. T. (2002b). Successful outpatient psychotherapy of chronic schizophrenic with a delusion based on borrowed guilt: A 50–year retrospective (discussion). In A. Morrison (Ed.), *A casebook of cognitive therapy for psychosis* (pp. 15–19). Hove, UK: Brunner-Routledge.

Beck, A. T., Brown, G., & Steer, R. A. (1989). Prediction of eventual suicide in psychiatric inpatients by clinical rating of hopelessness. *Journal of Consulting and Clinical Psychology, 57*(2), 309–310.

Beck, A. T., Butler, A. C., Brown, G. K., Dahlsgaard, K. K., Beck, N., & Beck, J. S. (2001). Dysfunctional beliefs discriminate personality disorders. *Behaviour Research and Therapy, 39*(10), 1213–1225.

Beck, A. T., & Emery, G., with Greenberg, R. L. (1985). *Anxiety disorders and phobias: A cognitive perspective.* New York: Basic Books.

Beck, A. T., Epstein, N., Brown, G., & Steer, R. A. (1988). An inventory for measuring clinical anxiety: Psychometric properties. *Journal of Consulting and Clinical Psychology, 56*(6), 893–897.

Beck, A. T., Freeman, A., Davis, D. D., Pretzer, J., Fleming, B., Arntz, A., Butler, A., Fusco, G., Simon, K., Beck, J. S., Morrison, A., Padesky, C., & Renton, J. (2004). *Cognitive therapy of personality disorders* (2nd ed.). New York: Guilford Press.

Beck, A. T., Freeman, A., Pretzer, J., Davis, D., Fleming, B., Ottaviani, R., Beck, J., Simon, K., Padesky, C. A., Meyer, J., & Trexler, L. (1990). *Cognitive therapy of personality disorders.* New York: Guilford Press.

Beck, A. T., & Hurvich, M. S. (1959). Psychological correlates of depression: 1. Frequency of "masochistic" dream content in a private practice sample. *Psychosomatic Medicine, 21*(1), 50–55.

Beck, A. T., Kovacs, M., & Weissman, A. (1975). Hopelessness and suicidal behavior: An overview. *Journal of the American Medical Association, 234,* 1146–1149.

Beck, A. T., Kovacs, M., & Weissman, A. (1979). Assessment of suicidal intention: The Scale for Suicidal Ideation. *Journal of Consulting and Clinical Psychology, 47*(2), 343–352.

Beck, A. T., Laude, R., & Bohnert, M. (1974). Ideational components of anxiety neurosis. *Archives of General Psychiatry, 31,* 319–325.

Beck, A. T., & Rector, N. A. (1998). Cognitive therapy for schizophrenic patients. *Harvard Mental Health Letter, 15*(6), 4–6.

Beck, A. T., & Rector, N. A. (2002). Delusions: A cognitive perspective. *Journal of Cognitive Psychotherapy: An International Quarterly, 16*(4), 455–468.

Beck, A. T., Rush, A. J., Shaw, B. F., & Emery, G. (1979). *Cognitive therapy of depression.* New York: Guilford Press.

Beck, A. T., Schuyler, D., & Herman, I. (1974). Development of suicidal intent scales. In A. T. Beck, H. L. P. Resnik, & D. J. Lettieri (Eds.), *The prediction of suicide* (pp. 45–56). Bowie, MD: Charles Press.

Beck, A. T., & Steer, R. A. (1990). *Beck Anxiety Inventory manual.* San Antonio, TX: Psychological Corporation.

Beck, A. T., & Steer, R. A. (1996). Beck Depression Inventory—II. *Behavioral Measurements Letter, 3*(2), 3–5.

Beck, A. T., Steer, R. A., & Shaw, B. F. (1984). Hopelessness in alcohol- and heroin-dependent women. *Journal of Clinical Psychology, 40*(2), 602–606.

Beck, A. T., Ward, C. H., Mendelson, M., Mock, J., & Erbaugh, J. (1961). An inventory for measuring depression. *Archives of General Psychiatry, 4,* 561–571.

Beck, A. T., Weissman, A., & Kovacs, M. (1976). Alcoholism, hopelessness and suicidal behavior. *Journal of Studies on Alcohol, 37*(1), 66–77.

Beck, A. T., Weissman, A., Lester, D., & Trexler, L. (1974). The measurement of pessimism: The Hopelessness Scale. *Journal of Consulting and Clinical Psychology, 42*(6), 861–865.

Beck, A. T., Wright, F. D., Newman, C. F., & Liese, B. S. (1993). *Cognitive therapy of substance abuse.* New York: Guilford Press.

Beck, J. S., & Beck, A. T., with Jolly, J. (2001). *Beck Youth Inventories of Emotional and Social Impairment manual.* San Antonio, TX: Psychological Corporation.

Blackburn, I. M., Bishop, S., Glen, A. I. M., Whalley, L. J., & Christie, J. E. (1981). The efficacy of cognitive therapy in depression: A treatment trial using cognitive therapy and pharmacotherapy, each alone and in combination. *British Journal of Psychiatry, 139,* 181–189.

Brown, G. K., Beck, A. T., Steer, R. A., & Grisham, J. R. (2000). Risk factors for suicide in psychiatric outpatients: A 20-year prospective study. *Journal of Consulting and Clinical Psychology, 68*(3), 371–377.

Clark, D. A., & Beck, A. T. (2002). *Clark–Beck Obsessive–Compulsive Inventory manual.* San Antonio, TX: Psychological Corporation.

Clark, D. A., & Beck, A. T., with Alford, B. A. (1999). *Scientific foundations of cognitive theory and therapy of depression.* New York: Wiley.

Minkoff, K., Bergman, E., Beck, A. T., & Beck, R. (1973). Hopelessness, depression and attempted suicide. *American Journal of Psychiatry, 130*(4), 455–459.

Morrison, A. (Ed.). (2002). *A casebook of cognitive therapy for psychosis.* Hove, UK: Brunner-Routledge.

Newman, C. F., Leahy, R., Beck, A. T., Reilly-Harrington, N., & Gyulai, L. (2002). *Bipolar disorder: A cognitive therapy approach.* Washington, DC: American Psychological Association.

Padesky, C. A., & Beck, A. T. (2003). Science and philosophy: Comparison of cognitive therapy (CT) and rational emotive behavior therapy (REBT). *Journal of Cognitive Psychotherapy: An International Quarterly, 17,* 211–224.

Pretzer, J. L., & Beck, A. T. (1996). A cognitive theory of personality disorders. In J. Clarkin & M. F. Lenzenweger (Ed.), *Major theories of personality disorder* (pp. 36–105). New York: Guilford Press.

Pretzer, J. L., Beck, A. T., & Newman, C. (1989). Stress and stress management: A cognitive view. *Journal of Cognitive Psychotherapy: An International Quarterly, 3,* 163–179.

Rector, N. A., & Beck, A. T. (2001). Cognitive behavioral therapy for schizophrenia: An empirical review. *Journal of Nervous and Mental Disease, 189*(5), 278–287.

Rector, N. A., & Beck, A. T. (2002). Cognitive therapy for schizophrenia: From conceptualization to intervention. *Canadian Journal of Psychiatry, 47*(1), 39–48.

Rush, A. J., Beck, A. T., Kovacs, M., & Hollon, S. D. (1977). Comparative efficacy of cognitive therapy and pharmacotherapy in the treatment of depressed outpatients. *Cognitive Therapy and Research, 1*(1), 7–37.

Task Force on Promotion and Dissemination of Psychological Procedures. (1995). Training in and dissemination of empirically-validated psychological treatments: Report and recommendations. *The Clinical Psychologist, 48,* 3–23.

Task Force on Psychological Intervention Guidelines. (1995). *Template for developing guidelines: Interventions for mental disorders and psychosocial aspects of physical disorders.* Washington, DC: American Psychological Association.

Warman, D., & Beck, A. T. (2003). Cognitive behavioral therapy of schizophrenia: An overview of treatment. *Cognitive and Behavioral Practice, 10,* 248–254.

Weishaar, M. E. (1993). *Aaron T. Beck*. Thousand Oaks, CA: Sage.

Weishaar, M. E. (1996). Cognitive risk factors in suicide. In P. Salkovskis (Ed.), *Frontiers of cognitive therapy* (pp. 226–249). New York: Guilford Press.

Weishaar, M. E. (2004). A cognitive-behavioral approach to suicide risk reduction in crisis intervention. In A. R. Roberts & K. Yeager (Eds.), *Evidence-based practice manual* (pp. 749–757). New York: Oxford University Press.

Weishaar, M. E., & Beck, A. T. (1992). Hopelessness and suicide. *International Review of Psychiatry, 4*, 185–192.

Weissman, A., Beck, A. T., & Kovacs, M. (1979). Drug abuse, hopelessness and suicidal behavior. *International Journal of the Addictions, 14*(4), 451–464.

Winterowd, C. L., Beck, A. T., & Gruener, D. (2003). *Cognitive therapy with chronic pain patients*. New York: Springer.

Wright, J., Thase, M., Beck, A. T., & Ludgate, J. W. (1993). (Eds.). *Cognitive therapy with inpatients: Developing a cognitive milieu*. New York: Guilford Press.

Part II

THEORETICAL AND CONCEPTUAL ISSUES

Chapter 2

Beck's Theory of Depression

Origins, Empirical Status, and Future
Directions for Cognitive Vulnerability

CHRISTINE D. SCHER
ZINDEL V. SEGAL
RICK E. INGRAM

According to the World Health Organization, when the "burden of ill health" imposed by all diseases worldwide is considered, unipolar major depression imposes the fourth greatest such burden of any disease (Murray & Lopez, 1996). The same investigators projected that by the year 2020, this burden will increase both absolutely and relatively—so that at that time depression will impose the second greatest burden of ill health, very close behind the top cause, ischemic heart disease. A major reason for the scale of the burden caused by major depressive disorder (MDD) is that, as well as having a high rate of incidence, it is a condition characterized by relapse, recurrence, and chronicity. Recent estimates project that people will experience an average of four lifetime major depressive episodes of 20 weeks' duration each (Judd, 1997). Within these projections, however, it appears that not all people are at equal risk. Prognosis significantly varies between patients with no past history of depression and those who have had multiple recurrences. Those with at least three prior episodes relapse at rates of 70–80% within 3 years, while those with no prior depression history relapse at rates between 20% and 30% over a comparable interval. Thus patients recovering from their first few episodes of depression are at a critical juncture in the development of the course of their disorder. On the one hand, the risk of future recurrence is thought to increase by 16% with each episode of MDD experienced; on the other hand, the risk of recurrence progressively decreases as a patient is able to stay well longer (Solomon et al., 2000).

In the late 1960s and early 1970s, Aaron Beck described a model of depression from the standpoint of cognition and phenomenology. This cognitive model accounted for many of the hallmark features of depression, and it outlined some ways in which individuals are at risk for the onset of depression—and, once depressed, remain at risk for its return. Although a broader awareness of the nature of depression had not yet been achieved, Beck's vision was far-reaching. He understood that vulnerability to depression is of paramount importance, and that comprehensive treatment of episodic MDD involves both recovery and prophylaxis. Beck's clinical insights were quickly translated into the procedures and processes of cognitive therapy for depression, while the premises underlying individuals' vulnerability to depression followed a slower course of empirical investigation and refinement. Currently, there is a general consensus that cognition is an important factor in depression, and that current treatments are very effective acutely but show much less efficacy over the long term. Thus Beck's seminal contributions continue to inform us about the nature of depression's onset, its relapse/recurrence, and in time its eventual prevention. This chapter reviews this body of theory and research, and outlines the current status of cognitive vulnerability in the context of depression.

VULNERABILITY DEFINED

Ingram, Miranda, and Segal (1998) note that there are few explicit definitions of "vulnerability" available in the literature. However, they argue that the theory and research on vulnerability suggest a number of features that are essential to the construct and can therefore be used to arrive at a suitable definition of vulnerability. The most fundamental of these features is that vulnerability is conceptualized as a *trait* rather than as the kind of state that characterizes the appearance of depression. That is, even as episodes of depression emerge and then disappear, vulnerability remains constant. It is important to note in this regard that even though vulnerability is seen as a trait, this does not mean that it is necessarily permanent or unalterable. Although psychological vulnerability may be resistant to change, corrective experiences (e.g., therapy) can occur that attenuate vulnerability. Vulnerability is also viewed as *endogenous* to the person (in contrast to risk, which is a function of external forces),[1] as well as typically being viewed as *dormant* unless it is activated in some fashion. Related to this notion of dormancy, *stress* can also be viewed as a central aspect of vulnerability, in that cognitive diatheses cannot precipitate depression without the occurrence of stressful life events. A number of depression theories incorporate notions of vulnerability—for example, the hopelessness theory of Abramson and colleagues (Abramson, Metalsky, & Alloy, 1989), Ingram's information-processing model (Ingram, 1984), and Teasdale's interacting cognitive sub-systems model (Teasdale & Barnard, 1993). Nonetheless, in the spirit of this volume, this chapter will focus on Beck's theory of depression as an exemplar of vulnerability principles.

BRIEF SUMMARY OF BECK'S THEORY OF DEPRESSION

Although encompassing a number of different aspects, Beck's theory of depression (Beck, 1963, 1967/1972, 1987; Kovacs & Beck, 1978) emphasizes cognitive structures as the critical elements in the development, maintenance, and recurrence of depression. These cognitive structures, or "schemas," can be conceptualized as stored bodies of knowledge that interact with incoming information to influence selective attention and memory search (Segal, 1988; Williams, Watts, MacLeod, & Mathews, 1997). They are hypothesized to develop from interactions with the environment, primarily those interactions that occur during childhood (Beck, 1967/1972, 1987; Kovacs & Beck, 1978). Thus, for example, if early experiences are characterized by negativity, schemas may develop that guide attention to negative rather than positive events, and that lead to the enhanced recall of negative experiences. Such preferential processing of information reinforces the knowledge contained in schemas and ultimately contributes to quite stable views of the world (Markus, 1977). Although all persons possess schemas that develop from life experiences and guide processing of information, the schemas of depression-prone individuals are considered dysfunctional, in that they contain knowledge about the self, the world, and the future that is both rigid and unrealistically negative (Beck, 1967/1972, 1987; Kovacs & Beck, 1978).

The mere presence of a negative self-schema is insufficient for the occurrence of depression; another major tenet of Beck's theory is that

---

[1]External forces are conceptualized in terms of risk factors (e.g., poverty) rather than vulnerability, because they do not specify the mechanisms of onset or maintenance; the term "vulnerability" refers to these mechanisms.

schemas are assumed to lie dormant until activated by relevant stimuli (Beck, 1967/1972, 1987; Kovacs & Beck, 1978; see Segal & Ingram, 1994). In the case of depression-prone individuals, schemas, once activated, are thought to provide access to a complex system of negative themes and give rise to a corresponding pattern of negative information processing that precipitates depression (Kovacs & Beck, 1978; Segal & Shaw, 1986). Segal and Ingram (1994) have further elaborated two ways in which such activation can occur. First, activation may occur when some stimulus corresponds to a partially activated schema. In this case, the stimulus may provide enough additional activation to exceed the threshold level required for the schema to become fully active and perform its functions. Second, a schema may become activated through its relationships to other, fully activated schemas. In essence, schemas are linked to various degrees with one another, based on similarity of content. When a schema becomes fully activated, it sends activation to associated schemas. If the link between the activated schema and an associated schema is strong, the associated schema may become fully activated as well. If the link is weak, the associated schema may become partially activated, but may not exceed the threshold required for full activation (see Bower, 1981; Ingram, 1984). For example, a man may be vulnerable to depression because of a belief that he is unlovable. When he has a negative encounter with an attractive neighbor, his "unlovability schema" may become partially activated through its relationship to a schema regarding attractive persons. However, it may take rejection by a current romantic partner to fully activate the schema and result in depressive thoughts that spiral into depression.

This example illustrates that, theoretically, many types of experiences can activate schemas. However, the types of experiences typically hypothesized to activate schemas fall under the general rubric of stress. Beck (1967/1972) suggested that both catastrophic occurrences (e.g., the death of a spouse) and taxing daily events (e.g., missing a doctor's appointment) can activate schemas. He also theorized that particular kinds of stressors may differentially activate schemas with particular kinds of content (Beck, 1987). We will discuss this aspect of Beck's theory in more detail in a later section, but for now we note that he proposed that dependent persons, whose schemas of self-worth are based on the support and admiration of others, may be more vulnerable to depression after interpersonal rejection than are autonomous persons, whose schemas of self-worth are based on independence from others and personal achievement. Thus the kinds of stressors one experiences interact with specific cognitive vulnerabilities to spur the occurrence of depression.

In sum, Beck (1967/1972, 1987; Kovacs & Beck, 1978) suggests that depression-prone individuals possess latent dysfunctional schemas characterized by negative content. When activated, these dysfunctional schemas give rise to negative cognitions and corresponding patterns of information processing that serve to precipitate depression. Although experiences of any kind may activate schemas, Beck (1987) emphasized the importance of stress as a primary source of activation. It is an understatement to suggest that Beck's theory has substantially influenced scientific inquiry on depression—both by inspiring additional theorizing about the nature of depression (see, e.g., Kuiper, Olinger, & MacDonald, 1988, Ingram et al., 1998; Segal, 1988), and by contributing to its treatment (see Blackburn & Moorhead, 2000, for a discussion of treatment outcome studies and meta-analyses evaluating cognitive therapy for depression). The major tenets of this theory with regard to vulnerability schemas have also inspired a great deal of empirical examination, with sometimes conflicting findings. Thus the remainder of this chapter is largely devoted to examining the empirical status of Beck's theory, with an emphasis on two key tenets with particular relevance to the notion of vulnerability: (1) that dysfunctional schemas give rise to negative cognitions and corresponding information processing only when sufficiently activated; and (2) that stressors will differentially activate dysfunctional schemas with matching content.

DIATHESIS–STRESS PERSPECTIVES IN BECK'S THEORY: SCHEMAS ARE LATENT UNTIL ACTIVATED

The earliest tests of Beck's ideas about cognitive mechanisms of depression relied on contrasting depressed versus nondepressed control groups on some cognitive variable. The implication of finding differences was that these cognitive variables reflected causal or vulnerability aspects of depression. Although informative in a number of respects, this approach has been largely discarded as it applies to vulnerability (Ingram et al., 1998; Ingram & Siegle, 2002). The reasons for this are reflected in a second generation of studies, which have examined individuals whose depression has remitted. Sometimes these designs compare individuals with remitted depression to currently depressed and nondepressed groups, but more frequently they examine cognitive variables in individuals in an episode and then again in remission (e.g., Gotlib & Cane, 1987). In general, these studies find that it becomes difficult to detect these cognitive variables, leading to suggestions that these cognitive factors are mere correlates or consequences of the depressed state (see Atchley, Ilardi, & Enloe, 2003, for an intriguing exception).

As Ingram and Siegle (2002) note, remission methodologies can also provide information about vulnerability factors. However, remission designs alone are poor methodological choices to test a model in which there is theoretical reason to believe that vulnerability factors may be stable, but not easily accessible. Such assumptions are inherent in diathesis–stress models, in which the diathesis is only accessed under stress. Hence, to test such a theory appropriately, studies must model the complexity of diathesis–stress models; investigators must therefore either find a way to assess such activating features naturalistically, or simulate the stress activation of vulnerability factors in the lab (Hollon, 1992). Beck's theory is clearly a diathesis–stress theory in suggesting that dysfunctional schemas give rise to negative cognitions and congruent information processing only when activated:

> An individual who has incorporated . . . [a negative] constellation of attitudes . . . has the necessary predisposition for the development of clinical depression in adolescence or adulthood. Whether he will ever become depressed depends on whether the necessary conditions are present at a given time to activate the depressive constellation. (Beck, 1967/1972, p. 278)

Priming Designs

A clear implication of this hypothesis is that in the absence of schema activation, persons with and without depressive schemas should appear similar on measures of maladaptive cognitions and information processing. However, under conditions of activation, vulnerable persons should evidence maladaptive cognitions and information processing, while nonvulnerable persons should not. The most widely used way of evaluating this hypothesis is through the use of priming designs with persons whose depression has remitted; such persons are assumed to be cognitively vulnerable because they possess latent depressive schemas. In such studies, a prime such as a negative mood induction, or sometimes the induction of a self-focused state, is used to activate negative schemas. Typically, the cognitive processes of presumably vulnerable individuals following a prime are compared to those of a control group.

Among those studies with adequate priming procedures, findings are generally quite consistent with Beck's schema activation hypothesis. Teasdale and Dent (1987) were among the first to conduct a priming study of formerly depressed individuals that included an adequate mood induction. These authors found that following a negative mood induction, recovered depressed persons were more likely to recall negative adjectives endorsed as self-descriptive compared to never-depressed persons. Similar results were found by Hedlund and Rude (1995), who examined incidental recall and intrusions of negative and positive words following a self-focus manipulation. They found that formerly depressed persons recalled more negative words and had fewer positive intrusions than never-depressed persons did.

Two studies have examined interpretive biases among formerly depressed and never-depressed persons. Using a scrambled-sentences task, Hedlund and Rude (1995) found that formerly depressed persons constructed more negative sentences than never-depressed persons following a self-focus manipulation. Gemar, Segal, Sagrati, and Kennedy (2001) examined self-evaluative bias using a negative mood induction and found that depressed individuals evidenced a negative self-evaluative bias following the induction, but that never-depressed individuals did not evidence such a shift. The postinduction negative bias demonstrated by the recovered depressed group was comparable to that evidenced by a currently depressed group.

In addition to studies examining recall and interpretive biases, several studies have used a priming procedure to examine attention in never-depressed and formerly depressed individuals. Ingram, Bernet, and McLaughlin (1994) used a modified dichotic listening paradigm to assess attention to irrelevant positive and negative stimuli. No differences between individuals in a normal mood control condition were found, but when induced into a sad mood, formerly depressed individuals made more tracking errors for negative stimuli than did never-depressed individuals. The number of tracking errors for the never-depressed group, however, was quite similar in both the normal and sad mood conditions. These results were replicated in a subsequent study by Ingram and Ritter (2000). McCabe, Gotlib, and Martin (2000) also examined the attentional biases of previously depressed and never-depressed persons following neutral or sad mood inductions. Following both neutral and sad mood inductions, never-depressed persons demonstrated biased attention to positive and/or neutral trait words relative to negative trait words. Formerly depressed persons demonstrated a similar bias toward positive and neutral words following a neutral mood induction, but attended to word types equally following a sad mood induction.

A number of studies have examined reports of dysfunctional attitudes and beliefs among formerly depressed and never-depressed persons. These studies either have used experimental primes such as mood inductions, or have examined relationships between reports of dysfunctional attitudes and naturally occurring sad mood. In these latter studies, sad mood is expected to bear a positive relationship with reports of dysfunctional attitudes among formerly depressed participants, but not among never-depressed participants. Consistent with Beck's hypothesis, Miranda and colleagues (Miranda & Persons, 1988; Miranda, Persons, & Byers, 1990) found that mood predicted the occurrence of dysfunctional attitudes only in people with a history of depression; as negative mood increased, people with a history of depression were more likely to endorse dysfunctional attitudes. In people without such a history, little evidence of a relationship between mood and dysfunctional attitude endorsement was found. Studies by Roberts and Kassel (1996) and Solomon, Haaga, Brody, Kirk, and Friedman (1998) support these findings. However, expected relationships between mood and dysfunctional attitudes among formerly depressed participants are not always found (Brosse, Craighead, & Craighead, 1999; Dykman, 1997). For example, Brosse et al.

(1999) found that increased endorsement of dysfunctional attitudes following a negative mood induction was unrelated to depression history. Dykman (1997) also found that shifts in dysfunctional attitudes following a mood induction were unrelated to depression history. Similarly, Solomon et al. (1998) failed to find differences in irrational beliefs between never depressed and recovered depressed persons following priming by negative sociotropic and autonomous event scenarios.

Finally, Segal, Gemar, and Williams (1999) conducted a retrospective assessment of a group of formerly depressed patients (n = 30) who had been treated to remission with either cognitive-behavioral therapy (CBT) or antidepressants. These patients participated in a mood induction task in which changes in dysfunctional attitudes were examined in both euthymic and induced, transient dysphoric moods. They were recontacted up to 30 months later and assessed for relapse status. Logistic regression indicated that the magnitude of mood-linked cognitive reactivity exhibited following, but not before, the mood induction significantly predicted relapse over this interval. *This was the first demonstration of a direct relationship between mood-linked changes in cognitive processing among formerly depressed patients and subsequent relapse.* Furthermore, some of the data suggested that this type of cognitive reactivity was differentially affected by the type of treatment patients had received. Patients recovered through CBT, which targets cognition, showed less reactivity than patients recovered through equally effective antidepressant medication, which does not engage these cognitive processes.

Although not all studies find support, the bulk of priming studies comparing formerly depressed and never-depressed persons support Beck's hypothesis that dysfunctional schemas lie dormant until sufficiently activated. Clearly, the general principle of schema activation can be considered now to be well established, even though some more specific aspects of schema activation appear to vary somewhat, depending on the process under investigation. For example, studies evaluating information-processing biases are remarkably consistent in their support, whereas studies investigating dysfunctional attitudes and beliefs tend to provide somewhat more mixed support.

Behavioral High-Risk Designs

Though priming designs with persons whose depression has remitted have provided a large amount of empirical information regarding Beck's cognitive vulnerability hypotheses, other designs are possible. One such design is the "behavioral high-risk" approach. This approach has several advantages compared to the priming approach, including the ability to demonstrate temporal antecedence of hypothesized cognitive vulnerability factors and the ability to examine the effects of naturally occurring stressors. The behavioral high-risk approach to depression vulnerability is exemplified by the Temple–Wisconsin Cognitive Vulnerability to Depression Project (Alloy & Abramson, 1999). This two-site longitudinal study has examined the proposals of both the hopelessness theory of depression and Beck's schema theory of depression. The project assessed a group of individuals who, upon entry into college, were identified as possessing negative inferential styles or dysfunctional attitudes; it then compared their outcomes over time with those of individuals who did not show these cognitive characteristics. Several reports based on this project have been published (e.g., Abramson et al., 1999; Alloy, Abramson, Murray, Whitehouse, & Hogan, 1997). These tend to support the validity of Beck's (and the hopelessness theory's) cognitive vulnerability proposals.

STRESSORS DIFFERENTIALLY ACTIVATE SCHEMAS WITH MATCHING CONTENT

As discussed earlier, a second major tenet of Beck's theory is that schemas may be differentially activated by stressors with matching content: " . . . life stressors, chronic or acute, primary or secondary, will have their greatest depressogenic effect if they impinge on . . . specific vulnerabilities" (Beck, 1987, p. 23). In discussing this stress–schema congruency hypothesis, Beck has focused on two categories of problematic schema content (see also Robins, 1990; Robins & Block, 1988; Robins & Luten, 1991). The first is interpersonal in nature ("sociotropy/dependency"); individuals with these schemas value positive interchange with others and focus on acceptance, support, and guidance from others. The second type of cognitive content is concerned with achievement ("autonomy/self-criticism"); these individuals rely on independence, mobility, and achievement, and are prone to be self-critical. According to this formulation, the experience of stressors congruent with these themes should activate these dysfunctional cognitive structures and precipitate depression. For example, disruptions in interpersonal relationships should be especially problematic for the person with a sociotropic schema, whereas problems in achievement situations (e.g., work) should activate depressive experiences for the person with an autonomous schema type.

Although most of the research evaluating the stress–schema congruency hypothesis is cross-sectional, evidence in support of this hypothesis has begun to accumulate (e.g., Robins, 1990; Segal, Shaw, Vella, & Katz, 1992). In a review of this literature, Nietzel and Harris (1990) concluded that the match between cognitive style and congruent life stress is more closely associated with depression than is the nonmatching of events of similar severity. They also found that some types of matches were especially problematic—for example, that the combination of elevated sociotropy/dependency interacting with negative social events led to greater depression than did the autonomy/ self-criticism matching or the other two mismatches. In a more recent appraisal of this literature, Coyne and Whiffen (1995) acknowledge that matches between personality and life stress have greater predictive power than mismatches between personality and life stress. However, because they do not believe that this model is complex enough to accommodate fluctuations in the course of people's lives, they are more skeptical about the relevance of this model to the study of depression vulnerability. This skepticism notwithstanding, the empirical findings are clearly supportive of Beck's stress–schema congruency hypothesis, which locates vulnerability in the activation of individuals' meaning and need structures, and in the ways these structures match up with life events.

Interestingly, these types of findings are now being extended to predict depression status following treatment. One recent example was reported by Mazure, Bruce, Maciejewski, and Jacobs (2000). They examined whether sociotropy and autonomy in interaction with congruent adverse life events predicted treatment outcome among persons receiving 6 weeks of pharmacotherapy for depression. Findings suggested that schemas of sociotropy and autonomy interacted with matched events to predict treatment outcome; persons whose depression onset followed a stress–schema match evidenced better outcome following pharmacotherapy. Such findings are open to a variety of interpretations, including the possibility that stress–schema matches contribute to the onset of depression but not to its maintenance. Regardless, future studies of this nature have great potential to extend Beck's work and further inform treatment outcomes. Additional directions for research centered on the role of interpersonal experience will be addressed next.

FUTURE DIRECTIONS: THE ROLE OF INTERPERSONAL EXPERIENCE AND VULNERABILITY

As supportive evidence mounts for Beck's vulnerability ideas, a number of researchers have turned their attention to identifying the developmental origins of the maladaptive schemas and the associated information processing that are thought to create risk. At first glance, such attention may seem misplaced, as most theoretical discussions and empirical evaluations devoted to Beck's model have been directed toward the development and course of depression in adults (see Engel & DeRubeis, 1993; Haaga, Dyck, & Ernst, 1991; Ingram & Holle, 1992; Ingram, Scott, & Siegle, 1999; Sacco & Beck, 1995). Nonetheless, at the core of Beck's model is the idea that vulnerability to depression develops through the acquisition of cognitive schemas concerning stressful or traumatic events in childhood and ado-lescence. Specifically, Beck (1967/1972) suggests that when such events oc-cur relatively early in an individual's development, the individual becomes sensitized to just these types of events. The corresponding generation of negative schemas to process information about these events leads to the subsequent activation of these schemas, and corresponding depression, if and when similar events occur in the future:

> In childhood and adolescence, the depression-prone individual becomes sensitized to certain types of life situations. The traumatic situations ini-tially responsible for embedding or reinforcing the negative attitudes that comprise the depressive constellation are the prototypes of the specific stresses that may later activate these constellations. When a person is sub-jected to situations reminiscent of the original traumatic experiences, he may then become depressed. The process may be likened to conditioning in which a particular response is linked to a specific stimulus; once the chain has been formed, stimuli similar to the original stimulus may evoke the conditioned response. (Beck, 1967/1972, p. 278)

Thus, although Beck's model is most commonly viewed as a theory of adult depression, is specifically and centrally incorporates the idea that vulnera-bility to depression develops early in life, during childhood and adoles-cence. While stressful early interactions with any number of people may be linked to the development of cognitive vulnerability to depression, data suggest that negative interactions with attachment figures may have an es-pecially pernicious effect on schema development. Thus we now turn to a discussion of attachment relationships and their implications for the development of maladaptive schemas.

Childhood Attachment

Many of Beck's ideas are paralleled by Bowlby's (1969/1982) attachment theory. Bowlby suggested that an attachment relationship—consisting of proximity-maintaining behaviors by the human infant, and caregiving be-haviors by his or her primary caregiver(s)—typically forms during the first year of an infant's life, with the goals of security and protection of the in-fant. These attachment relationships differ from many other types of social relationships in significant ways. First, attachment relationships are endur-ing: Attachment relationships formed during childhood frequently persist throughout the lifespan. Second, although a child may form more than one early attachment relationship, attachment figures are not interchangeable. For example, an attachment relationship with a deceased parent cannot be replaced by an attachment relationship with a surviving parent. Third, a child desires physical and emotional closeness with his or her attachment figure(s), and may become distressed upon uncontrollable separation. Finally, a child seeks security and comfort in attachment relationships; this latter component distinguishes attachment relationships from all other social relationships (Ainsworth, 1989; Bowlby, 1969/1982). In sum, attachment relationships are unique and, according to attachment theorists, long-lasting parts of most people's lives.

The longevity and uniqueness of attachment relationships suggest that they are fertile ground for the development of schemas, including maladaptive ones of the type that Beck has proposed lead to cognitive vulnerability. By their very nature, attachment relationships consist of repeated interactions, often over the course of a lifetime. During the course of a healthy (or secure) early attachment relationship, a child experiences consistently accessible and responsive caregiving on the part of the attachment figure (Bowlby, 1973, 1977). Through such experiences, a child may surmise that he or she is loved and valued. During the course of an unhealthy (or insecure) attachment relationship, however, a child finds his or her caregivers to be inaccessible or unresponsive; such caregiving may include hostility and rejection directed toward a child, and threats used as a means of control (Bowlby, 1973, 1977, 1980). Within the context of such relationships, a child may surmise that he or she is unlovable and unwanted. Moreover, the messages provided in the context of these relationships may be especially meaningful, in that they are coming from someone who is uniquely valued by the child and who functions as one of only a few sources of security and comfort. Thus the messages, whether positive or negative, are likely to be quite well established in a child's developing schemas.

Although investigation of the potential relationship between early attachment and depression vulnerability of the sort proposed by Beck is relatively new, several studies have emerged that support this possibility. For example, Whisman and colleagues (Whisman & Kwon, 1992; Whisman & McGarvey, 1995) and Randolph and Dykman (1998) have examined whether attachment experiences are related to dysfunctional attitudes in adulthood. These studies suggested that several negative parenting behaviors contribute to the development of dysfunctional attitudes, including criticism, rejection, and low care. Randolph and Dykman also conducted a path analysis and found that attachment experiences contributed to the development of dysfunctional attitudes, which in turn contributed to depression proneness as measured by the Depression Proneness Rating Scale (Zemore, Fischer, Garratt, & Miller, 1990). Also implicating attachment experiences in the development of depression vulnerability is a previously discussed study by Ingram and Ritter (2000). In addition to examining information processing as a function of depression history, these authors examined such processing as a function of childhood experiences with parents. They found that among formerly depressed individuals in a sad mood, low levels of perceived maternal care were related to increased attention to negative information. Never-depressed individuals did not evidence similar relationships between early experiences and attention. Ingram, Overby, and Fortier (2001) also found that low levels of maternal care in particular were linked to dysfunctional levels of automatic thinking (a presumed product of vulnerability schemas) in individuals who might be vulnerable to depression. Although largely cross-sectional, the findings of such studies clearly implicate childhood experiences in the development of presumably cognitive vulnerability to depression.

Adult Attachment

Beck suggests that vulnerability cognitions develop in childhood, and, as noted above, Bowlby (1969/1982, 1973, 1980) also focused much of his attention on the correlates and consequences of childhood attachment relationships. Beck and Bowlby both suggest that the effects of these early relationships are present throughout the lifespan. Though the immediate goals of attachment behavior may vary between adults and children (e.g., the immediate goal of attachment behavior for a toddler may be physical proximity, whereas the goal for an adult may be information that physical proximity can be achieved if needed), the overarching goal of such behavior—a sense of security and protection—remains the same (Bowlby, 1969/1982, 1973; see also Kobak, 1999, for a review of Bowlby's theorizing). The focus of these adult attachment relationships may also change or increase in number to include, for example, romantic partners. Such theorizing may have implications for Beck's schema theory. Most saliently, experiences within adult attachment relationships may affect schemas of significant others and of oneself in relation to others. Such schemas may then serve as vulnerability (or, conceivably, protective) factors in the development of depression.

Congruent with this thinking, researchers have begun to investigate relationships between adult attachment and depression. One of the most methodologically sound studies was conducted by Hammen et al. (1995). They examined whether attachment cognitions could predict both interviewer-assessed and self-reported psychopathology among female high school seniors. Attachment cognitions regarding adult romantic relationships predicted changes in interviewer-assessed depression, both as main effects and in interaction with interviewer-assessed interpersonal events. However, these findings were not unique to depression; attachment cognitions alone and in interaction with interpersonal events also predicted changes in general psychopathology. In an extension of this work, Hammen and colleagues (Burge et al., 1997) examined whether attachment cognitions regarding relationships with parents and peers as well as with romantic partners would predict psychopathology 1 year later. Again, attachment cognitions regarding romantic relationships predicted depressive symptoms, alone and in interaction with previous symptoms; and again, these relationships did not appear specific to depression. Attachment cognitions regarding current relationships with parents and peers did not predict depressive symptoms, although they predicted the occurrence of other types of symptoms (e.g., eating disorders). Thus attachment cognitions concerning romantic relationships appear particularly important in the development of depressive symptoms, at least among women making the transition from high school. The provocative findings of Hammen and colleagues, along with findings examining childhood attachment, suggest that continued examination of both cognitive and interpersonal factors in evaluating Beck's theory of depression may greatly contribute to our understanding of depression vulnerability.

FINAL COMMENTS

In this chapter, we have discussed Beck's proposals regarding vulnerability to depression. In so doing, we have examined definitions of vulnerability that were inspired by Beck's work, as well as diathesis–stress perspectives that researchers have only recently rediscovered from Beck's original proposals. We have also discussed research assessing Beck's vulnerability ideas, with a specific focus on priming in the laboratory context, and more general ideas revolving around the notion that the stressors that are particularly potent in causing depression are those that match the content of depressogenic schemas. Although priming designs serve as the focus of much of our discussion, we have also noted behavioral high-risk research designs that have been informative about the accuracy of Beck's ideas. Finally, we have examined future directions of theory and research pertaining to cognitive vulnerability that are in line with Beck's earliest proposals.

The three to four decades since Beck's original proposals (1963, 1967/ 1972) have witnessed an explosion of research testing his ideas. Indeed, hundreds of studies with thousands of participants have examined his proposals, and have generally supported his ideas. In specific regard to vulnerability, it is the case that some studies have failed to find evidence of cognitive vulnerability. A number of these studies, however, have failed to take into account the diathesis–stress nature of Beck's proposals. For those that have done so, not only do the clear majority find that vulnerable individuals appear to possess reactive dysfunctional cognitive schemas of the type Beck proposed (Ingram et al., 1998; Segal & Ingram, 1994), but recent data have also shown that this reactivity predicts future depression (Segal et al., 1999). Beck's theory is widely acknowledged as an achievement when it has been applied to the development of cognitive therapy, but it is no less so when applied to vulnerability. Beck's theories can thus clearly be considered to be a success when questions of basic cognitive processes underlying vulnerability have been tested. Few theorists in the history of psychology or psychiatry have had their proposals so clearly validated.

Beck understood before anyone else that vulnerability to depression was a key to understanding the most important processes in the disorder, and his views have been borne out by the data. It is thus worth reiterating what we noted at the beginning of this chapter: It is difficult to overstate Beck's contribution to our understanding of depression. But Beck's influence goes beyond tests of his own ideas; he has inspired virtually all cognitive models of depression in existence, and has served as the inspiration for related work springing from the core concepts of his theories (e.g., Ingram et al., 1998). Beck has therefore helped shaped the view of several generations of depression researchers, and we see no reason why these views will not shape generations to come.

REFERENCES

Abramson, L. Y., Alloy, L. B., Hogan, M. E., Whitehouse, W. G., Donovan, P., Rose, D., et al. (1999). Cognitive vulnerability to depression: Theory and evidence. *Journal of Cognitive Psychotherapy, 13,* 5–20.

Abramson, L. Y., Metalsky, G. I., & Alloy, L. B. (1989). Hopelessness depression: A theory-based subtype of depression. *Psychological Review, 96,* 358–372.

Ainsworth, M. D. S. (1989). Attachments beyond infancy. *American Psychologist, 44,* 709–716.

Alloy, L. B., & Abramson, L. Y. (1999). The Temple–Wisconsin Vulnerability to Depression Project: Conceptual background, design, and methods. *Journal of Cognitive Psychotherapy: An International Quarterly, 13,* 227–262.

Alloy, L. B., Abramson, L. Y., Murray, L. A., Whitehouse, W. G., & Hogan, M E. (1997). Self-referent information processing in individuals at high and low risk for depression. *Cognition and Emotion, 11,* 539–568.

Atchley, R., Ilardi, S. S., & Enloe, A. (2003). Hemispheric asymmetry in the processing of emotional content in word meanings: The effects of current and past depression. *Brain and Language, 84,* 105–119.

Beck, A. T. (1963). Thinking and depression: I. Idiosyncratic content and cognitive distortions. *Archives of General Psychiatry, 9,* 324–333.

Beck, A. T. (1972). *Depression: Causes and treatment.* Philadelphia: University of Pennsylvania Press. (Original work published 1967)

Beck, A. T. (1987). Cognitive models of depression. *Journal of Cognitive Psychotherapy, 1,* 5–37.

Blackburn, I., & Moorhead, S. (2000). Update in cognitive therapy for depression. *Journal of Cognitive Psychotherapy, 14,* 305–336.

Bower, G. H. (1981). Mood and memory. *American Psychologist, 36,* 129–148.

Bowlby, J. (1973). *Attachment and loss: Vol. 2. Separation.* New York: Basic Books.

Bowlby, J. (1977). The making and breaking of affectional bonds. *British Journal of Psychiatry, 130,* 201–210.

Bowlby, J. (1980). *Attachment and loss: Vol. 3. Loss.* New York: Basic Books.

Bowlby, J. (1982). *Attachment and loss: Vol. 1. Attachment.* New York: Basic Books. (Original work published 1969)

Brosse, A. L., Craighead, L. W., & Craighead, W. E. (1999). Testing the mood-state hypothesis among previously depressed and never-depressed individuals. *Behavior Therapy, 30,* 97–115.

Burge, D., Hammen, C., Davila, J., Daley, S. E., Paley, B., & Lindberg, N. (1997). The relationship between attachment cognitions and psychological adjustment in late adolescent women. *Development and Psychopathology, 9,* 151–167.

Coyne, J. C., & Whiffen, V. E. (1995). Issues in personality as diathesis for depression: The case of sociotropy–dependency and autonomy–self-criticism. *Psychological Bulletin, 118,* 358–378.

Dykman, B. M. (1997). A test of whether negative emotional priming facilitates access to latent dysfunctional attitudes. *Cognition and Emotion, 11,* 197–222.

Engel, R. A., & DeRubeis, R. J. (1993). The role of cognition in depression. In K. S. Dobson & P. C. Kendall (Eds.), *Psychopathology and cognition* (pp. 83–119). San Diego, CA: Academic Press.

Gemar, M. C., Segal, Z. V., Sagrati, S., & Kennedy, S. J. (2001). Mood-induced changes on the implicit association test in recovered depressed patients. *Journal of Abnormal Psychology, 110,* 282–289.

Gotlib, I. H., & Cane, C. B. (1987). Construct accessibility and clinical depression: A longitudinal investigation. *Journal of Abnormal Psychology, 96,* 199–204.

Haaga, D. A. F., Dyck, M. J., & Ernst, D. (1991). Empirical status of cognitive theory of depression. *Psychological Bulletin, 110,* 215–236.

Hammen, C. L., Burge, D., Daley, S. E., Davila, J., Paley, B., & Rudolph, K. D. (1995). Interpersonal attachment cognitions and prediction of symptomatic responses to interpersonal stress. *Journal of Abnormal Psychology, 104,* 436–443.

Hedlund, S., & Rude, S. S. (1995). Evidence of latent depressive schemas in formerly depressed individuals. *Journal of Abnormal Psychology, 104,* 517–525.

Hollon, S. D. (1992). Cognitive models of depression from a psychobiological perspective. *Psychological Inquiry, 3,* 250–253.

Ingram, R. E. (1984). Toward an information processing analysis of depression. *Cognitive Therapy and Research, 8,* 443–477.

Ingram, R. E., Bernet, C. Z., & McLaughlin, S. C. (1994). Attentional allocation processes in individuals at risk for depression. *Cognitive Therapy and Research, 18,* 317–332.

Ingram, R. E., & Holle, C. (1992). The cognitive science of depression. In D. J. Stein & J. E. Young (Eds.), *Cognitive science and clinical disorders* (pp. 187–209). Orlando, FL: Academic Press.

Ingram, R. E., Miranda, J., & Segal, Z. V. (1998). *Cognitive vulnerability to depression.* New York: Guilford Press.

Ingram, R. E., Overby, T., & Fortier, M. (2001). Individual differences in dysfunctional automatic thinking and parental bonding: Specificity of maternal care. *Personality and Individual Differences, 30,* 401–412.

Ingram, R. E., & Ritter, J. (2000). Vulnerability to depression: Cognitive reactivity and parental bonding in high-risk individuals. *Journal of Abnormal Psychology, 109,* 588–596.

Ingram, R. E., Scott, W., & Siegle, G. (1999). Depression: Social and cognitive aspects. In T. Millon, P. Blaney, & R. Davis (Eds.), *Oxford textbook of psychopathology* (pp. 203–226). Oxford: Oxford University Press.

Ingram, R. E., & Siegle, G. J. (2002). Methodological issues in depression research: Not your father's Oldsmobile. In I. Gotlib & C. Hammen (Eds.), *Handbook of depression* (3rd ed., pp. 86–114). New York: Guilford Press.

Judd, L. L. (1997). The clinical course of unipolar major depressive disorders. *Archives of General Psychiatry, 54,* 989–991.

Kobak, R. (1999). The emotional dynamics of disruptions in attachment relationships: Implications for theory, research, and clinical intervention. In J. Cassidy & P. R. Shaver (Eds.), *Handbook of attachment: Theory, research, and clinical applications* (pp. 21–43). New York: Guilford Press.

Kovacs, M., & Beck, A. T. (1978). Maladaptive cognitive structures in depression. *American Journal of Psychiatry, 135,* 525–533.

Kuiper, N. A., Olinger, L. J., & MacDonald, M. (1988). Vulnerability and episodic cognitions in a self-worth contingency model of depression. In L. B. Alloy (Ed.), *Cognitive processes in depression* (pp. 289–309). New York: Guilford Press.

Markus, H. (1977). Self-schemata and processing information about the self. *Journal of Personality and Social Psychology, 35,* 63–78.

Mazure, C. M., Bruce, M. L., Maciejewski, P. K., & Jacobs, S. C. (2000). Adverse life events and cognitive–personality characteristics in the prediction of major depression and antidepressant response. *American Journal of Psychiatry, 157,* 896–903.

McCabe, S. B., Gotlib, I. H., & Martin, R. A. (2000). Cognitive vulnerability for depression: Deployment of attention as a function of history of depression and current mood state. *Cognitive Therapy and Research, 24,* 427–444.

Miranda, J., & Persons, J. B. (1988). Dysfunctional attitudes are mood-state dependent. *Journal of Abnormal Psychology, 97,* 76–79.

Miranda, J., Persons, J. B., & Byers, C. (1990). Endorsement of dysfunctional beliefs depends on current mood state. *Journal of Abnormal Psychology, 99,* 237–241.

Murray, C. L., & Lopez, A. D. (1996). *The global burden of disease: A comprehensive assessment of mortality and disability from diseases, injuries and risk factors in 1990 and projected to 2020.* Cambridge, MA: Harvard University Press.

Nietzel, M. T., & Harris, M. J. (1990). Relationship of dependency and achievement/autonomy to depression. *Clinical Psychology Review, 10,* 279–297.

Randolph, J. J., & Dykman, B. M. (1998). Perceptions of parenting and depression-proneness in the offspring: Dysfunctional attitudes as a mediating mechanism. *Cognitive Therapy and Research, 22,* 377–400.

Roberts, J. E., & Kassel, J. D. (1996). Mood state dependence in cognitive vulnerability to depression: The roles of positive and negative affect. *Cognitive Therapy and Research, 20,* 1–12.

Robins, C. J. (1990). Congruence of personality and life events in depression. *Journal of Abnormal Psychology, 99,* 393–397.

Robins, C. J., & Block, P. (1988). Personal vulnerability, life events, and depressive symptoms: A test of a specific interactional model. *Journal of Personality and Social Psychology, 54,* 847–852.

Robins, C. J., & Luten, A. G. (1991). Sociotropy and autonomy: Differential patterns of clinical presentation in unipolar depression. *Journal of Abnormal Psychology, 100,* 74–77.

Sacco, W. P., & Beck, A. T. (1995). Cognitive theory and therapy. In E. E. Beckham & W. R. Leber (Eds.), *Handbook of depression* (2nd ed., pp. 329–351). New York: Guilford Press.

Segal, Z. V. (1988). Appraisal of the self-schema construct in cognitive models of depression. *Psychological Bulletin, 103,* 147–162.

Segal, Z. V., Gemar, M. C., & Williams, S. (1999). Differential cognitive response to a mood challenge following successful cognitive therapy or pharmacotherapy for unipolar depression. *Journal of Abnormal Psychology, 108,* 3–10.

Segal, Z. V., & Ingram, R. E. (1994). Mood priming and construct activation in tests of cognitive vulnerability to unipolar depression. *Clinical Psychology Review, 14,* 663–695.

Segal, Z. V., & Shaw, B. F. (1986). Cognition in depression: A reappraisal of Coyne and Gotlib's critique. *Cognitive Therapy and Research, 10,* 671–694.

Segal, Z. V., Shaw, B. F., Vella, D. D., & Katz, R. (1992). Cognitive and life stress predictors of relapse in remitted unipolar depressed patients: Test of the congruency hypothesis. *Journal of Abnormal Psychology, 101,* 26–36.

Solomon, A., Haaga, D. A. F., Brody, C., Kirk, L., & Friedman, D. G. (1998). Priming irrational beliefs in recovered-depressed people. *Journal of Abnormal Psychology, 107,* 440–449.

Solomon, D., Keller, M., Mueller, T., Lavori, P., Shea, T., Coryell, W., et al. (2000). Multiple recurrences of major depressive disorder. *American Journal of Psychiatry, 157,* 229–233.

Teasdale, J. D., & Barnard, P. J. (1993). *Affect, cognition, and change.* Hillsdale, NJ: Erlbaum.

Teasdale, J. D., & Dent, J. (1987). Cognitive vulnerability to depression: An investigation of two hypotheses. *British Journal of Clinical Psychology, 26,* 113–126.

Whisman, M. A., & Kwon, P. (1992). Parental representations, cognitive distortions, and mild depression. *Cognitive Therapy and Research, 16,* 557–568.

Whisman, M. A., & McGarvey, A. L. (1995). Attachment, depressotypic cognitions, and dysphoria. *Cognitive Therapy and Research, 19,* 633–650.

Williams, J. M .G., Watts, F. N., MacLeod, C., & Mathews, A. (1997). *Cognitive psychology and emotional disorders.* Chichester, UK: Wiley.

Zemore, R., Fischer, D. G., Garratt, L. S., & Miller, C. (1990). The Depression Proneness Rating Scale: Reliability, validity, and factor structure. *Current Psychology: Research and Reviews, 9,* 255–263.

Chapter 3

Effectiveness of Treatment for Depression

STEVEN D. HOLLON
ROBERT J. DERUBEIS

A cognitive model of psychopathology is based on the idea that erroneous beliefs and maladaptive information processing can lead to emotional distress and problems in behavioral adaptation (Beck, 1976). In depression, errors in thinking usually take the form of unrealistic pessimism and unjustifiably low confidence in the self (Beck, 1991). Errors in thinking frequently involve discrete automatic negative thoughts in specific situations (such as "I can't do this" or "I won't enjoy it anyway") that spring from more general and abstract underlying beliefs and assumptions (such as "I'm incompetent/unlovable" or "If I don't ask for anything, I won't get disappointed"). These beliefs are part of a larger cognitive schema that also includes the operation of logical errors (information processing heuristics) such as "all-or-none thinking" or "selective abstraction," which serve to keep the depressed individual from recognizing the inaccuracy of his or her beliefs (Kovacs & Beck, 1978).

Cognitive therapy for depression, then, aims to correct these erroneous beliefs and maladaptive information-processing strategies, with the goal of reducing distress and facilitating adaptive coping (Beck, 1970). In this approach, the therapist encourages clients to use their own behaviors to test their beliefs. A prototypic technique is the use of experiments, the aim of which is to gather information to test the accuracy of clients' negative beliefs (Beck, Rush, Shaw, & Emery, 1979). In its original incarnation, the emphasis was put on getting clients moving in early sessions and testing the accuracy of specific beliefs in specific situations. In recent years, cognitive therapy has evolved to incorporate an emphasis on core beliefs and underlying assumptions earlier in the course of treatment, plus greater attention to childhood antecedents and the therapeutic relationship, to go along with the traditional emphasis on current life problems (the combination of emphases is referred to as the "three-legged stool"). This expansion of the original approach, called "schema-focused therapy," evolved in response to efforts to treat more complicated patients with long-standing character disorders, given clinical observations that such patients had no healthy, nondepressed schema to activate (Beck, Freeman, & Associates, 1990).

EFFICACY AND EFFECTIVENESS OF COGNITIVE THERAPY FOR DEPRESSION

Early Context and Initial Evidence

By the time cognitive therapy first emerged in the early 1970s, the antidepressant medications had come to be considered the standard treatments for depression. As a group, the antidepressant medications had been shown to be superior to a pill placebo in about two-thirds of over 300 randomized controlled acute treatment trials (Morris & Beck, 1974). Moreover, patients who were kept on medications were less likely to relapse following successful treatment than patients withdrawn onto a pill placebo (Prien & Kupfer, 1986). By way of contrast, psychotherapy typically was less effective than (and did little to enhance the efficacy of) medications, and was no more effective than a pill placebo in several controlled trials in clinical populations (Covi, Lipman, Derogatis, Smith, & Pattison, 1974; Daneman, 1961; Friedman, 1975; Klerman, DiMascio, Weissman, Prusoff, & Paykel, 1974).

In this context, the publication of a study suggesting that cognitive therapy was more effective and longer-lasting than medications attracted real attention. In that trial, 41 depressed outpatients were randomly assigned to 12 weeks of treatment with either cognitive therapy or imipramine pharmacotherapy (Rush, Beck, Kovacs, & Hollon, 1977). By the end of acute treatment, patients treated with cognitive therapy showed greater symptom reduction and were less likely to drop out of treatment than patients treated with medication. Moreover, patients who responded to cognitive therapy were less likely to relapse or return to treatment over a subsequent 12-month naturalistic follow-up than were patients who responded to medications (Kovacs, Rush, Beck, & Hollon, 1981).

Publication of this article created quite a stir in the field, and it was soon joined by a second study in Edinburgh that appeared to confirm the efficacy of cognitive therapy. In that trial, depressed psychiatric outpatients treated with a combination of drugs and cognitive therapy did better than patients treated with either one alone, and cognitive therapy (with or without medications) did better than medications alone in the treatment of depressed patients in a general practice setting (Blackburn, Bishop, Glen, Whalley, & Christie, 1981). Moreover, patients in this second study who responded to cognitive therapy were again less likely to relapse following treatment termination than were patients who responded to medications (Blackburn, Eunson, & Bishop, 1986).

Studies with More Adequate Medication Implementation

These studies led some to conclude that cognitive therapy was superior to medications in the treatment of depression (Dobson, 1989). However, there were problems with each study that made drawing such a conclusion questionable (Meterissian & Bradwejn, 1989). In the study by Rush and colleagues, drug doses were low, and medication was withdrawn starting 2 weeks before the end of treatment. In Blackburn and colleagues' study, the advantage for cognitive therapy alone over drugs alone in the general practice sample occurred in the context of a drug response rate so low as to call into question the adequacy with which medication treatment was provided.

In this context, several studies sought to compare cognitive therapy to medications in trials in which drug treatment was adequately implemented. Our own work at the University of Minnesota is one example. In a controlled trial, 107 patients who met criteria for major depression were randomly assigned to 12 weeks of cognitive therapy, imipramine pharmacotherapy, or combined treatment (Hollon et al., 1992). At the end of acute treatment, patients who responded to either cognitive therapy or combined treatment were withdrawn from all treatment and followed over the next 2 years. Patients who responded to medications alone were randomly assigned either to continue on medications for the first year, or to be withdrawn from medications and followed over the 2 years. Patients were drawn from persons requesting treatment at existing outpatient treatment facilities, and the therapists in both conditions were drawn from the indigenous staffs at those sites.

Considerable effort went into making sure that medication treatment was adequately implemented. The prescribing clinicians were all board-certified psychiatrists with considerable experience in other controlled drug trials. Average daily dosage levels were more than adequate (over 300 mg/day from Week 6 on), and patients were continued at their maximally tolerated dose through the end of acute treatment. Plasma levels were used to monitor compliance and absorption, and several patients had their dosages raised above 300 mg/day when indicated (to a high of 450 mg/day). Finally, patients in continuation medication were kept on full active treatment doses through the first year of the 2-year follow-up. These strategies made for considerably stronger medication treatment than was provided during the earlier trials already described.

On the whole, all three treatments (cognitive therapy, medications, and their combination) showed considerable change over time, with the average patient showing a drop from moderate-to-severe depression at intake to the high end of the normal range by the end of treatment. Most of the change occurred across the first 6 weeks of treatment. Patients in combined treatment did somewhat better than patients in either single modality, although differences fell just short of significance (responses rates were in excess of 50% among either single condition and approached 70% among patients in combined treatment). On the whole, these findings suggested that cognitive therapy was about as effective as medication treatment (even when adequately implemented)—a finding that was essentially replicated in a trial conducted at another setting known for the rigor of its medication treatment (Murphy, Simons, Wetzel, & Lustman, 1984).

As in the earlier trials, there were also indications that cognitive therapy had an enduring effect that survived the end of treatment. As shown in Figure 3.1, patients who responded to cognitive therapy were about half as likely to relapse as treatment responders withdrawn from medication, and no more likely to relapse than patients continued on medications (Evans et al., 1992). The fact that patients who responded to combined treatment

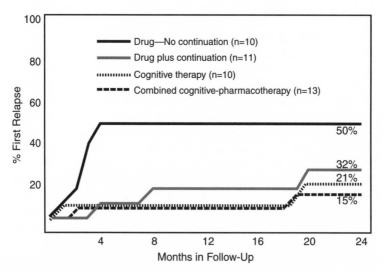

FIGURE 3.1. Relapse after successful treatment. From Evans et al. (1992, p. 805). Copyright 1992 by the American Medical Association. Reprinted by permission.

were no more likely to relapse than patients who responded to cognitive therapy alone suggests that this difference was not simply an artifact of medication withdrawal, since patients in combined treatment were withdrawn from medications on the same schedule as medication patients in the noncontinuation condition. This is also consistent with the fact that there was no marked increment in relapses among medication patients in the continuation condition when they were withdrawn from medications at the end on the first year of continuation. Again, findings from the study by Murphy and colleagues largely paralleled those just reported (Simons, Murphy, Levine, & Wetzel, 1986). On the whole, these two studies suggest that cognitive therapy is at least as effective as medications in the acute treatment of depressed outpatients, and quite possibly longer-lasting.

Cognitive Therapy and More Severely Depressed Patients

By this time (a decade after it was first introduced), cognitive therapy was gaining widespread acceptance as a treatment for depression and was being disseminated at a rapid rate. However, publication of the National Institute of Mental Health's Treatment of Depression Collaborative Research Program (TDCRP) raised new questions about the efficacy of cognitive therapy, at least for more severely depressed outpatients (Elkin et al., 1989). In that trial, 250 depressed outpatients were randomly assigned to treatment with cognitive therapy, interpersonal psychotherapy (IPT), medication treatment with imipramine, or a pill placebo control. At the end of 16 weeks of treatment, there were no differences among the treatments for the less severely depressed patients, but indications of an advantage for drug treatment or IPT over cognitive therapy (which did not differ from placebo) among more severely depressed patients (Elkin et al., 1995). Moreover, there were only minimal indications of any enduring effect for cognitive therapy following treatment termination, although such differences as were apparent did favor cognitive therapy (Shea et al., 1992).

Because of its size and the fact that it was the first such comparison to include a pill placebo control, the TDCRP exerted a considerable impact upon the field. Adherents of biological psychiatry had been disinclined to believe that psychotherapy alone could be as effective as medications with more severely depressed patients, and the TDCRP appeared to confirm that belief (Klein, 1996). The notion that medications were necessary for more severely depressed patients became a cornerstone of treatment guidelines, especially those promulgated by organized psychiatry (American Psychiatric Association, 2000). But the TDCRP was not without problems; there were differences between the sites that tracked their prior experience with cognitive therapy, leading to the claim that cognitive therapy was less than adequately implemented at two of the three sites (Jacobson & Hollon,

1996). DeRubeis and colleagues conducted a mega-analysis that focused on more severely depressed patients from the existing studies just described. As shown in Figure 3.2, cognitive therapy was no less effective than medications when data were aggregated across the available trials, and only the TDCRP appeared to show any advantage for medications (DeRubeis, Gelfand, Tang, & Simons, 1999).

These findings suggest that cognitive therapy is about as effective as medications when each is adequately implemented. However, no trial in the literature had as yet implemented both conditions adequately in the presence of a minimal treatment control. Against that backdrop, we launched a two-site, triple-blind, placebo-controlled comparison of drugs and cognitive therapy in the treatment of more severely depressed outpatients. Our study, designed to explore the questions raised in these earlier trials, included 240 depressed outpatients, all of whom met the same criteria used in the TDCRP to define severe depression. Patients were randomly assigned to 16 weeks of acute treatment with either cognitive therapy, medication treatment, or a pill placebo control. For ethical reasons, patients were kept on placebo for only 8 weeks; at that point the fact that they were on a placebo was revealed, and patients in that condition were provided humanitarian treatment. At the end of acute treatment, responders to cognitive therapy were withdrawn from treatment and followed over the subsequent 2-year interval. Responders to medication treatment were randomly assigned to either continuation medication (for

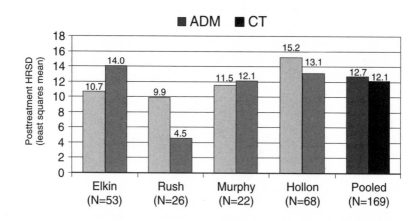

FIGURE 3.2. Average response as assessed via the Hamilton Rating Scale for Depression (HRSD) at posttreatment, to cognitive-behavioral therapy (CT) versus antidepressant medications (ADM) in severe depression. These severely depressed patients had HRSD scores of ≥20 at intake. From DeRubeis, Gelfand, Tang, and Simons (1999, p. 1010). Copyright 1999 by the American Psychiatric Association. Reprinted by permission.

1 year) or withdrawal onto a pill placebo (again triple-blind) and were followed across that same interval.

Given the concerns raised about the previous trials, we went to considerable lengths to ensure that each modality was adequately implemented. Highly trained research psychiatrists at each site who met to review patient progress on a weekly basis provided medication treatment. Paroxetine was used as the medication of choice, and dosing was quite aggressive, usually reaching a maximally tolerated dose (up to 50 mg/day) within the first 8 weeks. Patients who had shown a less than full response to paroxetine by the middle of treatment received augmentation with either lithium or desipramine (and in one instance venlafaxine) across the rest of the active treatment period. Those patients who were continued on medications after the end of acute treatment were kept at full dosage levels, and dose was increased or augmentation was initiated as needed to ward off an impending relapse.

Similar efforts were made with respect to cognitive therapy. One of our two sites (the University of Pennsylvania) was the birthplace of cognitive therapy and the setting in which the original trial by Rush and colleagues was conducted. Both the Center for Cognitive Therapy and the Beck Institute are located in Philadelphia, and the respective institutions are home to a number of highly trained and experienced therapists who split their time between clinical research and training. If cognitive therapy can be done well for depression, it can be done well in Philadelphia. Therapists at our other site (Vanderbilt University) were somewhat less experienced with cognitive therapy and more representative of what happens when this modality is exported to other sites. Potential therapists were selected from practitioners in the community who had some experience with the approach, and they were provided additional training, but it was clear from ratings of tapes sent back to the Beck Institute that they entered the trial with a lower level of competence than therapists at the Penn site. As a consequence, all three Vanderbilt therapists received additional training through the extramural program offered by the Beck Institute, and their scores on competence ratings improved over the course of the trial (as did patient outcomes). Our sense is that much of the variability in patient outcomes in the literature reflects variability in therapist competence. It is not that cognitive therapy does not work when it is done well; it is just that it is harder to do well (at least with more difficult patients) than the early literature would lead one to believe.

Both cognitive therapy and medication treatment outperformed the pill placebo in terms of acute response by midtreatment, with response rates of 43% and 50%, respectively, versus 25% for the control condition. By the end of acute treatment (16 weeks), response rates were virtually identical between the two active modalities (58.3% vs. 57.5%, respectively). Attrition was low in both conditions (15% and 16%, respectively) and was largely accounted for by dislike for the amount of work involved in the case of cognitive therapy, or side effects in the case of medications. Overall, this pattern of findings suggests that cognitive therapy is about as effective as medications in the treatment of even more severely depressed outpatients, and that both treatments are essentially well received. The drug–placebo differences also indicate that the sample as a whole was drug-responsive and that medication treatment was adequately implemented.

There were differences between the sites in the pattern of response. In essence, patients at Penn did better in cognitive therapy than they did in medication treatment, whereas patients at Vanderbilt did better in medication treatment than they did in cognitive therapy. These differences between the sites could be attributed in part to differences in experience between the cognitive therapists, and there were indications that these differences shrank over time as the Vanderbilt therapists received additional training. They also appeared to reflect a difference in medication augmentation strategy between the sites; at Penn, when nonresponsive patients received augmentation at midtreatment, the prescribing psychiatrists often reduced the dosage of the main antidepressant, whereas the prescribing psychiatrists at Vanderbilt did not. Dropping the dosage when augmenting an antidepressant is a widespread practice, but not perhaps the most efficacious thing to do. In that regard, it is noteworthy that response rates continued to increase among patients treated with medication from mid- to posttreatment at the Vanderbilt site, but not at Penn. (Response rates also increased in cognitive therapy at both sites.)

Patients who responded to cognitive therapy were withdrawn from treatment at the end of 16 weeks and followed across a subsequent 2-year period. These patients could receive up to three booster sessions over that first year, but no more than one in any given month. For all intents and purposes, they approached the follow-up as if treatment was over. They were on their own to use the skills they had learned during treatment. Patients who responded to medications were randomly assigned to either continuation medication (for the first year of the 2-year follow-up) or withdrawn onto a pill placebo. As was the case for patients assigned to the pill placebo during acute treatment, placebo withdrawal was accomplished triple-blind; that is, neither the patients nor the therapists nor the independent evaluators knew whether the pills provided contained active medication.

Patients previously treated with cognitive therapy were less likely to relapse following treatment termination than patients withdrawn from medication (31% vs. 76%), and no more likely than patients continued on medications (47%). This is wholly consistent with the earlier studies already described, which suggest that cognitive therapy has an enduring effect that protects patients against subsequent relapse, and that this effect is at least as great as that produced by keeping patients on medications. Differences between medication continuation and medication withdrawal were consistent with what is typically found in the literature and fully significant when noncompliance was taken into account. Moreover, patients who showed only partial response, or who had earlier ages of onset or more prior episodes, were at greater risk of relapse if not protected by either prior exposure to cognitive therapy or ongoing medication. This suggests that not all patients may require the protection afforded by exposure to cognitive therapy or ongoing medication, but those who do can have their risk reduced to that of low-risk patients.

Cognitive therapy costs more to provide initially than does medication treatment, but may be more cost-effective over the long run. Cognitive therapy cost about $2,000 to provide per patient in the current study (20 sessions at $100 per session), whereas medication treatment only cost about $1,000 (12 sessions at $75 per session, and $125 per month for medications). However, by the eighth month of the follow-up, the costs of continuing to keep patients on medications had passed those associated with prior cognitive therapy. Since current practice is moving toward keeping patients with a history of recurrence on medications indefinitely, cognitive therapy may prove to be considerably less expensive than medication treatment (at least to the extent that it has an enduring effect).

At the end of the first 12 months of continuation, patients were withdrawn from any ongoing medication and followed (along with patients previously treated with cognitive therapy) over 12 additional months of naturalistic conditions. These patients could be considered to have recovered from their initial episodes by virtue of the fact that they had gone more than 6 months without relapse following initial remission (Frank et al., 1991). Half of the patients withdrawn from medications experienced a recurrence (onset of a new episode) over the subsequent year, compared to only 25% of the patients with prior exposure to cognitive therapy.

Cognitive Therapy and the Prevention of Recurrence

These data, although suggestive, do not prove that cognitive therapy's enduring effect extends to the prevention of recurrence. The sample size was too small to inspire real confidence, and too large a proportion of the patients initially assigned were lost to attrition, nonresponse, or prior relapse to rule out differential retention as a rival alternative to the notion of an enduring effect. If too high a proportion of patients are lost along the way, then it is possible that initial treatment acts like a "differential sieve," screening high-risk patients out of one modality while retaining them in another (Klein, 1996). To preclude or limit the operation of a differential sieve, what is needed is a study that maximizes the number of patients who meet criteria for full recovery and does so by minimizing the differences between prior treatment conditions.

This is precisely our aim in the study that we are currently conducting. In our ongoing trial, patients who meet criteria for major depression are randomly assigned to either medication treatment alone or combined treatment with drugs and cognitive therapy. Patients are first treated to the point of remission (1 month with minimal symptoms) and then to recovery (6 months without relapse). At that point, all recovered patients in the combined condition are withdrawn from cognitive therapy, and recovered patients in both conditions are randomly assigned to either maintenance medication or medication withdrawal and followed over the next 3 years with respect to recurrence. The project is a three-site study, adding Rush Medical Center in Chicago to the ongoing collaboration between Penn and Vanderbilt.

Because our goal is to bring as many patients to full recovery, medication treatment is designed to be both flexible and aggressive. Patients typically are started on a serotonin–norepinephrine reuptake inhibitor (e.g., venlafaxine), and receive augmentation (in the case of partial response) or are switched to another medication (if unable to tolerate the initial medication, or in the event of subsequent nonresponse). Patients are given up to a year to meet criteria for remission, which allows sufficient time to try each patient on at least three different medication classes, including the older tricyclic antidepressants and monoamine oxidase inhibitors. Levels are raised aggressively to the maximally tolerated dose, and augmenting and ancillary medications are allowed if they are likely to boost response or help deal with side effects.

Similarly, our choice of combined treatment over cognitive therapy alone was driven by a desire to minimize differences between the conditions other than the actual contrast of interest. Since we were interested in seeing whether cognitive therapy's enduring effect extends to the prevention of recurrence, and prior studies suggest that this effect is robust regardless of whether cognitive therapy is accompanied by medications, choosing combined treatment should serve to minimize differences between the conditions related solely to medication taking. Moreover, by taking patients off all pills in the medication withdrawal condition (rather than withdrawing them onto pill placebos), we increase the external validity of the findings, since this is what would happen in actual clinical practice.

The study is still ongoing, and it would be premature to present findings; however, attrition is low (about 15%), and the vast majority of the patients appear to be meeting criteria for remission (some on their second or third medication). If current rates hold, we should be able to get 75–80% of the patients originally assigned into full recovery and eligible for the second randomization (and subsequent medication withdrawal). Such a rate would be considerably higher than those in most previous studies, which typically got only about half of the patients initially assigned into their maintenance phase (e.g., Frank et al., 1990).

As previously mentioned, cognitive therapy's enduring effect appears to be robust whether cognitive therapy is provided alone or in combination with medications (Evans et al., 1992). Moreover, it also appears to be robust regardless of whether cognitive therapy is provided during acute treatment or after patients are first brought to remission with medications (Paykel et al., 1999). Similarly, well-being therapy, an extension of cognitive therapy that incorporates attention to positive activities and self-perceptions, has been shown to reduce risk for recurrence when added to continuation medication treatment (Fava, Rafanelli, Grandi, Conti, & Belluardo, 1998). In the same vein, mindfulness-based cognitive therapy (which incorporates training in meditation) has been shown to reduce risk for relapse/recurrence when provided to patients first treated until remission with medications (Teasdale et al., 2000). Finally, there are indications that cognitive-behavioral interventions can be used to reduce risk for depression in children and adolescents and young adults at risk but not currently in an episode (Clarke et al., 2001; Jaycox, Reivich, Gillham, & Seligman, 1994; Seligman, Schulman, DeRubeis, & Hollon, 1999).

In summary, there are converging lines of evidence that cognitive therapy is about as effective as drugs in the treatment of depression (regardless of severity), and that it has an enduring effect that appears to reduce risk. Moreover, this enduring effect appears to be robust regardless of whether cognitive therapy is provided with medications (and if so, when), and of whether it incorporates additional techniques or foci not part of the standard approach. In the section to follow, we next turn to a consideration of just how cognitive therapy exerts its effects.

ACTIVE INGREDIENTS AND MECHANISMS OF ACTION

The first question of interest is whether cognitive therapy works (when it works) by virtue of the particular strategies specified by theory. All cognitive therapists are trained to do certain things with depressed patients, and it seems reasonable to ask whether those strategies and techniques really contribute to the change process; that is, are they the active ingredients driving therapeutic change? The notion that theoretically specified ingredients play a causative role in change is not universally supported; some have argued that nonspecific relationship factors found in all human interactions are in fact the true agents of change.

In fact, the quality of the working alliance has been found to be predictive of response in numerous studies across a number of different treatments, including cognitive therapy (Gaston, Marmar, Gallagher, & Thompson, 1991; Krupnick et al., 1994). The problem with the bulk of this research is that it has failed to control for temporal antecedence; that is, simply correlating measures of process with measures of change does not tell us whether good alliance precedes subsequent change, or whether positive change leads to the perception of good alliance.

DeRubeis and colleagues have addressed this issue in a pair of studies (DeRubeis & Feeley, 1990; Feeley, DeRubeis, & Gelfand, 1999). In each, measures of therapy process were taken across the course of treatment and related to both prior and subsequent change in depression. They found that the early implementation of specific cognitive-behavioral strategies predicted subsequent change in depression, whereas early change in depression predicted subsequent quality of alliance. In brief, therapists who engaged in strategies specified by theory got their patients better, whereas patients who got better grew to like their therapists.

Although plots of treatment outcome in most studies show group means that decrease in a smooth and negatively decelerated fashion, change for individual patients is often anything but gradual. In examining the course of individual change from the TDCRP and the Minnesota studies cited earlier, Tang and DeRubeis (1999) found that nearly half of the patients in cognitive therapy showed "sudden gains" of at least a standard deviation in depression scores from one session to the next. Further examination revealed that these "sudden gains" were not just transient noise; in most instances, they were maintained and accounted for about half of the overall change across the course of therapy. Moreover, patients who experienced sudden gains were more likely to show a full response to treatment and to maintain it longer than patients who showed a more gradual pattern of change. Finally, an examination of the preceding sessions showed a much higher incidence of cognitive change in the sessions just prior to the sudden gains than in other sessions.

This leads logically to the question of whether cognitive therapy works by virtue of changing beliefs and information processing. In most studies, medication treatment will produce as much change in most measures of cognition as does cognitive therapy (Imber et al., 1990; Simons, Garfield, & Murphy, 1984). However, the relevant question is not whether change in cognition is specific to cognitive therapy, but whether the pattern of change over time is consistent with causal agency. In the Minnesota study already described, change in cognition predicted later change in depression in cognitive therapy, but not in medication treatment (DeRubeis et al., 1990). This is exactly the pattern that would be expected if cognitive change was a mechanism of change in depression in cognitive therapy, but a consequence in other types of treatment.

One class of cognition tends to show nonspecific change. Whereas "stream-of-consciousness" beliefs tend to show nonspecific change over time (people become less negative as they become less depressed), more stable patterns of underlying information processing show a different pattern of change. In the Minnesota trial, explanatory style tended to change more slowly than measures of surface cognition (following change in depression rather than leading it), and showed greater change in cognitive therapy than it did in medication treatment (despite comparable changes in depression). Moreover, difference in explanatory style at the end of treatment was one of the better predictors of subsequent risk for relapse following treatment termination (Hollon, Evans, & DeRubeis, 1990). This suggests that the way in which an individual processes information about negative life events may play a role in how he or she responds to those events. It further suggests that cognitive therapy may exert its preventive effect (in part) through changing the way that people process information about those negative life events.

In that regard, it is of interest that Teasdale et al. (2001) have found that cognitive therapy tends to make people less extreme in their judgments, and that this reduction in extremity predicts subsequent reductions in risk. In our own most recent two-site study, explanatory style again showed greater change in cognitive therapy than it did in medication treatment, and again predicted risk for relapse in that latter condition. However, unlike our previous Minnesota trial, a small number of patients in cognitive therapy became unduly positive in their explanatory style; that is, they went from being unduly negative to being unduly positive. As was found by Teasdale and colleagues, these patients were as likely to relapse as patients with a more negative explanatory style were. This suggests that accuracy in thinking is the key, not just becoming more positive or optimistic.

CONCLUSIONS

It appears that cognitive therapy is about as effective as medications (even for more severely depressed outpatients), and that it has an enduring affect that reduces subsequent risk. Quality of implementation does appear to matter (especially for more challenging patients), just as it does for medication treatment, and there are indications that theoretically specific ingredients drive the change in depression by virtue of inducing change in existing beliefs and information-processing strategies. None of these statements have been proven, but the accumulating evidence is highly suggestive and in some instances persuasive. Nearly 40 years after it was first proposed (and 25 years after it was first tested), it appears that cognitive therapy is a viable alternative (or complement) to antidepressant medications in the treatment of most depressions—one that may confer certain advantages in terms of long-term costs and the reduction of subsequent risk.

ACKNOWLEDGMENTS

Preparation of this chapter was supported by Grants No. MH55875 (R10) and No. MH01697 (K02) (Steven D. Hollon) and No. MH50129 (Robert J. DeRubeis) from the National Institute of Mental Health.

REFERENCES

American Psychiatric Association (2000). Practice guideline for the treatment of patients with major depressive disorder (revision). *American Journal of Psychiatry, 157*(Suppl. 4).

Beck, A. T. (1970). Cognitive therapy: Nature and relation to behavior therapy. *Behavior Therapy, 1,* 184–200.

Beck, A. T. (1976). *Cognitive therapy and the emotional disorders.* New York: International Universities Press.

Beck, A. T. (1991). Cognitive therapy: A 30-year retrospective. *American Psychologist, 46,* 368–375.

Beck, A. T., Freeman, A., & Associates. (1990). *Cognitive therapy of personality disorders.* New York: Guilford Press.

Beck, A. T., Rush, A. J., Shaw, B. F., & Emery, G. (1979). *Cognitive therapy of depression.* New York: Guilford Press.

Blackburn, I. M., Bishop, S., Glen, A. I. M., Whalley, L. J., & Christie, J. E. (1981). The efficacy of cognitive therapy in depression: A treatment trial using cognitive therapy and pharmacotherapy, each alone and in combination. *British Journal of Psychiatry, 139,* 181–189.

Blackburn, I. M., Eunson, K. M., & Bishop, S. (1986). A two-year naturalistic follow-up of depressed patients treated with cognitive therapy, pharmacotherapy and a combination of both. *Journal of Affective Disorders, 10,* 67–75.

Clarke, G. N., Hornbrook, M. C., Lynch, F., Polen, M., Gale, J., Beardslee, W. R., et al. (2001). Offspring of depressed parents in a HMO: A randomized trial of a group cognitive intervention for preventing adolescent depressive disorder. *Archives of General Psychiatry, 58,* 1127–1134.

Covi, L., Lipman, R., Derogatis, L., Smith, J., & Pattison, I. (1974). Drugs and group psychotherapy in neurotic depression. *American Journal of Psychiatry, 131,* 191–198.

Daneman, E. A. (1961). Imipramine in office management of depressive reactions (a double-blind study). *Diseases of the Nervous System, 22,* 213–217.

DeRubeis, R. J., Evans, M. D., Hollon, S. D., Garvey, M. J., Grove, W. M., & Tuason, V. B. (1990). How does cognitive therapy work?: Cognitive change and symptom change in cognitive therapy and pharmacotherapy for depression. *Journal of Consulting and Clinical Psychology, 58*, 862–869.

DeRubeis, R. J., & Feeley, M. (1990). Determinants of change in cognitive therapy for depression. *Cognitive Therapy and Research, 14*, 469–482.

DeRubeis, R. J., Gelfand, L. A., Tang, T. Z., & Simons, A. D. (1999). Medications versus cognitive behavioral therapy for severely depressed outpatients: Mega-analysis of four randomized comparisons. *American Journal of Psychiatry, 156*, 1007–1013.

Dobson, K. (1989). A meta-analysis of the efficacy of cognitive therapy for depression. *Journal of Consulting and Clinical Psychology, 57*, 414–419.

Elkin, I., Gibbons, R. D., Shea, M. T., Sotsky, S. M., Watkins, J. T., Pilkonis, P. A., et al. (1995). Initial severity and differential treatment outcome in the National Institute of Mental Health Treatment of Depression Collaborative Research Program. *Journal of Consulting and Clinical Psychology, 63*, 841–847.

Elkin, I., Shea, M. T., Watkins, J. T., Imber, S. D., Sotsky, S. M., Collins, J. F., et al. (1989). NIMH Treatment of Depression Collaborative Research Program: I. General effectiveness of treatments. *Archives of General Psychiatry, 46*, 971–982.

Evans, M. D., Hollon, S. D., DeRubeis, R. J., Piasecki, J. M., Garvey, M. J., Grove, W. M., et al. (1992). Differential relapse following cognitive therapy, pharmacotherapy, and combined cognitive–pharmacotherapy for depression. *Archives of General Psychiatry, 49*, 802–808.

Fava, G. A., Rafanelli, C., Grandi, S., Conti, S., & Belluardo, P. (1998). Prevention of recurrent depression with cognitive behavioral therapy: Preliminary findings. *Archives of General Psychiatry, 55*, 816–820.

Feeley, M., DeRubeis, R. J., & Gelfand, L. A. (1999). The temporal relation of adherence and alliance to symptom change in cognitive therapy for depression. *Journal of Consulting and Clinical Psychology, 67*, 578–582.

Frank, E., Kupfer, D. J., Perel, J. M., Cornes, C., Jarrett, D. B., Mallinger, A. G., et al. (1990). Three-year outcomes for maintenance therapies in recurrent depression. *Archives of General Psychiatry, 47*, 1093–1099.

Frank, E., Prien, R. F., Jarrett, R. B., Keller, M. B., Kupfer, D. J., Lavori, P. W., et al. (1991). Conceptualization and rationale for consensus definitions of terms in major depressive disorder: Remission, recovery, relapse, and recurrence. *Archives of General Psychiatry, 48*, 851–855.

Friedman, A. S. (1975). Interaction of drug therapy with marital therapy in depressive patients. *Archives of General Psychiatry, 32*, 619–637.

Gaston, L., Marmar, C., Gallagher, D., & Thompson, L. (1991). Alliance prediction of outcome beyond in-treatment symptomatic change as psychotherapy processes. *Psychotherapy Research, 1*, 104112.

Hollon, S. D., DeRubeis, R. J., Evans, M. D., Wiemer, M. J., Garvey, M. J., Grove, W. M., et al. (1992). Cognitive therapy, pharmacotherapy and combined cognitive–pharmacotherapy in the treatment of depression. *Archives of General Psychiatry, 49*, 774–781.

Hollon, S. D., Evans, M. D., & DeRubeis, R. J. (1990). Cognitive mediation of relapse prevention following treatment for depression: Implications of differential risk. In R. E. Ingram (Ed.), *Psychological aspects of depression* (pp. 114–136). New York: Plenum Press.

Imber, S. D., Pilkonis, P. A., Sotsky, S. M., Elkin, I., Watkins, J. T., Collins, J. F., et al. (1990). Mode-specific effects among three treatments for depression. *Journal of Consulting and Clinical Psychology, 58,* 352–359.

Jacobson, N. S., & Hollon, S. D. (1996). Prospects for future comparisons between drugs and psychotherapy: Lessons from the CBT-versus-pharmacotherapy exchange. *Journal of Consulting and Clinical Psychology, 64,* 104–108.

Jaycox, L. H., Reivich, K. J., Gillham, J., & Seligman, M. E. P. (1994). Prevention of depressive symptoms in school children. *Behaviour Research and Therapy, 32,* 801–816.

Klein, D. F. (1996). Preventing hung juries about therapy studies. *Journal of Consulting and Clinical Psychology, 64,* 74–80.

Klerman, G. L., DiMascio, A., Weissman, M., Prusoff, B., & Paykel, E. S. (1974). Treatment of depression by drugs and psychotherapy. *American Journal of Psychiatry, 131,* 186–191.

Kovacs, M., & Beck, A. T. (1978). Maladaptive cognitive structures in depression. *American Journal of Psychiatry, 135,* 525–533.

Kovacs, M., Rush, A. T., Beck, A. T., & Hollon, S. D. (1981). Depressed outpatients treated with cognitive therapy or pharmacotherapy: A one-year follow-up. *Archives of General Psychiatry, 38,* 33–39.

Krupnick, J., Collins, J., Pilkonis, P. A., Elkin, I., Simmens, S., Sotsky, S. M., et al. (1994). Therapeutic alliance and clinical outcome in the NIMH Treatment of Depression Collaborative Research Program: Preliminary findings. *Psychotherapy, 31,* 28–35.

Meterissian, G. B., & Bradwejn, J. (1989). Comparative studies on the efficacy of psychotherapy, pharmacotherapy, and their combination in depression: Was adequate pharmacotherapy provided? *Journal of Clinical Psychopharmacology, 9,* 334–339.

Morris, J. B., & Beck, A. T. (1974). The efficacy of the anti-depressant drugs: A review of research (1958–1972). *Archives of General Psychiatry, 30,* 667–674.

Murphy, G. E., Simons, A. D., Wetzel, R. D., & Lustman, P. J. (1984). Cognitive therapy and pharmacotherapy, singly and together, in the treatment of depression. *Archives of General Psychiatry, 41,* 33–41.

Paykel, E. S., Scott, J., Teasdale, J. D., Johnson, A. L., Garland, A., Moore, R., et al. (1999). Prevention of relapse in residual depression by cognitive therapy. *Archives of General Psychiatry, 56,* 829–835.

Prien, R. F., & Kupfer, D. J. (1986). Continuation drug therapy for major depressive episodes: How long should it be maintained? *American Journal of Psychiatry, 143,* 18–23.

Rush, A. J., Beck, A. T., Kovacs, M., & Hollon, S. D. (1977). Comparative efficacy of cognitive therapy and pharmacotherapy in the treatment of depressed outpatients. *Cognitive Therapy and Research, 1,* 17–38.

Seligman, M. E. P., Schulman, P., DeRubeis, R. J., & Hollon, S. D. (1999, December 21). The prevention of depression and anxiety. *Prevention and Treatment,*

2, Article 8. Retrieved from *http://journals.apa.org/prevention/volume2/pre0020008a.html*

Shea, M. T., Elkin, I., Imber, S. D., Sotsky, S. M., Watkins, J. T., Collins, J. F., et al. (1992). Course of depressive symptoms over follow-up: Findings from the National Institute of Mental Health Treatment of Depression Collaborative Research Program. *Archives of General Psychiatry, 49,* 782–787.

Simons, A. D., Garfield, S. L., & Murphy, G. E. (1984). The process of change in cognitive therapy and pharmacotherapy in depression: Changes in mood and cognition. *Archives of General Psychiatry, 41,* 45–51.

Simons, A. D., Murphy, G. E., Levine, J. L., & Wetzel, R. D. (1986). Cognitive therapy and pharmacotherapy for depression: Sustained improvement over one year. *Archives of General Psychiatry, 43,* 43–48.

Tang, T. Z., & DeRubeis, R. J. (1999). Sudden gains and critical sessions in cognitive-behavioral therapy for depression. *Journal of Consulting and Clinical Psychology, 67,* 894–904.

Teasdale, J. D., Scott, J., Moore, R. G., Hayhurst, H., Pope, M., & Paykel, E. S. (2001). How does cognitive therapy prevent relapse in residual depression: Evidence from a controlled trial. *Journal of Consulting and Clinical Psychology, 69,* 347–357.

Teasdale, J. D., Segal, Z. V., Williams, J. M. G., Ridgeway, V. A., Soulsby, J. M., & Lau, M. A. (2000). Prevention of relapse/recurrence in major depression by mindfulness-based cognitive therapy. *Journal of Consulting and Clinical Psychology, 68,* 615–623

Chapter 4

Cognitive Theory and Research on Generalized Anxiety Disorder

JOHN H. RISKIND

Generalized anxiety disorder (GAD) is associated with excessive and uncontrollable worry, as well as significant somatic complaints, lost productivity at work, impaired social relationships and role functioning, and increased medical service cost (e.g., Greenberg et al., 1999). Moreover, the course of GAD appears to be chronic and relatively unremitting (Noyes et al., 1992), with the majority of patients reporting an early age of onset (e.g., Hoehn-Saric, Hazlett, & McLeod, 1993). Epidemiological studies using *Diagnostic and Statistical Manual of Mental Disorders,* third edition, revised (DSM-III-R) criteria have estimated the current and lifetime prevalence rates of GAD in the United States to be 1.6% and 5.1%, respectively (Wittchen, Zhao, Kessler, & Eaton, 1994). The prevalence of GAD seems to be even higher in primary care settings and among high utilizers of medical care (Greenberg et al., 1999).

Beck's cognitive theory of anxiety continues to have a profound impact on our understanding of GAD. In this chapter, I briefly describe Beck's pivotal role in the study of GAD, and then discuss some offshoots and recent research. I begin by discussing basic tenets of Beck's cognitive formulation of anxiety; I then consider some central issues that have been studied in research on cognitive aspects of GAD, and discuss the extent to which research upholds Beck's formulation. Next, I discuss several paths of inquiry that recent investigators have pursued, including (1) an emphasis on worry and its role in GAD; and (2) the particular phenomenology of the danger cognitions and images in anxiety that stimulate compensatory overprotective responses such as worry in GAD, as proposed by the model of "looming vulnerability" in anxiety. The chapter concludes with a brief summary.

GENERAL BACKGROUND: BECK'S COGNITIVE MODEL OF ANXIETY

The impact of Beck's cognitive formulation of anxiety is best understood in the context of the existing alternative theoretical models of GAD (or its rough equivalent in the existing nomenclature) at the time. The diagnostic classification system of that era (DSM-II) had not yet distinguished GAD and panic disorder as separate disorders, and labeled them both as "neurotic anxiety." Implicit to this labeling was a psychoanalytic approach to conceptualizing these phenomena as "free-floating anxiety." Such anxiety was believed to stem from unconscious causes, unrelated to the individual's consciously accessible ideational content. Behavioral theories shared little sympathy for the psychoanalytic perspective but also deemphasized the role of consciously accessible ideation. Anxiety was conceptualized by behaviorists in simple stimulus–response (S-R) terms as a conditioned response to external stimuli.

A pioneering seminal study that was conducted by Beck, Laude, and Bohnert (1974) marked a turning point, because it showed the way to a new way of conceptualizing the causes of GAD. Beck et al. interviewed a consecutive series of patients who were admitted for treatment for "anxiety neurosis" (which would often correspond to GAD by DSM-IV standards). The evidence of these interviews was remarkable. Consistent with a cognitive theory, but less so with psychoanalytic and simple S-R models, Beck et al. demonstrated that patients with neurotic anxiety identified threat-related automatic thoughts and/or pictorial images at times when their anxiety intensified. These results made it possible to explain the anxiety symptoms of clinical patients by means of their consciously accessible verbal thoughts and pictorial images.

In the 1980s, Beck and colleagues' ground-breaking book (Beck & Emery with Greenberg, 1985) elaborated the cognitive theory of anxiety and pointed the way to developing effective treatments. The importance of this book is that it helped to extend the cognitive formulations and treatments that had already been so fruitfully applied to depression (Beck, 1967; Beck, Rush, Shaw, & Emery, 1979).

Turning Anxiety on Its Head: Beck's Original Cognitive Model of Anxiety Disorders

The important theme of the Beck et al. (1985) landmark volume is that anxiety disorders can be better understood if we "turn anxiety on its head." That is, an adequate account of what we call GAD today must address its characteristic cognitive content and profile.

Beck's "cognitive content specificity hypothesis" argued that each distinct form of affective disturbance is related to its own "disorder-specific cognitive profile." For example, the specific core cognitive themes of hopelessness and irreversible loss characterize depression. In contrast, the disorder-specific themes in anxiety center on future-oriented vulnerability to possible harm. The future-oriented content of anxiety is related to overestimations of perceived threat and underestimations of one's personal resources for coping with threat. Including the theoretical ideas of social psychologist Richard Lazarus (e.g., Lazarus, 1966), Beck et al. (1985) suggested that automatic, involuntary "primary" cognitive appraisals of the magnitude and severity of potential threat are at the heart of anxiety.

Beck et al. (1985) suggested that the concept of "fear" refers to a cognitive process that centers on the "primary appraisal" of threat. Such appraisal of threat, or fear, will be central to any anxiety response or disorder, and so will also be central to GAD. In addition to the concept of primary appraisal of threat, which they drew from Lazarus (1966), they also drew on Lazarus's concept of "secondary appraisals" of resources for coping with threat. For example, a patient who is diagnosed with GAD will be likely both to overestimate the magnitude of future threat *and* to underestimate his or her capacity to cope with the threat.

Multiple Levels of Cognitive Phenomena in GAD

In Beck's model, the cognitive phenomena associated with anxiety occur at multiple levels. Threat ideation, in the form of thoughts or images in the stream of consciousness, is caused by an interaction between basic cognitive processes (e.g., memory, attention, interpretation) and a person's underlying belief structures or cognitive structures/schemas concerned with personal vulnerability to threat. The interaction between basic processes and structures or schemas produces cognitive biases in selective attention (or avoidance), memory, and exaggerated interpretation of threat stimuli. The same interaction leads anxious individuals to interpret ambiguous events as threatening, even though they can be interpreted in more than one way (some of which are even neutral or positive). For example, the perception that another person who is present has a remote look will tend to be interpreted as a sign of rejection, rather than as a sign of the other person's preoccupation.

Individuals who are highly prone to anxiety have developed maladaptive variants of cognitive structures called "danger schemas" that guide information processing (e.g., attention, interpretation, and memory for threat stimuli). The danger schemas in GAD, in contrast to those in what is now called specific phobia, tend to encompass multiple broad spheres—such as fears of negative social evaluation, disability, and death. Patients with GAD have acquired danger schemas that bias them to (1) overestimate the degree of threat that is represented by a wide range of given stimuli; (2) underestimate personal control; and (3) experience heightened levels of threat-related stream-of-consciousness thoughts and pictorial images (e.g., concerned with the presence of threats of injury, social embarrassment, or other aversive events).

Research on Cognitive Aspects of GAD

Evidence from a considerable number of studies tends to uphold Beck's view that typical threat-related thoughts/images are reported by patients with GAD (see Beck & Clark, 1997, for a review). Many studies have found evidence for systematic biases in the ways patients with GAD process threat-related information (Beck & Clark, 1997), particularly in the early phases of selective attention to threatening material (Mogg & Bradley, in press) and on implicit memory tasks (Coles & Heimberg, 2002). Contrary to what would have been expected from Beck's early formulation, cognitive biases in GAD are not so clearly found on explicit memory tasks—that is, on tasks that make explicit reference to the material to be remembered (Coles & Heimberg, 2002). This research suggests that there are defensive processes in GAD operating at a more controlled or deliberate level that override automatic biases for threat information posited by Beck's cognitive formulation.

Beck and Clark (1997) have refined the cognitive model to take account of the role of compensatory, self-protective processes (e.g., cognitive avoidance, avoidance of negative affect). To generalize from this, it appears that even compulsive checking behaviors are associated with GAD (Schut, Castonguay, & Borkovec, 2001). Among these compensatory protective processes, one of the most investigated in recent years is the phenomenon of "pathological worry" in GAD (Borkovec, Ray, & Stoeber, 1998).

Research on Worry in GAD

DSM-IV stipulates that excessive and uncontrollable worry is a hallmark of the GAD syndrome. The worry in GAD has both temporal and content requirements. A GAD diagnosis requires worry about four or more life circumstances that occur over a minimum of 6 months. The worry is particularly protracted and difficult to terminate voluntarily, and individuals with GAD compound the problem by "worrying about their own worry"—a type of worry that Adrian Wells labels "metaworry" (see Wells, Chapter 9, this volume).

The DSM-IV identifies excessive worry as a characteristic symptom of GAD, but does not theoretically explain the functions of the excessive worry. Borkovec has formulated an avoidance theory of the nature and functions of worry. The pathological worry of GAD is seen as a maladaptive tactic for cognitively avoiding internally generated aversive images of danger and intense feelings of fear. It appears that worry may contribute to faulty emotion regulation more broadly (Mennin, Heimberg, Turk, & Fresco, 2002) and to experiential avoidance (e.g., Roemer & Orsillo, 2002), which includes the avoidance of other unpleasant emotions as well (Freeston, Rheaume, Letarte, Dugas, & Ladouceur, 1994). According to Borkovec, worry will usually involve an active form of predominantly verbal/linguistic thought (an activity of the left-hemisphere of the brain). This predominance of verbal/linguistic processing shifts the person's attention away from vivid and concrete threatening mental images (a right-hemisphere activity), which otherwise would provoke intense fear (Borkovec & Inz, 1990) and autonomic reactivity (Borkovec et al., 1998). It has been suggested by Borkovec et al. (1998) that pathological worry in GAD is maintained through negative reinforcement contingencies (i.e., the avoidance of somatic anxiety, emotional distress, and aversive imagery).

Beck and colleagues suggest that worry is an attempt to cope with the fear (Beck & Clark, 1997; Beck et al., 1985). This conception is in line with Borkovec's avoidance theory of worry, as well as with recent evidence suggesting that worry cycles may be triggered by threatening thoughts or images, and maintained as a defensive response to cognitively avoid the fear and other unpleasant emotions they produce. Other recent evidence likewise indicates that individuals with GAD attempt to control or avoid negative emotional experience more generally (e.g., Roemer & Orsillo, 2002).

Summary of Theory and Research on Beck's Cognitive Model

Beck's cognitive model made an important contribution by providing a fundamental theoretical foundation for a cognitive-behavioral understanding of GAD. Considerable research has amassed that directly tests and often upholds many components of the model, but several paths of inquiry and sets of findings suggest the needs to refine and elaborate the fundamental model in new directions. Examples are the work on worry (Borkovec et al., 1998; Wells, Chapter 9, this volume) and experiential avoidance (e.g.,

Roemer & Orsillo, 2002). Another path of such inquiry, to which we turn now, is the model of "looming vulnerability" (e.g., Riskind, 1997; Riskind & Williams, in press-a). The purpose of this model is to pinpoint specific fear-provoking threat cognitions and cognitive styles that will be important in inducing anxiety and worry.

WHY IS IT NECESSARY TO BETTER IDENTIFY SPECIFIC THREAT COGNITIONS IN ANXIETY?

There has been considerable attention to the maladaptive compensatory and neutralizing responses (e.g., worry, affect avoidance) in GAD, but a dearth of attention to the specific cognitive underpinnings of the driving appraisals of threat in the disorder. However, an adequate understanding of the specific cognitive underpinnings of the perception of threat is necessary for developing the most effective treatment and prevention interventions.

The score card for cognitive-behavioral interventions, assessments, and conceptualizations of anxiety is strong, but far from the optimum that might be expected or hoped. Although cognitive-behavioral interventions are highly successful for some disorders (such as social anxiety disorder and panic disorder), for other disorders (such as GAD) they are only modestly successful. Many researchers and clinicians recognize that there is substantial room for improvement in the cognitive-behavioral treatment of these latter disorders. Beyond this, even when GAD is successfully treated, there are "treatment-resistant" patients who don't seem to respond to the usual cognitive-behavioral protocols.

One possible explanation for the current uneven success rate of cognitive-behavioral interventions for GAD is that the specific details of the cognitive phenomena in the disorders need to be better worked out. A possible sign of this possible lack of precision in understanding these details is the difficulty in empirically distinguishing the putative cognitive phenomena that are specific to anxiety from those that are discernible in depression (Riskind, 1997). R. Beck and Perkins (2001) conducted a recent meta-analysis indicating that anxiety-related cognitive phenomena are often identified just as strongly in individuals with depression as in those with anxiety. Both threat-related automatic thoughts and the phenomenon of worry were not unique to anxiety and did not differentiate anxiety from depression. The R. Beck and Perkins findings echo similar findings that have been obtained for decades (e.g., Butler & Mathews, 1983). The extent of such overlap in both cognitions and symptoms has suggested to some that anxiety and depression are essentially the same construct and syndrome, and that they are not usefully distinguished. Such findings challenge cognitive models to achieve greater precision in identifying the specific threat cognitions that are important in GAD and other forms of anxiety

THE TIME–DISTANCE RELATIONSHIP IN THREAT: THE MODEL OF LOOMING VULNERABILITY

The formulation of the model of looming vulnerability originally grew out of an attempt to determine what can cognitively distinguish anxiety and depression from one another (Riskind, 1997; Riskind, Williams, Gessner, Chrosniak, & Cortina, 2000; Riskind & Williams, in press-a). The model was drawn from an analysis of the possible evolutionary functions of responses to danger in fear and anxiety, as compared to responses to helplessness and hopeless in sadness and depression. It unified this analysis with ethological observations of animals responding to threat stimuli; developmental observations of young children; and cognitive and social-cognitive concepts about the nature of mental representations of meaningful and emotionally relevant stimuli and events in the environment.

As a preview of this analysis, the perception of danger has a functional role in the adaptive behavior of humans and other animals. When individuals can anticipate what has not yet occurred or been encountered, preparations can be made to bring about or facilitate good events or to avoid or avert negative events. Cognitive representations of danger reflect this reality constraint. In this context, the fact that danger varies with time is inherent to the logic of the danger posed by any frightening situation. An external environmental threat (e.g., a predator in the wild, an interpersonal rejection) or an internal threat (e.g., a serious illness, a prospect of loss of mental or physical control) is a more extreme source of danger when it is successively rising or increasing in danger than when it is falling or decreasing.

In accord with other research that underscores the role of mental imagery in anxiety, the model of looming vulnerability emphasizes that the perceptions of danger that instigate worry and other maladaptive neutralizing compensatory responses are related to a specific maladaptive imaging and appraisal process. This imaging process is not just focused on the static capacity of a threatening situation to harm, but portrays dynamic, variable properties, such as how quickly it is changing. A stimulus (e.g., a threat of potential injury, rejection, or emotional harm) will elicit more intense fear and compensatory need for neutralizing responses when there is a predominant impression in images or appraisals of looming vulnerability to a threat whose risk is intensifying and rising, either in time or in space.

The Need to Distinguish Concepts of Fear, Anxiety, Worry, and Panic

Any endeavor to explore the psychological underpinnings of threat perceptions must start with a recognition that the concept of "anxiety" refers to a class of interrelated but conceptually distinct phenomena. Despite common features of fear, anxiety, worry, and panic as responses to perceptions of threat, these terms do not refer to interchangeable phenomena. The term "fear" is used to refer to a fundamental emotion, observed in humans and many other species of animals, that is an integral aspect of the "fight or flight" response. A threatening stimulus that is perceived or is vividly imagined as possessing immediacy in its implications for well-being will elicit fear. A more intense fear reaction will occur when the threatening situation or event is perceived as, or portrayed in mental images as, rapidly rising in risk.

The term "anxiety" is a multilayered complex of elements that comprises fear, worry, and several other psychological processes. The trigger for anxiety is often a perception of threat that generates recurring instants of fear (see above), which then alternate with the more abstract and verbal/conceptual thinking activity that is referred to as "worry." Because worry is a predominantly lexical activity, it shifts attentional resources from vivid imagery of a concrete threat to more abstract verbal representations and ideas; it thus results in less intense fear.

The model of looming vulnerability holds that anxiety is initiated and maintained by fear-provoking mental images and appraisals that portray threats as rapidly intensifying. Such images are the catalysts for maladaptive neutralizing strategies such as worry or experiential avoidance. The greater the extent to which images and perceptions portray the threat as rapidly intensifying in risk, the greater the fear, and the greater the consequent self-protective response of worry. Individuals with GAD frequently alternate between fear reactions and neutralizing responses such as worry or experiential avoidance. Both types of reactions are dependent on perceptions or mental images of rapidly intensifying threat. Persons with GAD also sometimes experience "panic" reactions, which are maximum fear reactions that cannot be neutralized because the threat is already so close at hand.

The "Looming Cognitive Style"

Although great strides have been made in the past decade in understanding the nature and function of faulty neutralizing responses (e.g., worry, affect avoidance), relatively little research or theory has addressed their potential cognitive antecedents. The "looming cognitive style" (LCS) is believed to be a psychological antecedent. It is a negative cognitive style that functions as a danger schema and involves primarily imagery-based mental representations of the intensification of threats.

Basic experimental and perceptual research informs us that all perceptions as well as visualizations are "tricks" played by the mind, reflecting the fact that perceptions/images are to a large degree self-constructed. Perception is the result of a person-by-environment interaction. Any complete understanding of anxiety and fear must take account of both the person characteristics and the environmental stimuli that provoke these reactions to threat. Although an impression that threats are rapidly intensifying is sometimes accurate and adaptive, a problem in pathological anxiety is that a sense of looming vulnerability is not flexibly stimulus-driven in a "bottom-up" fashion by environmental cues, but is rigidly imposed in a "top-down" fashion by maladaptive mental representations. The ability to mentally simulate the potential progression of threat through time and space may become generalized into a broad and pervasive tendency to mentally represent potential threats as rapidly intensifying in risk and danger.

According to the model of looming vulnerability, some individuals develop a distinct danger schema, the LCS, which produces unique cognitive risk for anxiety states and disorders by inducing individuals to formulate mental representations or expectations that portray threats as rapidly intensifying and rising in risk (Riskind et al., 2000). The LCS functions as a danger schema that leads to an automatic stereotypic depiction of threats as characterized by rapidly rising risk. As noted, the LCS is hypothesized to consist of primarily imagery-based mental representations of the developmental progression(s) of potential threat over time (i.e., dynamic or kinetic rather than static and lifeless fear-related imagery) (Riskind & Williams, in press-a, in press-b; Williams, McDonald, Owens, & Lunt, 2003). Consequently, individuals who develop the LCS are likely to have difficulty habituating to potential threats, to demonstrate increased vigilance and anxiety, to perceive a sense of time urgency and imperative need for action, and to overutilize cognitive and behavioral avoidance strategies (Riskind, 1997; Riskind & Williams, in press-a). In functioning as a danger schema, the LCS is held to be implicated in a variety of phenomena—ranging from conditioning and sensitization to threat stimuli and impedance of habituation, salience and biased processing of threat information, cognitive phenomenology of experiences of anxiety and fear, and cognitive vulnerability for threat (Riskind, 1997).

A central goal of work on the LCS is to address the dearth of attention that has been given to developing questionnaire measures of the peculiar danger schemas and cognitive vulnerabilities in GAD and other anxiety disorders. The looming model also attempts to specify with greater precision the critical component of danger schemas and perceived threat that discriminates anxiety from depression. As noted, past studies have not reliably distinguished anxiety from depression via standard measures of threat appraisal (e.g., probability) or threat-related automatic thoughts (R. Beck & Perkins, 2001). The model of looming vulnerability portrays the concept of looming vulnerability as unique and disorder-specific to anxiety.

The Model of Looming Vulnerability and GAD

The model of looming vulnerability model postulates that GAD and the tendency to worry and avoid unpleasant emotions (Freeston et al., 1994; Roemer & Orsillo, 2002) are often based in the LCS. According to the model, individuals who have this maladaptive cognitive style will be more likely to generate mental images that portray danger as rapidly intensifying and provide an impetus to engage in compensatory self-protective responses such as worry or experiential avoidance (e.g., Riskind & Williams, in press-a, in press-b). Figure 4.1 depicts these proposed relationships.

There are several pathways through which the LCS is hypothesized to function as both a cognitive antecedent to and a maintaining factor in GAD. First, the LCS may lead individuals to generate a continuing stream of threatening, catastrophic image-based mental representations of even relatively mundane potential threats, which motivate the need to utilize lexically based cognitive avoidance strategies such as worry. Second, since the LCS involves the generation of animated fear-inducing mental scenarios, images, and expectations of being overtaken by rapidly escalating risks and

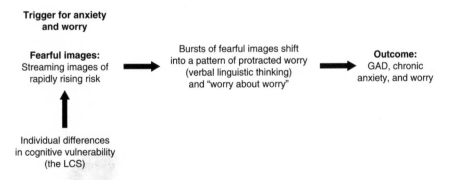

FIGURE 4.1. Proposed relations among individual differences, fearful imagery, and GAD.

dangers, it may lead to higher levels of intensity of emotional experience and subsequent difficulties regulating negative emotion. In this way, it leads to affect avoidance and faulty emotion regulation strategies. Third, the LCS fosters a schematic processing bias for threatening material. For instance, the LCS can lead individuals with GAD to interpret ambiguous material in threatening ways, and show a bias to attend to and remember such material. Fourth, when the LCS is activated, it may absorb the attentional control resources that cognitively vulnerable individuals need to cope optimally with negative emotion. In consequence, the LCS impairs the mental control mechanisms that are required to deal effectively with threatening images and affect.

The following sections briefly summarize the evidence for the model of looming vulnerability. First they summarize evidence for the broader model, and then they cover specific evidence bearing on the relationship between the LCS and GAD.

Overview of Studies on the General Model of Looming Vulnerability

The looming model stipulates that the sense of looming vulnerability can occur either as a state elicitation, or as a characterological feature of cognitive organization (i.e., the LCS). At any given moment, one can have a subjective sense of looming vulnerability (e.g., when standing in the street in front of a speeding automobile). As we have seen, however, people who have the LCS characteristically conjure up scenarios that distort and exaggerate the degree to which threats are rapidly mounting and rising in risk; such persons are prone to anxiety.

Numerous studies have examined the validity of the model of looming vulnerability with specific focal forms of anxiety and fear (e.g., Riskind, 1997; Riskind et al., 2000; Riskind & Maddux, 1993; Riskind, Moore, & Bowley, 1995; Riskind & Wahl, 1992; Riskind & Williams, 1999a, 1999b). This research has used a variety of methodologies, including self-report assessments, computer-simulated movement of objects (e.g., moving spiders vs. moving rabbits), the presentation of videotaped scenarios (e.g., a campus mugging, possible contamination scenarios, etc.), and the presentation of moving and static visual images. These studies have also investigated a range of cognitive clinical processes (e.g., thought suppression, worry, coping styles, uncontrollability, catastrophizing, attachment styles, memory bias, etc.) across a wide range of stimuli (e.g., individuals with mental illness, individuals with HIV, spiders, contamination, weight gain, social and romantic rejection, performance mistakes, etc.) and a diversity of populations (e.g., college students and individuals with GAD, panic disorder, obsessive–compulsive disorder [OCD], or specific animal phobias).

As a whole, this body of studies provides remarkably consistent evidence for the model of looming vulnerability (for reviews, see Riskind, 1997; Riskind, Williams, & Joiner, in press; Riskind & Williams, in press-a). Many studies have examined focal or highly specific forms of looming vulnerability in relation to stimulus-specific fears of spiders (e.g., Riskind, Kelly, Harman, Moore, & Gaines, 1992; Riskind & Maddux, 1993; Riskind et al., 1995), AIDS or HIV (Riskind & Maddux, 1994), toxic contaminants (Riskind, Wheeler, & Picerno, 1997; Riskind, Abreu, Strauss, & Holt, 1997), and social rejection (e.g., Riskind & Mizrahi, 1994). For instance, symptoms of OCD are associated with mental representations that portray the threat of spreading contamination as rapidly intensifying (Riskind et al., 1995; Tolin, Worhunsky, & Maltby, in press). OCD symptoms are also associated with mental representations that portray the risk of losing control of aggressive impulses (e.g., stabbing someone) as rapidly rising (Riskind & Williams, 2004). Importantly, measures of the subjective sense of looming vulnerability contribute to OCD symptoms (Riskind, Wheeler, & Picerno, 1997; Riskind, Abreu, et al., 1997), and fears of HIV infection (Riskind & Maddux, 1994), as well as to social performance anxiety (Riskind & Mizrahi, 2004), even when studies have controlled for other facets of perceived (or appraised) threat-stimulus-specific fear (e.g., predominantly verbal and static estimates of the likelihood or unpredictability of harm).

Validity of the LCS Measure

A self-report questionnaire was developed to assess the LCS, defined as the characteristic extent to which individuals generate images that portray risk as rapidly rising (Riskind et al., 1992, 2000). Participants are presented with six brief vignettes describing different types of stressful situations (e.g., threat of illness, risk of physical injury, romantic rejection), and are asked to complete a three-item list of questions for each vignette. A long series of our studies provides evidence for both the internal consistency (alpha = .91) and temporal stability of the LCS measure over 4 months (Riskind et al., 2000).

A considerable number of studies have supported the convergent and discriminant validity of the LCS measure, indicating that higher scores on this "Looming Maladaptive Style Questionnaire" are related to higher levels of anxiety as assessed by a variety of measures, and have found unusually consistent evidence that the LCS is significantly associated with several correlates of anxiety, including worry, thought suppression, and behavioral avoidance (e.g., Riskind et al., 2000; for a review, see Riskind & Williams, in press-a). However, as expected from the model, the LCS is not consistently related to depression. As will be mentioned below, there is also evidence that the LCS is incrementally predictive of future anxiety when initial anxiety is controlled for (Riskind et al., 2000), and that it predicts anxiety even when such variables as neuroticism, anxiety sensitivity, negative affectivity, and dysfunctional attitudes are controlled for (Riskind, Williams, Joiner, Black, & Cortina, 2003).

Additional convergent validity data come from a study using a homophone task. The LCS was significantly and uniquely related to the tendency to process and encode ambiguous verbal information—recordings of homophones, such as "dye" versus "die"—in a threatening manner. Individuals who had the LCS were significantly more biased than other individuals to choose the more threatening spelling of the homophones (Riskind et al., 2000, Study 3). This effect, on a measure of implicit memory for threat, was unique to the LCS and was not related to anxiety itself or to an alternative approach to cognitive vulnerability assessed by static likelihood estimates of threat.

Other studies of memory bias also support the validity of the LCS and the hypothesis that it is associated with schematic processing bias. We (Riskind et al., 2000, Study 4) tested the effects of the LCS on memory for pictorial threat-related stimuli, using a laboratory task in which pictorial images were presented (e.g., threatening pictorial images of a house fire or auto crash, or neutral or positive images such as a table or flower). Structural equation modeling revealed that the LCS was significantly and uniquely related to a measure of implicit memory for threat (a word stem completion task). Individuals who had the LCS were significantly more biased than other individuals to complete word stems with threatening words. This effect, on the word stem completion task of implicit memory for threat, was again unique to the LCS and was not related to anxiety itself. The LCS was also significantly and uniquely related to two measures of explicit memory for threat (a free-recall task and a frequency estimation task).

Specificity of LCS to Anxiety versus Depression

As previously noted, research has also demonstrated with remarkable consistency that the LCS is specific to anxiety and not depression. Studies to date have produced a body of evidence for the discriminant validity of the LCS, suggesting that scores on the LCS can differentiate between anxiety and depression—despite the high overlap and correlation commonly found between these syndromes. Typically, we find that significant correlations between the LCS and anxiety remain significant even after the effects of variance in depression scores are statistically removed. But any correlation between LCS and depression is reduced to nonsignificance after the effects of variance in anxiety scores are controlled for. All of these findings are consistent with the model of looming vulnerability, which hypothesizes that the LCS is specific to anxiety and not depression.

Does the LCS Incrementally Predict Anxiety beyond Other Powerful Variables?

One can also wonder whether the LCS also *incrementally predicts* scores for anxiety beyond other potentially powerful variables such as negative affectivity, anxiety sensitivity, neuroticism, or dysfunctional attitudes. The answer is yes. There is now compelling evidence that the LCS predicts significant unique variance in current and future anxiety, even after anxiety-relevant variables that might be potential confounds are controlled for.

First, we (Riskind et al., 2000) demonstrated with structural equation modeling that although the LCS and anxiety are correlated, their measurement properties clearly distinguish them. Next, studies have shown that the LCS, though correlating with measures of neuroticism, negative affectivity, anxiety sensitivity, or negative life events, is distinct from and can clearly be distinguished from these variables, and that it predicts distinct variance in scores for anxiety over and above that predicted by these measures (Riskind et al., 2000; Riskind, Williams, et al., 2003). For example, the strong relationship between LCS and both trait anxiety and state anxiety remains significant, even after controlling for neuroticism scores as well as negative affectivity (a measure of neuroticism). These findings support the incremental value of the LCS in predicting additional significant and distinct variance in scores for anxiety, above the effects of neuroticism or negative affectivity.

Several studies using structural equation modeling and confirmatory factor analysis provide additional strong support for the discriminant validity and incremental value of the LCS. One of these studies used structural equation modeling with 142 college students and showed that the LCS is psychometrically distinct from anxiety sensitivity and negative affectivity, and that it offers additional significant prediction of variance in scores for trait anxiety over and above these variables. Moreover, tests comparing the correlations showed that anxiety sensitivity and negative affectivity were significantly more strongly correlated with each other than they were with the LCS. Results for the incremental validity of the LCS beyond the effect of negative affectivity were confirmed by another study, which examined these variables in relation to both anxiety and depression. Results demonstrated that the LCS was specific to anxiety, whereas negative affectivity was nonspecifically related to scores for both anxiety and depression.

In another recent study on 206 college students, confirmatory factor analyses showed that LCS was distinct from dysfunctional attitudes on the Dysfunctional Attitudes Scale and from the pessimistic explanatory style (e.g., Abramson, Metalsky, & Alloy, 1989). The LCS was significantly and uniquely related to anxiety, and the pessimistic explanatory style was significantly and uniquely related to depression. The results also showed that the LCS and pessimistic explanatory style, but not dysfunctional attitudes, were better predictors of anxiety and depression symptoms than a trait anxiety measure (Riskind, Williams, et al., 2003).

The incremental value of the LCS is also upheld by the fact that it predicts significant variance in anxiety measures beyond the effects accounted for by predominantly static verbal predictions of unpredictability, uncontrollability, likelihood, or imminence of threat (e.g., Riskind et al., 2000; Riskind & Williams, in press-a). In general, then, these results have importantly confirmed that the LCS is not simply another measure or proxy for other variables, including standard threat appraisals, trait anxiety, anxiety sensitivity, neuroticism or negativism, or dysfunctional attitudes.

Cognitive Vulnerability to the Development of GAD

Abramson and Alloy (Abramson et al., 1989; Alloy, Abramson, Raniere, & Dyller, 1999; Riskind & Alloy, in press) have defined a "cognitive vulnerability factor" as a potential antecedent cause (*distal* cause) that operates toward the beginning of the temporal sequence, distant in time from the first occurrence (or recurrence) of the disorder. A putative cognitive vulnerability factor is thought to increase the likelihood that a disorder such as GAD will arise after exposure to stressful events. In this context, the LCS is hypothesized to be in place and to create a liability for GAD long before the earliest signs or symptoms of GAD appear. The LCS purportedly creates a specific liability to an anxiety disorder such as GAD after individuals encounter stressful events, and maintains the problems after their onset. Of course, only by addressing the LCS with high-risk prospective designs can its status as a putative vulnerability factor be tested.

The LCS as a Predictor of the Occurrence of Future Anxiety and Worry

Although no studies have examined the development of GAD over time, there is other evidence that the LCS is a cognitive vulnerability factor. Support for the putative status of the LCS as such a factor is provided by evidence that it incrementally predicts scores for future anxiety, beyond the effects of initial scores for anxiety. Several longitudinal studies with follow-ups ranging in duration from 1 week to 4 months demonstrate that the LCS significantly predicts residualized gains in anxiety scores when anxiety at Time 1 is controlled for (e.g., Riskind et al., 2000, Study 2; Williams & Riskind, 2004b). The LCS also predicts residualized gains in worry as assessed by the Penn State Worry Questionnaire (Meyer et al., 1990) over a 1-week time interval (Riskind, Williams, et al., 2003).

Combined with the preceding studies, there is also evidence that the LCS increases cognitive vulnerability to stressful life events. A longitudinal study conducted with 160 subjects tested 6 weeks apart (Williams & Riskind, 2004b) has demonstrated this. As would be expected from the model of looming vulnerability, a highly significant interaction was found between the LCS and negative life events in predicting increases in anxious symptoms at the follow-up session. Stressful life events only predicted future onset or increases in anxiety symptoms when subjects had elevated LCS scores.

Evidence of the LCS in GAD

The hypothesis that there is an elevated level of the LCS in GAD has been supported in three studies, using both nonclinical and clinical subject samples (Riskind & Williams, in press-b; Riskind, Gessner, & Wolzon, 2003). In one study (Riskind & Williams, in press-b) an analogue sample of students with and without a probable GAD diagnosis was used to examine whether the group with probable GAD demonstrated elevated levels of the LCS, and what the relative contribution of the LCS was in discriminating between the groups with and without probable GAD. When strict scoring criteria for the Generalized Anxiety Disorder Questionnaire–IV (GADQ-IV; Newman et al., 2002), were used, 19 individuals were identified as having probable GAD (20.4% of the sample), and 70 individuals were identified as not having GAD (79.6% of the sample). We chose more stringent scoring criteria than Newman et al. to minimize the rate of false-negative diagnoses of GAD, even though these more stringent criteria may have resulted in reduced sensitivity of the GADQ-IV to detect probable cases of GAD. The group with probable GAD consisted of 14 women and 5 men, while the group without GAD consisted of 42 women and 32 men. Results of the study provide consistent evidence for elevated scores for the LCS in the group with GAD, and for the contribution of the LCS to discriminate the two groups.

Two natural follow-up studies with community clinical samples have replicated these findings and confirmed that the LCS is elevated in GAD in psychiatric populations (Riskind & Williams, in press-b; Riskind, Gessner, & Wolzon, 2003). In the Riskind, Gessner, and Wolzon study, the

GADQ-IV was used in a sample of persons with substance abuse who were in a detoxification program. Thirty-three individuals were identified as having probable GAD (34% of the sample), and 72 individuals were identified as not having GAD (66% of the sample). Results with this sample in a detoxification unit confirmed that those with probable GAD had LCS scores that were significantly elevated in comparison to the scores of those without GAD.

In another study (Riskind & Williams, in press-b, Study 2), the Structured Clinical Interview for DSM-IV (SCID) was used in a clinical sample to identify 19 individuals who were diagnosed with GAD and 9 individuals who were diagnosed with unipolar depression (major depressive disorder and/or dysthymia). These two clinical groups were compared to each other and to 28 individuals in a nonpsychiatric control group who were disorder-free. The results of this study replicated and extended those of the previous two studies: They confirmed that persons with stringent SCID diagnoses of GAD had LCS scores that were significantly elevated in comparison to those of the other groups. Importantly, the group with GAD had LCS scores that were significantly elevated in comparison to those of the group with unipolar depression, which in turn did not significantly differ from the scores of the nonpsychiatric control group.

It is also notable that recent studies have shown that the LCS is strongly predictive of faulty emotion regulation strategies (Riskind, Mann, & Ployhart, 2004), worry (Riskind et al., 2000; Riskind, Williams, et al., 2004), and thought suppression (Riskind et al., 2000; Riskind & Williams, in press-b). All of these factors are central to current cognitive-behavioral theories of GAD.

The research discussed to this point has shown that the LCS is elevated in GAD. However, research using high-risk prospective designs has not yet addressed whether the LCS is a putative antecedent or a cognitive vulnerability factor.

Studies of the Developmental Origins of the LCS

According to the model of looming vulnerability, the LCS can be rooted in faulty modeling and parenting, unresolved childhood fears, or insecure attachment experiences. To date, three studies have investigated attachment and parenting and found evidence that they help mold the LCS (Riskind, Williams, et al., 2004; Williams & Riskind, 2004a). The Williams and Riskind (2004a) study found that LCS scores were positively associated with increased anxiety and higher levels of attachment insecurity, and that the LCS partially mediated the relationship between adult attachment and anxious symptoms. That is, the LCS is a significant mediator of the effects of attachment relationships on anxiety, indicating that the link between the intermediary cognitive style and prior attachment patterns is a significant pathway for the effects of attachment patterns. Another study (Riskind, Williams, et al., 2004, Study 2) provided evidence of an independent link between the LCS and retrospective reports of parents' attachment styles, and this relationship continued to be significant even when current anxiety and depression were statistically controlled for.

Paternal overprotection as well as problematic attachment styles may contribute to the development of the LCS. We (Riskind, Williams, et al., 2004, Study 1) found that paternal overprotection predicted LCS scores in college women, even after anxiety and depression scores were controlled for. Women whose fathers had been overprotective had higher cognitive vulnerability to anxiety, as assessed by the LCS.

Studies Suggesting That the LCS Is a Broader Common Vulnerability Factor in Anxiety Disorders

Although the focus of this chapter is on GAD, the LCS is hypothesized to be a common vulnerability factor in anxiety disorders. The actual anxiety disorder that emerges is hypothesized to depend on the interaction of the LCS with other factors (e.g., environmental factors, particular kinds of stressors, or the specific compensatory self-protective responses that are learned). Evidence that the LCS is a common factor in many anxiety syndromes has been found in two studies using structural equation modeling (Riskind, Shahar, et al., 2003; Williams, Shahar, Riskind, & Joiner, in press).

The Williams, Shahar, et al. (2003) study examined the supposition that this cognitive phenomenology of rapidly rising risk underlies the common features of numerous anxiety disorder symptoms. We found evidence for the hypothesis that when depressive symptoms were controlled for, the LCS would predict a latent factor comprising indicators of five anxiety disorder symptoms: OCD, posttraumatic stress disorder, GAD, social phobia (or fear of negative social evaluation), and specific phobic fears. Structural equation modeling analyses on measures of these symptoms that were administered to 123 undergraduates provided support for the hypothesis that the LCS is an overarching dimension of vulnerability to anxiety. Our construction of a latent anxiety disorder symptoms factor enabled us to partition the variance of the various anxiety symptom scales, and to examine the effect of LCS scores on the variance associated with the latent factor versus that associated with specific anxiety indicators. Results indicated that LCS scores were strongly related to the latent anxiety disorder symptoms factor, whereas a measure of threat perception based on likelihood estimates was not.

A limitation of the Williams, Shahar, et al. (in press) study pertains to the reliance on a strictly cross-sectional design, which limits the ability to examine causal relations between variables. Evidence that the LCS incrementally predicts future levels over time for a latent factor based on multiple anxiety syndromes, beyond initial levels, has been provided by another recent study with more than 200 college student subjects (Riskind, Shahar, et al., 2003).

Implications of the LCS for Clinical Case Conceptualization and Intervention

The model of looming vulnerability stipulates a series of possible points for therapeutic or preventive intervention (Riskind & Williams, 1999a; Riskind & Williams, in press-a). Immediate, temporary relief may be provided by cognitive interventions that target the *proximal* aspects of the subjective sense of looming vulnerability. However, more durable improvement may be provided by changing the underlying cognitive vulnerability factor (the LCS) (Riskind & Williams, 1999a). The model implies that only by addressing this cognitive vulnerability factor can long-term therapeutic improvements be maintained, and the risk of recurrences or relapse be reduced. Examples of theory-based techniques are the use of mental imagery or other cognitive-behavioral techniques to modify perceptions of the speed with which threat is intensifying, the distance from threat (either physical or temporal), or the forward movement of perceived rapidly intensifying danger (see Riskind & Williams, 1999a, for details of such "looming management").

Case Study Illustration

A useful illustration of such interventions is a recent case study of a young woman who suffered from severe social performance anxiety about tap dancing in a classroom performance (Riskind, Long, Duckworth, & Gessner, in press). This young woman was first asked to imagine herself performing in the dance recital at extremely slow speeds (a "slow-world" intervention), followed by gradual and incremental increases in mentally generated performance until "real-time" velocity was achieved. The purpose of this first phase of the intervention was to build confidence and greater mastery beliefs—both by bolstering her confidence that she could keep up with the rest of her peers, and by creating enough "mental space and time" with which to plan her subsequent steps in the performance. After the young woman reported that she was able to perform at "real time" with minimal anxiety, she was then instructed to imagine performing at exaggerated speeds. With her confidence bolstered, the purpose was to inoculate her via exposure to even more exaggerated mental images that caused a subjective sense of looming vulnerability in her dance performance. Using these techniques, the client reported a greater sense of mastery and confidence that she would be *able* to perform in her upcoming recital, and her anxiety was greatly reduced.

CONCLUSIONS

Beck's seminal theory of GAD has spawned a considerable body of empirical research on its cognitive underpinnings. It has also served as the impetus for several recent paths of inquiry that widen the theory by focusing on faulty information processing (e.g., Mogg & Bradley, in press) and on neutralizing and defensive processes in GAD, such as worry (Borkovec et al., 1998; Wells, Chapter 9, this volume) or experiential avoidance (Roemer & Orsillo, 2002).

A major goal of research on the model of looming vulnerability is to address the dearth of attention that has been given to developing a questionnaire measure of the peculiar danger schemas and cognitive vulnerabilities to GAD and other anxiety disorders (e.g., Riskind, 1997; Riskind et al., 2000; Riskind & Williams, in press-a, in press-b). The model also attempts to specify with greater precision the exact nature of the components of danger schemas and perceived threats that discriminate anxiety from depression. Past studies have not reliably distinguished anxiety from depression via standard measures of threat appraisal (e.g., probability) or threat-related automatic thoughts (see the meta-analysis by R. Beck & Perkins, 2001).

The model of looming vulnerability emphasizes that danger schemas are related to a specific maladaptive imaging and appraisal process, and rooted in a negative cognitive style that functions as a danger schema (the LCS). The LCS is hypothesized to be a primarily imagery-based system that portrays threats as rapidly intensifying over time. Evidence has demonstrated that the LCS is specific to anxiety and not depression; that it incrementally predicts anxiety and schematic biases in memory over the effects of other variables; and that it functions as a cognitive vulnerability factor for future anxiety after stress. Research also shows that the LCS is elevated in persons with GAD. The worry and experiential avoidance in GAD are believed to be triggered by periodic instants of fear caused by dynamic or kinetic (rather than static or lifeless) fear-related imagery. Extensive empirical evidence has now accrued that shows the construct, discriminant, predictive, and incremental validity of the LCS. Scores for the LCS are elevated in persons with GAD compared to persons without GAD as well as to those with unipolar depression. As a closing note, the research summarized in this chapter seems to justify the conclusion that it may be just as necessary to devote careful attention to the specific imaging and threat appraisal process in GAD as to defensive processes such as worry and experiential avoidance.

REFERENCES

Abramson, L. Y., Metalsky, G. I., & Alloy, L. B. (1989). Hopelessness depression: A theory-based subtype of depression. *Psychological Review, 96,* 358–372.

Alloy, L. B., Abramson, L. Y., Raniere, D., & Dyller, I. (1999). Research methods in adult psychopathology. In P. C. Kendall, J. N. Butcher, & G. N. Holmbeck (Eds.), *Handbook of research methods in clinical psychology* (2nd ed.). New York: Wiley.

Beck, A. T. (1967). *Depression: Clinical, experimental, and theoretical aspects.* New York: Harper & Row.

Beck, A. T., & Emery, G., with Greenberg, R. L. (1985). *Anxiety disorders and phobias: A cognitive perspective.* New York: Basic.

Beck, A. T., & Clark, D. A. (1997). An information processing model of anxiety: Automatic and strategic processes. *Behaviour Research and Therapy, 35,* 49–58.

Beck, A. T., Laude, R., & Bohnert, M. (1974). Ideational components of anxiety neurosis. *Archives of General Psychiatry, 31,* 319–325.

Beck, A. T., Rush, A. J., Shaw, B. F., & Emery, G. (1979). *Cognitive therapy of depression.* New York: Guilford Press.

Beck, R., & Perkins, T. S. (2001). Cognitive content-specificity for anxiety and depression: A meta-analysis. *Cognitive Therapy and Research, 25,* 651–663.

Borkovec, T. D., & Inz, J. (1990). The nature of worry in generalized anxiety disorder: A predominance of thought activity. *Behaviour Research and Therapy, 28,* 153–158.

Borkovec, T. D., Ray, W. J., & Stoeber, J. (1998). Worry: A cognitive phenomenon intimately linked to affective, physiological, and interpersonal behavioral processes. *Cognitive Therapy and Research, 22,* 561–576.

Butler, G., & Mathews, A. (1983). Cognitive processes in anxiety. *Advances in Behavioural Research and Therapy, 5,* 51–62.

Coles, M. E., & Heimberg, R. G. (2002). Memory biases in the anxiety disorders. *Clinical Psychology Review, 22,* 587–627.

Freeston, M. H., Rheaume, J., Letarte, H., Dugas, M. J., & Ladouceur, R. (1994). Why do people worry? *Personality and Individual Differences, 17,* 191–802.

Greenberg, P. E., Sisitsky, T., Kessler, R. C., Finkelstein, S. N., Berndt, E. R., Davidson, J. R. T., et al. (1999). The economic burden of anxiety disorders in the 1990s. *Journal of Clinical Psychiatry, 60,* 427–435.

Hoehn-Saric, R., Hazlett, R. L., & McLeod, D. R. (1993). Generalized anxiety disorder with early and late onset of anxiety symptoms. *Comprehensive Psychiatry, 34,* 291–298.

Lazarus, R. S. (1966). *Psychological stress and the coping process.* New York: McGraw-Hill.

Mennin, D. S., Heimberg, R., G. Turk, C. L., & Fresco, D. M. (2002). Applying an emotion regulation framework to integrative approaches to generalized anxiety disorder. *Clinical Psychology: Science and Practice, 9,* 85–90.

Meyer, T. J., Miller, M. L., Metzger, R. L., & Borkovec, T. D. (1990). Development and validation of the Penn State Worry Questionnaire. *Behaviour Research and Therapy, 28,* 487–496.

Mogg, K., & Bradley, B. P. (in press). Attentional bias in generalized anxiety disorder versus depressive disorder. *Cognitive Therapy and Research.*

Newman, M. G., Zuellig, A. R., Kachin, K. E., Costantino, M. J., Przeworski, A., Erickson, T., et al. (2002). Preliminary reliability and validity of the Generalized Anxiety Disorder Questionnaire—IV: A revised self-report diagnostic measure of generalized anxiety disorder. *Behavior Therapy, 33,* 215–233.

Noyes, R., Woodman, C., Garvey, M. J., Cook, B. L., Suelzer, M., Clancy, J., et al. (1992). Generalized anxiety disorder versus panic disorder: Distinguishing characteristics and patterns of comorbidity. *Journal of Nervous and Mental Disease, 180,* 396–370.

Riskind, J. H. (1997). Looming vulnerability to threat: A cognitive paradigm for anxiety. *Behaviour Research and Theory, 35,* 685–702.

Riskind, J. H., Abreu, K., Strauss, M., & Holt, R. (1997). Looming vulnerability to spreading contamination in subclinical OCD. *Behaviour Research and Therapy, 35,* 405–414.

Riskind, J. H., & Alloy, L. B. (in press). Cognitive vulnerability to emotional disorders: Theory, design, and methods. In L. B. Alloy & J. H. Riskind (Eds.), *Cognitive vulnerability to emotional disorders.* Mahwah, NJ: Erlbaum.

Riskind, J. H., Gessner, T. D., & Wolzon, R. (2003). *Negative cognitive style for anxiety, generalized anxiety disorder, and restraint, in an alcohol detoxification program.* Unpublished manuscript.

Riskind, J. H., Kelly, K., Harman, W., Moore, R., & Gaines, H. (1992). The loomingness of danger: Does it discriminate focal fear and general anxiety from depression? *Cognitive Therapy and Research, 16,* 603–622.

Riskind, J. H., Long, D., Duckworth, R., & Gessner, T. (in press). A case study of social performance anxiety: Cognitive interventions originating from the model of looming vulnerability. *Journal of Cognitive Psychotherapy: An International Quarterly.*

Riskind, J. H., & Maddux, J. E. (1993). Loomingness, helplessness, and fearfulness: An integration of harm-looming and self-efficacy models of fear and anxiety. *Journal of Social and Clinical Psychology, 12,* 73–89.

Riskind, J. H., & Maddux, J. E. (1994). The loomingness of danger and the fear of AIDS: Perceptions of motion and menace. *Journal of Applied Social Psychology, 24,* 432–442.

Riskind, J. H., Mann, B., & Ployhart, R. (2004). *Looming cognitive style and emotion regulation.* Manuscript in preparation.

Riskind, J. H., & Mizrahi, J. (2004). *Fearful distortion in musical performance anxiety: Mental scenarios of looming vulnerability and rapidly rising risk.* Manuscript submitted for publication.

Riskind, J. H., Moore, R., & Bowley, L. (1995). The looming of spiders: The fearful perceptual distortion of movement and menace. *Behaviour Research and Therapy, 33,* 171–178.

Riskind, J. H., Shahar, G., Mann, B., Black, D., Williams, N. L., & Joiner, T. E., Jr. (2003, November). *The looming cognitive style predicts shared variance in anxiety disorder symptoms: A longitudinal study.* Poster presented at the annual meeting of the Association for Advancement of Behavior Therapy, Boston.

Riskind, J. H., & Wahl, O. (1992). Moving makes it worse: The role of rapid movement in fear of psychiatric patients. *Journal of Social and Clinical Psychology, 11,* 349–365.

Riskind, J. H., Wheeler, D. J., & Picerno, M. R. (1997). Using mental imagery with subclinical OCD to "freeze" contamination in its place: Evidence for looming vulnerability theory. *Behaviour Research and Therapy, 35,* 757–768.

Riskind, J. H., & Williams, N. L. (1999a). Cognitive case conceptualization and the treatment of anxiety disorders: Implications of the looming vulnerability model. *Journal of Cognitive Psychotherapy: An International Quarterly, 13*(4), 295–316.

Riskind, J. H., & Williams, N. L. (1999b). Specific cognitive content of anxiety and catastrophizing: Looming vulnerability and the looming maladaptive style. *Journal of Cognitive Psychotherapy: An International Quarterly, 13*(1), 41–54.

Riskind, J. H., & Williams, N. L. (2004). *Looming cognitive style and focal looming of aggressive urges and contamination: Effects on OCD symptoms and thought suppression.* Manuscript under review.

Riskind, J. H., & Williams, N. L. (in press-a). A unique vulnerability common to all anxiety disorders: The looming maladaptive style. In L. B. Alloy & J. H. Riskind (Eds.), *Cognitive vulnerability to emotional disorders.* Mahwah, NJ: Erlbaum.

Riskind, J. H., & Williams, N. L. (in press-b). The looming cognitive style in generalized anxiety disorder: Distinct danger schema and phenomenology. *Cognitive Therapy and Research.*

Riskind, J. H., Williams, N. L., Altman, M. D., Black, D. O., Balaban, M. S., & Gessner, T. (2004). Parental bonding, attachment, and development of the looming maladaptive style. *Journal of Cognitive Psychotherapy: An International Quarterly, 18,* 43–52.

Riskind, J. H., Williams, N. L., Gessner, T., Chrosniak, L. D., & Cortina, J. (2000). The looming maladaptive style: Anxiety, danger, and schematic processing. *Journal of Personality and Social Psychology, 79,* 837–852.

Riskind, J. H., Williams, N. L., & Joiner, T. (in press). A unique overarching vulnerability for the anxiety disorders: The looming maladaptive style. *Journal of Social and Clinical Psychology.*

Riskind, J. H., Williams, N. L., Joiner. T., Black, D., & Cortina, J. (2003). *Incremental value of the looming cognitive style as a cognitive vulnerability construct.* Manuscript in preparation.

Roemer, L., & Orsillo, S. M. (2002). Expanding our conceptualization of and treatment for generalized anxiety disorder: Integrating mindfulness/acceptance-based approaches with existing cognitive behavioral models. *Clinical Psychology: Science and Practice, 8,* 54–68.

Schut, A. J., Castonguay, L. G., & Borkovec, T. D. (2001). Compulsive checking behaviors in generalized anxiety disorder. *Journal of Clinical Psychology, 57,* 705–715.

Tolin, D. F., Worhunsky, P., & Maltby, N. (in press). Sympathetic magic in contamination-related OCD. *Journal of Behavior Therapy and Experimental Psychiatry.*

Williams, N. L., McDonald, T., Owens, T., & Lunt, M. (2003, November). *The anxious anticipatory style: A predominance of mental imagery.* Poster presented at the annual meeting of the Association for Advancement of Behavior Therapy, Boston.

Williams, N. L., & Riskind, J. H. (2002). *Vulnerability–stress interaction in the prediction of future anxiety: A test of the looming maladaptive style.* Manuscript in preparation.

Williams, N. L., & Riskind, J. H. (2004a). Adult romantic attachment and cognitive vulnerabilities to anxiety and depression: Examining the interpersonal basis of vulnerability models. *Journal of Cognitive Psychotherapy: An International Quarterly, 18,* 7–24.

Williams, N. L., Shahar, G., Riskind, J. H., & Joiner, T. (in press). The looming style has a general effect on an anxiety disorders factor: Further support for a cognitive model of vulnerability to anxiety. *Journal of Anxiety Disorders.*

Wittchen, H.-U., Zhao, S., Kessler, R. C., & Eaton, W. W. (1994). DSM-III-R generalized anxiety disorder in the National Comorbidity Survey. *Archives of General Psychiatry, 51,* 355–364.

Chapter 5

Evidence on Cognitive-Behavioral Therapy for Generalized Anxiety Disorder and Panic Disorder

The Second Decade

DIANNE L. CHAMBLESS
MICHAEL PETERMAN

In 1993, we (Chambless & Gillis, 1993) reported the results of meta-analyses of cognitive-behavioral therapy (CBT) for several anxiety disorders, including panic disorder and generalized anxiety disorder (GAD). Covering roughly the first decade of controlled research on CBT for these conditions, we concluded that CBT's efficacy was clearly superior to comparison conditions comprising waiting-list control conditions, nondirective therapy, or pill placebos. Controlled follow-up data were sparse, but we found that uncontrolled pretest–follow-up effect sizes, compared to uncontrolled pretest–posttest effect sizes, were generally stable; this indicated that on average, patients retained their gains. In addition, CBT had salutary effects on symptoms of depression, which are common among patients with anxiety disorders. A decade has now passed, and the purpose of the current chapter is to examine the efficacy of CBT in these conditions once again. A new treatment's effects often drop in size over the years as the treatment is applied by investigators not involved in its inception and to more difficult treatment samples. How has CBT for GAD and panic disorder fared in its second decade?

It has become the custom to divide research on psychotherapy into "efficacy" studies and "effectiveness" studies (Moras, 1998). In truth, these are not neat categories; often studies are blends of these two approaches. Nonetheless, the distinction is worth noting, and we will organize our presentation around it, pointing out blends when they occur. In brief, efficacy studies represent an emphasis on internal validity. Almost always, patients are randomly assigned to treatment conditions, and studies are conducted in research centers with selected therapists, who were trained to criterion in the protocol before beginning with study patients. Therapists usually follow treatment manuals meant to standardize the treatments and are supervised regularly to maintain the quality of treatment and its integrity to the protocol. Depending on the given study, restrictions may be placed on the types of comorbid conditions patients may have if they are to enter the trial, and patients on medication are typically required to stop medication or hold it constant during treatment. In general, the studies we reviewed met these standards for high internal validity.

Effectiveness studies, on the other hand, emphasize external validity in one or more regards. For example, they may be conducted in community settings with the therapists who ordinarily practice there; they may use a sample that has refused randomization or was not recruited for a controlled study; or they may focus on the effects of treatment for the kinds of patients who do not ordinarily participate in research trials, such as ethnic minorities, patients with high rates of comorbidity, or patients in primary care practices. Effectiveness research is in its infancy, but we will cover what is known to date about the generalization of CBT for anxiety disorders beyond the research clinic. Clearly, such research is of great importance to cognitive-behavioral therapists in practice.

META-ANALYSIS STRATEGY

To form the pool of studies for the meta-analysis, we conducted searches with PsycINFO using the search terms "cognitive therapy and panic disorder," "cognitive therapy and generalized anxiety disorder," "cognitive-behavior therapy and panic disorder," and "cognitive-behavior therapy and generalized anxiety disorder." In addition, we scanned by hand the major journals publishing research in CBT from 1992 to 2001, including *Behavior Therapy, Behaviour Research and Therapy, Cognitive Therapy and Research, Journal of Anxiety Disorders,* and *Journal of Consulting and Clinical Psychology.* We corresponded with CBT researchers regarding their latest work. Finally, we searched the reference sections of articles located as described for additional citations.

Typically, authors of the studies included in the meta-analysis used outcome measures that tapped several different, if related, problem areas for GAD or panic disorder—for example, measures of anxiety, panic, depression, and maladaptive cognitions. Separate effect sizes are reported in the tables for these different problem areas. When authors used multiple measures of a given problem area, these were standardized and averaged before inclusion in the meta-analysis, so that each study in a given analysis is represented by only one data point. Effect sizes from controlled studies were calculated as Cohen's d ([CBT M – comparison M]/pooled SD) and presented so that a positive effect size represents a better response to CBT than to the comparison condition. If authors did not provide means and standard deviations but did report inferential statistics such as t, formulas provided by Rosenthal (1991) were used to translate these statistics to d. Because effect sizes such as d are not intuitively interpretable, we have translated d into its equivalent in differences in success rates according to Rosenthal and Rubin's binomial effect size display (Rosenthal, 1991).

EFFICACY

Generalized Anxiety Disorder

CBT for GAD takes a variety of forms. Cognitive restructuring is, by definition, always included. However, investigators vary as to whether they include applied relaxation training as part of the treatment. Cognitive work always includes a focus on worry, but some investigators include problem-solving training and exposure to worrisome thoughts as part of the treatment, whereas others do not. Earlier CBT studies generally included relaxation training as part of the treatment, whereas some researchers presently eschew such training in order to provide a clearer focus on cognitive aspects of the treatment. Where relevant, we will point out some of this heterogeneity in reviewing the outcome of treatment studies.

Comparisons to Waiting List, Minimal Contact,
or Treatment as Usual

We located five randomized controlled trials conducted since our last meta-analysis in which CBT was compared to a waiting-list control condition (Dugas et al., 2003; Ladouceur et al., 2000; Wetherell, Gatz, & Craske, 2003) or a limited-contact condition (Linden, Zubrägel, Bär, Wendt, & Schlattmann, in press; Stanley, Beck, et al., 2003). In a second small-scale study, Stanley, Hopko, et al. (2003) compared CBT to treatment as usual. In effect, this condition was a minimal-contact control condition, because clients in this group received very little treatment. Effect sizes for these six studies are presented in Table 5.1, with the final row of the table giving the average effect size weighted by sample sizes, so that studies with larger sample sizes are given relatively more weight.

Three of these studies used individual therapy, whereas the other three used group therapy. The number of treatment hours appears large for the clients treated in groups, but of course this is not hours per client. Ladouceur et al. (2000) used fairly standard treatment lengths for individual therapy in a research trial, and Stanley, Hopko, et al. (2003) used a brief treatment designed to increase effectiveness, whereas Linden et al.'s (in press) clients were permitted up to 25 hours of treatment. Linden et al. did not report the actual amount of treatment clients received. This study was conducted in Germany in therapists' private practices, and the treatment clients received was paid for by their health insurance, which allowed up to 25 sessions. Another source of heterogeneity among the studies is the clients' age. The last three studies in Table 5.1 all involved treatment of GAD in elderly individuals.

On average, the weighted average effect sizes in Table 5.1 demonstrate what Cohen (1988) would term a large effect (0.80) for CBT compared to control conditions on measures of worry and anxious thinking, anxiety, and depression. The average d of 0.885 for the primary outcome measures of anxiety and worry/anxious thinking is equivalent to a difference in improvement rate of 30% for control groups to 70% for CBT groups (Rosenthal, 1991). These results were achieved in an average of 22 hours of therapy after pretest assessment.

Table 5.1 also presents figures for the percentage of clients in each study who achieved "high end-state functioning" (HEF) or "clinically significant change" (CSC; Jacobson & Truax, 1991). Authors used varying definitions for this designation, but typically this is intended to convey that clients have largely returned to the normal range of functioning on the measure(s) chosen to determine this status. Note that clients might no longer meet diagnostic criteria for GAD, but still might not achieve CSC/HEF status. Inclusion of these data is intended to help the reader determine how many individual clients did very well—a different matter than what the average change was for the group of clients in the study. On average, very few clients achieved CSC/HEF in control conditions (<6%). In studies of CBT with younger adults, 45–65% of clients achieved CSC/HEF. Elderly clients appeared to do less well. Whether this is due to the very long duration of their disorder (>30 years on average), the need to adapt CBT to better suit the needs of older clients, or some other factor(s) is yet to be determined. Wetherall et al. (2003) have suggested that the group therapy used with the elderly clients in their study and by Stanley, Beck, et al. (2003) may have

TABLE 5.1. GAD: CBT versus Waiting List, Minimal Contact, or Treatment as Usual

Study	Comparison condition	n CBT	n Control	# of session hours	Unweighted ES anxiety	Unweighted ES depression	Unweighted ES cognitive & worry	% CSC/HEF CBT	% CSC/HEF Control	% dropouts CBT	% dropouts Control
Dugas et al. (2003)[a]	WL	25	27	28	1.06	0.93	0.86	65	—	8	7
Ladouceur et al. (2000)	WL	14	12	16	1.24	1.51	2.07	62	—	0	0
Linden et al. (2002)	MC	36	36	25[b]	0.50	—	—	45	17	14	11
Stanley, Hopko, et al. (2003)	TAU	5	5	8	0.86	1.76	1.20	40	25	17	17
Stanley, Beck, et al. (2003)[a]	MC	29	35	18.9	0.92	0.78	0.51	3	0	26	10
Wetherall et al. (2003)[a]	WL	18	21	18	0.94	0.74	0.72	22	0	31	9
Weighted		21.17	22.67	21.54	0.87	0.96	0.90	37.87	5.42	16.54	8.89

Note. ES, effect size (Cohen's d); CSC, clinically significant change; HEF, high end-state functioning; WL, waiting-list control group; MC, minimal-contact control; TAU, treatment as usual. A positive ES means that clients receiving CBT fared better than those receiving the comparison treatment.
[a]Group therapy.
[b]Up to 25 sessions allowed. Actual amount received not reported.

been less efficacious than individual therapy. However, Dugas et al. (2003) also used group therapy and reported the highest percentages of CSC/HEF of all studies. The low rates of clinically significant change for elderly participants are particularly sobering when we take into account their relative physical health. Nonetheless, given the prevalence of GAD in elderly individuals, it is encouraging that CBT leads to substantial benefit, even if elderly clients remain somewhat anxious.

On the whole, CBT was well tolerated among younger adults, with dropout rates ranging from 0% to 14%. Dropout rates were higher among elderly clients; reported problems interfering with treatment included physical health problems, transportation difficulties, and the like. In light of the difficulties elderly clients have in keeping appointments, group therapy may not be the best vehicle for CBT. Greater flexibility of appointment times is likely with individual therapy.

The largest effect sizes and highest rates of CSC/HEF were obtained by Ladouceur et al. (2000) and Dugas et al. (2003). It is premature to draw conclusions, but it is worth noting that both of these studies were based on an innovative model of CBT for GAD incorporating current research on cognitive aspects of the disorder and developed by these Canadian researchers. Relaxation training is omitted, and the treatment focuses heavily on increasing patients' tolerance for uncertainty, as well as on reevaluation of patients' beliefs that there are benefits to worry, training to benefit problem-solving orientation, and exposure via a loop tape to a scenario involving patients' worst fear.

A frequent criticism of efficacy research is that authors are said to exclude most forms of comorbidity (Westen & Morrison, 2001), making results difficult to generalize to clinical practice. On the whole, this was not the case in this set of studies. Only Linden et al. (in press) eliminated all participants with comorbid conditions. Other researchers followed clinically reasonable and responsible procedures in ruling out those with organic brain syndrome, substance abuse, psychosis, medical complications that might interfere with treatment or cause symptoms like GAD, severe depression, and acute suicidality. The most common comorbid disorders reported were other anxiety disorders and depression, with over half of the participants having one or more comorbid diagnoses in studies for which authors reported these data. Stanley, Hopko, et al. (2003) conducted their study in a primary care clinic, accepting patients with medical as well as psychiatric comorbidity. Thus, so long as GAD was the primary problem for which clients sought treatment, clients with a wide range of comorbid disorders were included in most of this set of studies.

CBT for GAD seems to benefit clients' comorbid conditions. For example, we found a large effect size (see Table 5.1) for depression for CBT versus control conditions, and Ladouceur et al. (2000) reported a significant decline in the number of post-CBT comorbid diagnoses. Similarly, Borkovec, Abel, and Newman (1995) found that successful treatment of GAD led to a reduction in the number of clients who had comorbid diagnoses (a drop from 45% to 14%), with further reductions at a 1-year follow-up, even among those who received no additional treatment in the follow-up interval. Certainly it is reasonable to ask whether CBT is beneficial for clients with GAD as a secondary disorder or with GAD in those who are cognitively impaired. To date, the available data do not speak to these issues.

CBT versus Nonbehavioral Treatment

In three studies, CBT was compared to a nonbehavioral form of psychotherapy—either supportive group therapy (Stanley, Beck, & Glassco, 1996; Wetherell et al., 2003) or psychodynamic psychotherapy (Durham et al., 1994). The last two studies in Table 5.2 involved group treatment of elderly individuals, whereas the first concerned individual treatment of younger adults. Not surprisingly, effect sizes are smaller here than in Table 5.1, where comparisons are made to conditions not involving comparable amounts of treatment. Comparison conditions in this table controlled for support and expectancy as well as the passage of time and effects of assessment procedures. On average, CBT was superior to other treatments, with close to a medium effect size (defined as ≥ 0.50 and <0.80) for anxiety and for cognitive and worry measures, and a medium effect size for depression. The average effect size of 0.45 for the primary measures of anxiety and worry/anxious thinking is equivalent to a difference in improvement rates of 39% in the nonbehavioral treatment groups versus 61% in the CBT groups.

It is possible that the obtained effect size is exaggerated by expectancy differences between CBT and psychodynamic therapy in the study by Durham et al. (1994). These authors reported that clients in the CBT condition had a higher expectation for improvement than those in psychodynamic therapy did, and expectancy is often linked to better outcome for CBT (Borkovec, Newman, Pincus, & Lytle, 2002; Wetherell et al., 2003). In contrast, Wetherall et al. (2003) and Stanley et al. (1996) reported equivalent expectancy/credibility for their comparison groups. In addition, internal validity controls were generally looser in Durham et al.'s study than in the other two (e.g., no adherence measures or treatment manuals). Thus the small positive effect sizes for the two studies with elderly clients may be more trustworthy than the average medium effect size statistic.

Dropout rates were comparable to those in Table 5.1, and again higher in elderly individuals than in younger adults. The apparent superiority for CBT in the weighted average of the percentage of clients achieving CSC/HEF is misleading, in that it is entirely due to the Durham et al. (1994) study comparing CBT to psychodynamic therapy with younger adults.

TABLE 5.2. GAD: CBT versus Nonbehavioral Treatments

Study	Comparison condition	n		# of session hours	Unweighted ES anxiety	Unweighted ES depression	Unweighted ES cognitive & worry	% CSC/HEF		% dropouts	
		CBT	Control					CBT	Control	CBT	Control
Durham et al. (1994)	PD	35	29	13.5	0.73	1.00	0.58	37	10	10	24
Stanley et al. (1996)[a]	ST	18	13	21	0.10	−0.08	0.32	11	15	31	35
Wetherall et al. (2003)[a]	ST	18	18	18	0.29	0.31	0.29	22	22	31	31
Weighted		23.67	20.00	16.54	0.46	0.55	0.44	26.61	14.68	20.65	28.48

Note. ES, effect size (Cohen's *d*); CSC, clinically significant change; HEF, high end-state functioning; PD, psychodynamic psychotherapy; ST, supportive group therapy. A positive ES means that clients receiving CBT fared better than those receiving the comparison treatment.
[a]Group therapy.

Among elderly clients, supportive group therapy and CBT yielded comparable rates. This might be interpreted to mean that supportive group therapy is particularly efficacious for elderly clients; however, this does not appear to be the case. Rather, CBT and supportive therapy are similar on this variable because neither was very successful in helping clients to reach a normative level of functioning. Nonetheless, there does seem to be a small edge for CBT with anxious elderly persons, but the small sample of studies limits our confidence in this conclusion.

CBT versus Other Behavioral Treatments

In three studies (Borkovec et al., 2002; Durham et al., 1994; Öst & Breitholtz, 2000), CBT has been compared to other treatments in the behavior therapy family, all pairing relaxation with anxious responses and worrisome thoughts, although with slightly different approaches. None of these studies involved treatment of elderly clients. Note that although data from Durham et al. are presented in Table 5.2, the findings reported in Table 5.3 differ in being based on a brief version of CBT including only 9 hours of treatment. Borkovec et al. ran two CBT conditions—one a pure cognitive therapy and the other a cognitive therapy combined with self-control desensitization. Effect sizes for the former are reported in Table 5.3. In all three studies, clients' expectancy for improvement was equivalent across treatment conditions; Borkovec et al. also demonstrated that the therapeutic relationship was equally positive for CBT and behavior therapy.

Effect sizes of comparisons between the two types of treatment are all small, whether they be for anxiety, depression, or measures of worry and cognitive aspects of GAD. The average effect size for the primary outcome measures of anxiety and worry/anxious thinking (–0.15) is equivalent to a difference in improvement rates of 46.5% for CBT versus 53.5% for behavior therapies. Findings for CSC/HEF are in the low end of the range for nonelderly subjects reported in Table 5.1 and are roughly equivalent for CBT and other behavior therapies. Although the sample of studies is too small for firm conclusions, it is clear that there is no evidence of superiority of CBT over other behavioral treatments. One might have hypothesized that CBT would have been more beneficial than behavior therapy for depression, given its efficacy for treatment of mood disorders (Dobson, 1989). This proved not to be the case, perhaps because depression in anxious patients is often secondary to their anxiety.

Follow-Up

We have not included a table of follow-up effect sizes for the following reasons: (1) Controlled effect sizes for Table 5.1 data are not available, be-

TABLE 5.3. GAD: CBT versus Behavior Therapies

Study	Comparison condition	n CBT	n BT	# of session hours	Unweighted ES anxiety	Unweighted ES depression	Unweighted ES cognitive & worry	% CSC/HEF CBT	% CSC/HEF BT	% dropouts CBT	% dropouts BT
Borkovec et al. (2002)	SCD	23	23	16	0.15	0.08	−0.21	43	57	8	15
Durham et al. (1994)	AMT	20	16	9	0.37	0.72	−0.84	37	31	10	27
Öst and Breitholtz (2000)	AR	18	15	12	−0.10	−0.23	0.18	—	—	5	12
Weighted		20.33	18.00	12.52	0.15	0.19	−0.30	40.21	46.33	7.77	17.72

Note. BT, behavior therapies; ES, effect size (Cohen's *d*); CSC, clinically significant change; HEF, high end-state functioning; SCD, self-control desensitization; AMT, anxiety management training; AR, applied relaxation. A positive ES means that clients receiving CBT fared better than those receiving the comparison treatment.

cause for ethical reasons, clients in the non-CBT conditions were offered treatment after posttest; and (2) effect sizes for studies in Tables 5.2 and 5.3 are difficult to interpret with precision, because clients often received more treatment (pharmacological or psychological) in the follow-up period. For example, even though Linden et al.'s (in press) clients could receive up to 25 sessions (a generous number by present U.S. standards), nearly half obtained more treatment in the 8-month follow-up period. Perhaps this is not surprising, given the many clients who do not achieve CSC/HEF status at the end of treatment. However, a number of authors did not report assessing the amount of treatment received during follow-up; most authors did not compare treatment groups on the amount of treatment received during follow-up; and none controlled for such treatment's effects in the analysis of follow-up data. Accordingly, we provide only a brief narrative summary of follow-up data.

In all studies reporting follow-up data, clients as a group maintained or improved upon their pretest–posttest gains during follow-ups lasting up to 2 years (Borkovec et al., 2002; Dugas et al., 2003; Durham et al., 1999; Ladouceur et al., 2000; Linden et al., in press; Öst & Breitholtz, 2000; Stanley et al., 1996; Stanley, Beck, et al., 2003; Wetherall et al., 2003). Whether this would be the case if no clients had received additional treatment cannot be determined, although relatively few clients (17%) in Borkovec et al.'s study obtained treatment during follow-up. Compared to supportive therapy, CBT may lead to less need for treatment during the follow-up period (Borkovec & Costello, 1993; Stanley et al., 1996). Similarly, Durham et al. (1999) reported that fewer clients who received CBT took medication during the follow-up period than clients who received psychodynamic therapy (38% vs. 82%). If confirmed with additional studies, this would convey an important advantage for treatment with CBT compared to nonbehavioral treatments.

Summary

The results of efficacy studies on CBT of GAD in the past decade are consistent with the conclusions we drew in our first meta-analysis (Chambless & Gillis, 1993): CBT appears to be superior to waiting-list conditions, minimal-contact conditions, and nonbehavioral therapies, and equivalent to other behavior therapies. Dropout rates are less than 15% for young and middle-aged adults, indicating that treatment is well tolerated. Dropout is more of a problem for elderly clients (from 17% to 31%), but this problem was not unique to CBT.

In interpreting these results, let us keep in mind that in the majority of these studies, clients were allowed to continue on medication while in CBT (Borkovec et al., 2002; Dugas et al., 2003; Durham et al., 1994;

Ladouceur et al., 2000; Öst & Breitholtz, 2000; Stanley, Hopko, et al., 2003; Wetherall et al., 2003), typically with instructions to keep their dosage constant throughout treatment. This strategy was designed to enhance external validity by retaining in the sample clients who might have had difficulty withdrawing from medication before they were offered alternative treatment. Are the results reported here inflated because of clients' medication use? In our view, this is of greatest concern when it comes to interpreting CSC/HEF rates, in that clients had to reach an absolute threshold here, and their scores might have been boosted by their medication use. In their meta-analysis of CBT compared to pharmacotherapy, Gould, Otto, Pollack, and Yap (1997) found no evidence that effect sizes were larger in studies wherein clients were permitted to remain on versus being withdrawn from medication. Unfortunately, our sample of studies in which medication was not permitted is too small to replicate this analysis here.

Finally, the small number of studies including measures of quality of life did not justify inclusion of this measure in Tables 5.1–5.3. Some authors have questioned whether treatment with CBT leads to enhanced quality of life or just change in so-called "symptoms" (e.g., Kovacs, 1996). Authors of three of the studies included in our meta-analysis incorporated measures of quality of life in their assessment batteries. Stanley and colleagues (Stanley, Beck, et al., 2003; Stanley, Hopko, et al., 2003) found that CBT led to significantly greater increases in quality of life in their elderly patients than did a treatment-as-usual or a minimal-contact control condition. Durham et al. (1994) found improvements in quality of life that were comparable to those found with psychodynamic therapy and anxiety management training. Routine inclusion of quality-of-life measures in research on GAD would be desirable, but so far the available data indicate that CBT leads to positive changes, both in the direct focus of treatment (anxiety and worry) and in quality of life.

Panic Disorder

By definition, CBT for panic disorder always includes a focus on the catastrophic cognitions typical of this disorder. Education and challenges to beliefs are employed. Beyond this common element, treatments vary in their inclusion of relaxation training and exposure to fear-eliciting stimuli. The exposure may be interoceptive (exposure to induced bodily sensations associated with panic) or *in vivo* (exposure to actual phobic situations) for those with agoraphobic avoidance. In practice, those with expertise in treating panic disorder will almost always include exposure, at least in minimal amounts, to facilitate challenging beliefs about the dangerous consequences of panic, if not more extensively. However, in some of the research trials we report below, treatment was limited to cognitive restructuring without exposure for research purposes.

CBT versus Waiting List, Pill Placebo, or Attention Control Treatment

Table 5.4 reports the results of 13 studies in which CBT was compared to a waiting-list control group ($n = 8$), a pill placebo ($n = 4$), or an attention control treatment (associative therapy, $n = 1$). Effect sizes were large for panic, phobia, cognitive measures, and anxiety, and close to large for depression. The average effect size for panic and phobia (0.93) is equivalent to a difference in improvement rate of 29% for control conditions versus 71% for CBT. The rates of clients who reported no panic attacks in the posttreatment monitoring period (29% for control vs. 71% for CBT) were comparable to the percentages of clients who achieved CSC/HEF status (22% for controls vs. 72% for CBT). These results were achieved in an average of a little over 10 therapy hours after pretest assessment. Dropout rates were similar for CBT versus the control conditions as well. Effect sizes were comparable for individual versus group therapy. The one study yielding discrepant effect sizes for panic and cognition was that by Beck, Stanley, Baldwin, Deagle, and Averill (1994). For research purposes, these investigators issued antiexposure instructions for the first half of treatment and gave no systematic instruction for interoceptive or *in vivo* exposure for the second half. Possibly, if clients do not test their new thinking strategies during exposure, treatment is less efficacious.

Also included in Table 5.4 is a column describing the percentage of clients in each study who suffered from agoraphobic complications to panic disorder. Because clients with significant agoraphobic avoidance improve less than those who are not as avoidant (Williams & Falbo, 1996), effect sizes might vary substantially, depending on the number of avoidant clients in a sample. Unfortunately, we found this information difficult to ascertain. Some investigators reported excluding clients with more than mild agoraphobic avoidance (represented as 0% agoraphobic in the tables); others reported accepting those with and without agoraphobic avoidance, but neglected to provide data on the percentage of each (missing in the tables). Yet other investigators reported the percentage of clients who had any degree of agoraphobic avoidance in one figure, including those with mild avoidance. Accordingly, the figures in the tables for agoraphobic avoidance are a very rough guide to this important feature of samples. It is desirable that in future studies authors report the percentage of clients with mild, moderate, and severe agoraphobic avoidance.

Were clients in these studies suffering purely from panic disorder with no comorbidity? Rarely. Sharp et al. (1996) had extensive exclusion criteria

TABLE 5.4. Panic Disorder: CBT versus Waiting List, Pill Placebo, or Attention Control Treatment

Study	Comparison condition	n CBT	n Control	# of session hours	%Ag	Unweighted ES panic	Unweighted ES phobia	Unweighted ES cognitive	Unweighted ES depression	Unweighted ES anxiety	% panic-free CBT	% panic-free Control	% CSC/HEF CBT	% CSC/HEF Control	% dropouts CBT	% dropouts Control
Arntz & van den Hout (1996)[a]	WL	18	18	12	0	—	—	—	—	—	78	28	—	—	0	0
Barlow et al. (2000)[b]	PL	101[c]	14	10	0	—	—	—	—	—	—	—	73	39	28	42
Beck et al. (1994)[d]	WL	17	22	13.2	—	0.32	0.66	0.32	0.58	0.14	—	—	65	36	23	0
Black et al. (1993)	PL	25	25	8	72	—	—	—	0.15	0.03	53	29	—	—	36	28
Carter et al. (2003)[d]	WL	14	11	16.5	—	1.80	—	1.97	1.32	1.70	57	9	64	9	17	27
Clark et al. (1999)[e]	WL	29	14	8.5	85	1.66	1.65	1.77	1.45	1.8	75	8	75	0	3	0
Gould et al. (1993)	WL	9	11	8	0	0.74	0.52	-0.58	0.41	—	56	35	—	—	0	8
Lidren et al. (1994)[d]	WL	12	12	12	83	0.76	0.45	1.49	0.26	—	83	25	42	8	0	0
Sharp et al. (1996)	PL	62[c]	20	7	—	—	—	—	—	—	73	61	83	48	20	24
Shear et al. (2001)[a]	PL	22	14	12	0	0.74	—	—	—	—	—	—	—	—	39	39
Telch et al. (1993)[d]	WL	34	33	18	—	0.73	1.15	1.84	0.76	1.39	85	30	64	9	—	—
van den Hout et al. (1994)	AC	9	9	4	100	0.84	—	—	—	—	—	—	—	—	—	—
Williams and Falbo (1996)[f]	WL	27	9	8	92	0.79	0.58	1.15	1.10	—	63	11	—	—	0	0
Weighted		19.64	16.308	10.31	37.99	0.91	0.95	1.29	0.75	0.98	70.952	28.912	71.915	22.119	19.51	15.88

Note. % Ag, percentage of sample with agoraphobic avoidance; ES, effect size (Cohen's d); CSC, clinically significant change; HEF, high end-state functioning; AC, attention control treatment; PL, pill placebo. A positive ES means that clients receiving CBT fared better than those receiving the comparison treatment.

[a]Denotes a quasi-experiment.

[b]Data reported are based on the intention-to-treat sample (all those who started treatment).

[c]Data are combined for participants who received CBT alone and those who received CBT plus placebo.

[d]Denotes group treatment.

[e]Results were combined for a brief cognitive intervention (6.5 hours) and full cognitive therapy (12 hours).

[f]Results were combined for a pure cognitive therapy group and a cognitive therapy group that included homework exposure instructions.

for their subjects, and Lidren et al. (1994) excluded those with major depressive disorder. Most other investigators (Arntz & van den Hout, 1996; Barlow, Gorman, Shear, & Woods, 2000; Beck et al., 1994; Black, Wesner, Bowers, & Gabel, 1993; Carter, Sbrocco, Gore, Marin, & Lewis, 2003; Clark et al., 1999; Shear, Houck, Greeno, & Masters, 2001; Telch et al., 1993; Williams & Falbo, 1996) used similar exclusion criteria to those that would be used in clinical practice, omitting clients with psychosis, organicity, substance dependence, and significant medical illness that would interfere with treatment. So long as panic disorder was the primary diagnosis, these investigators included those with other comorbid disorders (typically depression, other anxiety disorders, and, less often, hypochondriasis), with one team reporting that approximately half of the clients had comorbid disorders (Arntz & van den Hout, 1996); other authors unfortunately neglected to provide these data. The other two teams of investigators failed to report exclusion criteria (Gould, Clum, & Shapiro, 1993; van den Hout, Arntz, & Hoekstra, 1994).

CBT versus Supportive–Experiential Psychotherapy

In three investigations, authors compared CBT to education plus a form of supportive, nondirective, experiential psychotherapy developed by Shear and colleagues and designed to help clients identify and resolve underlying life problems and feelings believed to contribute to panic attacks (Craske, Maidenberg, & Bystritsky, 1995; Shear et al., 2001; Shear, Pilkonis, Cloitre, & Leon, 1994). Thus clients in both conditions received the education about panic disorder that is more typical of CBT than of nondirective psychotherapy. Shear and colleagues reported that the two treatment conditions were equivalent in expectancy/credibility in both of their studies; Craske et al. did not provide these data. Table 5.5 provides the results for these three studies.

Unfortunately, data on all variables of interest were not available for each of the three studies. The effect size for panic, for which we have data from all three studies, is equivalent to a difference in improvement rates of 38% for nonbehavioral treatment versus 62% for CBT. For reasons that are not clear, Shear et al.'s (1994) data are discrepant with those of the other two studies, for which large effect sizes in favor of CBT were obtained despite the brevity of Craske et al.'s (1995) treatment. Given the heterogeneity of the effects sizes in this small pool of studies, the conclusion that CBT is moderately more efficacious than nonbehavioral psychotherapy must be held tentatively. Whether differences between the two types of treatment would have been sharper had education not been included in the supportive–experiential therapy (which is atypical for such an approach) cannot be determined from these studies.

TABLE 5.5. Panic Disorder: CBT versus Supportive–Experiential Psychotherapies

Study	n CBT	n SEP	# of session hrs.	% Ag	Unweighted ES panic	Unweighted ES phobia	Unweighted ES cognitive	Unweighted ES depression	Unweighted ES anxiety	% panic-free CBT	% panic-free SEP	% CSC/HEF CBT	% CSC/HEF SEP	% dropouts CBT	% dropouts SEP
Craske et al. (1995)	16	13	3.5	67	1.19	0.51	0.78	0.12	0.18	53	23	—	—	0	7
Shear et al. (1994)	24	21	15	94	-0.3	-0.22	0.06	-0.05	-0.01	66	78	—	—	35	28
Shear et al. (2001)[a]	22	23	12	[b]	0.81	—	—	—	—	—	—	—	—	35	28
Weighted	20.67	19	10.97	83.41	0.48	0.07	0.34	0.02	0.06	61	57	—	—	27	21

Note. % Ag, percentage of sample with agoraphobic avoidance; ES, effect size (Cohen's *d*); CSC, clinically significant change; HEF, high end-state functioning; SEP, supportive–experiential psychotherapy. A positive ES means that clients receiving CBT fared better than those receiving the comparison treatment.
[a]A quasi-experiment.
[b]No more than mild avoidance; % with avoidance not reported.

CBT versus Other Behavior Therapies

In comparison to the paucity of studies comparing CBT to nonbehavioral treatments, we located seven studies in which CBT was contrasted to another behavioral approach. In five of these (Arntz, 2002; Bouchard et al., 1996; Burke, Drummond, & Johnston, 1997; Hecker, Fink, Vogeltanz, Thorpe, & Sigmon, 1998; Williams & Falbo, 1996), that approach was interoceptive exposure (exposure to bodily sensations associated with panic), *in vivo* exposure to phobic situations, or both. In the other two (Arntz & van den Hout, 1996; Beck et al., 1994), the comparison treatment was relaxation training, although Arntz and van den Hout also included two sessions of *in vivo* exposure to facilitate practice of applied relaxation. Typically, interoceptive exposure is included as part of CBT for panic disorder, with *in vivo* exposure added for those with extensive agoraphobic avoidance. For research purposes, in these studies the exposure elements were omitted from CBT, other than an occasional behavioral experiment. The exception to this rule was the study by Burke et al., who included equivalent and extensive amounts of therapist-assisted exposure in both conditions. All authors except Arntz (2002) and Arntz and van den Hout (1996) assessed expectancy for change with treatment or credibility of treatment. In most cases, the CBT and other behavior therapy conditions were equivalent on expectancy/credibility. The exception was the study by Hecker et al. (1998), in which clients had a higher expectation for change in the CBT condition.

As may be seen in Table 5.6, the effect sizes were at best small (≥ 0.20 and < 0.50), and indicated no consistent advantage for CBT over behavior therapy without the explicit cognitive component, whether the measure was panic, phobia, depression, or cognitive measures. Not surprisingly, the percentages of clients achieving panic-free and CSC/HEF status were also similar in the two conditions. Dropout rates were low and comparable for both types of treatment.

Follow-Up

Of the 19 studies on panic disorder reviewed here, all but 6 (Black et al., 1993; Carter et al., 2003; Craske et al., 1995; Gould et al., 1993; Hecker et al., 1998; van den Hout et al., 1994) provide follow-up data useful for our purposes. (In some studies, follow-up data were collected, but only after clients had received another treatment in a second part of the protocol.) Follow-up intervals ranged from 6 months to 2 years. Almost all authors reported that on average, clients maintained their treatment gains or improved further during follow-up. Although these results are very positive, the difficulties in interpreting follow-up data have already been discussed in

TABLE 5.6. Panic Disorder: CBT versus Behavior Therapies

Study	n CBT	n BT	# of session hrs.	% Ag	Unweighted ES panic	Unweighted ES phobia	Unweighted ES cognitive	Unweighted ES depression	Unweighted ES anxiety	% panic-free CBT	% panic-free BT	%CSC/HEF CBT	%CSC/HEF BT	% dropouts CBT	% dropouts BT
Arntz (2002)[a]	29	29	12	0.00	0.16	—	—	—	-0.11	78	75	—	—	12	19
Arntz and van den Hout (1996)	18	18	12	0.00	0.82	—	—	—	—	78	50	—	—	0	5
Beck et al. (1994)[a]	17	19	13.2	—	0.22	0.56	0.16	-0.24	-0.64	—	—	65	47	23	5
Bouchard et al. (1996)[a]	14	14	22.5	10 / 0.00	0.03	-1.15	-0.28	-0.43	-0.46	64	79	64	86	0	0
Burke et al. (1997)	12	14	30	59.00	—	0.28	-0.02	0.45	-0.17	—	—	73	39	37	30
Hecker et al. (1998)	8	8	4	56.00	—	-0.39	-0.13	-0.78	-0.76	—	—	44	33	11	11
Williams and Falbo (1996)	27	12	8	92.00	-0.09	-0.15	-0.51	0.05	—	63	58	—	—	0	0
Weighted	17.8571	16.2857	13.69	43.44	0.22	-0.12	-0.17	-0.13	-0.36	71	67	63	53	10	11

Note. BT, behavior therapy; n, sample size; % Ag, percentage of sample with agoraphobic avoidance; ES, effect size (Cohen's d); CSC, clinically significant change; HEF, high end-state functioning. The BT comparison treatment was always exposure except in the studies by Arntz and van den Hout (1996) and Beck et al. (1994), who used relaxation training. A positive ES means that clients receiving CBT fared better than those receiving the comparison treatment.
[a]Group therapy.

the "Follow-Up" section for GAD. Few researchers reported whether individual clients' improvement held steady over follow-up. There were two exceptions: Shear et al. (2001) indicated that no clients in the CBT group relapsed, and Telch et al. (1993) reported that only 7% of clients who received CBT relapsed during follow-up.

Sharp et al. (1996) provide unique data, in that they reported the percentage of clients meeting criteria for CSC/HEF status at follow-up who had received no treatment at all in the intervening 6 months (60% of the sample of follow-up attenders). These authors indicated that clients treated with CBT had maintained their gains better than those who received medication alone or placebo, but that the CSC/HEF rate was lower at follow-up than at posttest. For example, at posttest 90% of the CBT group met criteria for CSC on anxiety, whereas at follow-up this figure dropped to 52% among those who had received no further treatment. Brown and Barlow (1995) raised a further caveat: Analyses of follow-up data for their sample of patients treated with CBT indicated better outcome at 24-month than at 3-month follow-up. However, when they queried patients about their experiences during the follow-up interval, some instability in patients' clinical status was apparent, with some patients experiencing panic attacks between follow-up assessments, even though they were panic-free at the time of assessments. Nonetheless, from a cognitive model, occasional panic attacks should not be cause for alarm among researchers or clients. Rather, patients' becoming fearful of panic attacks and resuming a life of anxiety and avoidance is the critical issue.

Summary

The results of efficacy studies on CBT of panic disorder in the past decade are consistent with the conclusions we drew in our first meta-analysis (Chambless & Gillis, 1993): CBT is consistently superior to waiting-list conditions, pill placebos, and attention control treatments, and appears to be equivalent to other behavior therapies. The results of several studies also indicate that CBT is modestly superior to supportive–experiential psychotherapy that includes an education component; additional studies are needed for a more confident conclusion.

Dropout rates were highly variable. The sample of studies in Table 5.4 is large enough to permit examination of one correlate of dropout. On average, 30.75% of clients dropped out of treatment when the CBT was conducted in the context of a trial involving a comparison with medication (Barlow et al., 2000; Black et al., 1993; Sharp et al., 1996; Shear et al., 2001), versus 6.14% when this was not the case (Mann–Whitney test, $z = 2.52, p < .02$). Whether this is due to differences in the kinds of clients who will consent to random assignment to medication, placebo, or CBT, or to other unknown variables, cannot be determined from the available data. According to one study (Hofmann et al., 1998), a substantial proportion of clients (30–47%) applying for treatment of panic disorder are unwilling to enter medication trials.

In the set of studies we examined, authors did not determine whether CBT for panic disorder reduced comorbid disorders, although it is clear that symptoms of depression and general anxiety were reduced (see Tables 5.4–5.6). In addition, Carter et al. (2003) reported that interviewer ratings of the severity of comorbid conditions decreased more in the CBT group than in the waiting-list group. In two other investigations, researchers have addressed CBT's effects on comorbid diagnoses. Brown, Antony, and Barlow (1995) and Tsao, Mystkowski, Zucker, and Craske (2002) both found that rates of comorbidity fell from pretreatment to posttest and from pretreatment to 3- or 6-month follow-up, respectively. However, Brown et al.'s report on a small group of patients who participated in a 24-month follow-up sounds a cautionary note. At this long-term follow-up point, the rate of comorbidity was no longer significantly lower than at pretest. Moreover, although the number of patients who had comorbid disorders in Tsao et al.'s sample was stable from posttest to follow-up, at an individual level the diagnoses were more fluid—with some patients developing additional disorders not present at posttest, and other patients losing diagnoses at follow-up that were observed at posttest. It seems likely that to the degree that another disorder, such as depression, is caused by the restrictions or demoralization associated with panic disorder, treatment of the panic disorder will be sufficient. Otherwise, in the long run, many patients with comorbid disorders will require treatment targeting those problems.

A caveat raised in our interpretation of the GAD data also pertains here. In 9 of the 19 studies we reviewed on treatment of panic disorder, patients were allowed to take medications they were already taking at the time of intake, so long as they continued on a stable dose throughout treatment (Arntz, 2002; Bouchard et al., 1996; Burke et al., 1997; Clark et al., 1999; Gould et al., 1993; Hecker et al., 1998; Lidren et al., 1994; Telch et al., 1993; Williams & Falbo, 1996). van den Hout et al. (1994) did not report their approach to clients on medication, but authors of the remaining 9 studies required clients taking medication to withdraw before participation in their trials. Unfortunately, few of those permitting medications reported the percentage of clients taking drugs (27.5%, Arntz, 2002; 42–50%, Burke et al., 1997) or analyzed the relationship of medication use to treatment outcome. Arntz (2002) and Telch et al. (1993), the only authors to test the effects of medication, reported that outcome was the same for clients who used medication versus those who did not. Interpretation of the controlled effect sizes is not imperiled by medication use (because random assignment should distribute clients on medication equally to the CBT and control conditions), but it is possible that the percentage of clients achieving panic-free or CSC/HEF status might have been inflated by studies wherein clients were possibly benefiting from medication effects as well as effects of CBT. The number of studies in Table 5.1 is large enough for us to conduct a rough test of this hypothesis. Using a Mann–Whitney test, we compared the effects of CBT on CSC/HEF for the 9 studies eschewing medication to those for the 9 studies in which medication was permitted, and found no trend for a boost for studies including medicated clients ($z = 0.89$, $p = .40$). However, the results for a comparable analysis for panic-free status were equivocal, with a nonsignificant tendency for studies permitting medication to fare better ($z = 1.55$, $p = .167$).

Finally, investigators have only recently begun to include measures of quality of life as well as measures of symptoms and disability. Telch, Schmidt, Jaimez, Jacquin, and Harrington (1995) found that clients treated with CBT in the study by Telch et al. (1993) showed significantly more improvement than waiting-list clients on measures of global adjustment. These tapped adjustment in work, social and leisure activities, and family life. At 6-month follow-up, these results were maintained. In contrast, Black et al. (1993) found CBT no better than placebo in this regard—perhaps not surprisingly so, given the poor performance of CBT overall in that investigation. Decreases in disability were comparable for CBT and other active treatments (supportive–experiential psychotherapy or exposure) in three other investigations (Bouchard et al., 1996; Craske et al., 1995; Shear et al., 1994). Thus it appears overall that CBT leads to improvement in quality of life, although no more so than other treatments.

EFFECTIVENESS

Based upon available research, it seems clear that within controlled research settings, CBT significantly reduces the symptoms of both GAD and panic disorder. Accordingly, the next critical step is to determine whether these results generalize to CBT for these disorders in practice settings. Some authors have argued that various features of research trials, such as random assignment to treatment, use of highly trained therapists, and homogeneity of the client sample, militate against transfer of findings to the clinical setting (Seligman, 1995; Westen & Morrison, 2001). Effectiveness studies, which examine interventions in actual clinical settings, allow researchers to directly evaluate the generalizability of a given treatment by removing many of the methodological constraints found in highly controlled research environments.

Generalized Anxiety Disorder

Effectiveness studies for CBT of GAD are sorely lacking. We located only three in our review. White, Keenan, and Brooks (1992) employed a quasi-experimental design to evaluate CBT for GAD in a primary care setting. A total of 109 patients were allocated, in the order of referral, to one of five treatment conditions: behavior therapy, cognitive therapy, CBT, a placebo treatment (listening to ersatz subliminal antianxiety messages), or a waiting-list control condition. Treatment consisted of six 2-hour sessions and, in contrast to efficacy trials, was administered to large groups of more than 20 patients each. The active therapies, which did not differ from one another, led to greater decreases in anxiety than the waiting-list control condition, but were not significantly more effective than the placebo treatment. However, power was low for these comparisons. Moreover, the impact of the active therapies may have been diminished by the large-group format, as clients probably received limited individual attention. Indeed, a group of more than 20 patients is more akin to psychoeducation than to group therapy.

The effectiveness of individual CBT for GAD has also been explored. We included the study by Linden et al. (in press) in Table 5.1, because the authors randomly assigned patients to CBT or a minimal-contact control group. However, in other respects this was an effectiveness trial, in that CBT was administered in practice settings by psychologists working full-time as private practitioners. Therapists were trained and supervised by the authors. CBT produced significantly and clinically meaningful reductions in anxious symptomatology and on a more global measure of clinical functioning. After the waiting period, patients in the control group also received CBT for their generalized anxiety. As a group, these patients achieved gains similar in magnitude to those of the initial treatment group. Because of the exclusion criteria used (e.g., no comorbid conditions), the sample from this study was probably more homogeneous than is typical in clinical settings, and it is unclear whether the positive findings of the study would generalize to a more diverse group of patients.

Finally, Stanley, Hopko, et al. (2003) have conducted a small investigation into the effectiveness of CBT for GAD as administered to elderly medical patients in primary care practices. Again, this was a hybrid efficacy–effectiveness trial, in that patients were randomly assigned to treatment (CBT vs. treatment as usual), and research-trained therapists were used. However, the setting and the nature of the sample took this study into the effectiveness realm. The results of this investigation are included in Table 5.1. Relative to the treatment-as-usual group, the CBT group improved more on measures of GAD severity, worry, and depression.

Clearly, additional effectiveness research on CBT for GAD is acutely needed. To date, the studies suggest that CBT for these clients can be effectively delivered in practice settings, at least when therapists are well trained.

Panic Disorder

Progress in effectiveness research on panic disorder has far outstripped that for GAD. In the first major study in the United States, Wade, Treat, and Stuart (1998) evaluated the effectiveness of CBT for panic disorder in a community mental health center (CMHC). Using a benchmarking research strategy, the authors compared treatment outcome results from the CMHC to those obtained in two controlled outcome studies (Barlow, Craske, Cerny, & Klosko, 1989; Telch et al., 1993). The CMHC sample included 110 clients who satisfied the *Diagnostic and Statistical Manual of Mental Disorders*, third edition, revised (DSM-III-R) diagnosis of panic disorder with agoraphobia or panic disorder without agoraphobia. Exclusionary criteria were kept to a minimum to better assess the generalizability of the therapy. Therapists were trained and supervised for the duration of the trial. Clients completing therapy improved significantly on almost every outcome measure and achieved gains comparable in magnitude to those obtained by participants in the controlled comparison studies. In addition, clients reduced their use of both antidepressant and anxiolytic medications. Improvements on all variables were maintained or enhanced over a 1-year follow-up period (Stuart, Treat, & Wade, 2000).

Two studies from Great Britain also speak to the effectiveness of CBT for panic disorder. Sharp, Power, and Swanson (2003) investigated the effects of CBT for panic disorder in primary care practices. Although this study had elements of an efficacy trial (e.g., random assignment to treatment, control over medication), it represented an effectiveness study in its setting and participants. Standard CBT (6 hours of therapist contact) proved more efficacious than a minimal-contact CBT condition (2 hours of therapist contact plus a manual) and than bibliotherapy (manual only). Clients in all three treatment groups improved from pretest to posttest. Similarly, Burke et al. (1997) blended elements of efficacy and effectiveness studies in their comparison of CBT to exposure for agoraphobia (see Table 5.6). Random assignment to treatment was used, but clients were seen in ordinary clinical settings by National Health Service therapists. The therapists were, however, trained before the trial and received supervision for its duration. Although Arntz's studies in the Netherlands (Arntz, 2002; Arntz & van den Hout, 1996) were largely efficacy trials (see Table 5.6), the author emphasizes the effectiveness nature of the samples, which were drawn from a CMHC. In a final Dutch study, Bakker, Spinhoven, van Balkom,

Vleugel, and van Dyke (2000) directly tested one of the assertions of critics of efficacy trials (e.g., Seligman, 1995)—namely, that clients who refuse random allocation to treatments in a research study will have a different outcome than those who accept randomization will. These authors compared the effects of CBT for clients in a randomized controlled trial of CBT versus medication to those of clients who refused random assignment because they were unwilling to take medication. Both groups improved, and there were no differences between conditions.

Another dimension of effectiveness is CBT's benefit for ethnically diverse clients. Sanderson, Raue, and Wetzler (1998), working in a large urban medical center, used a manual-based cognitive-behavioral intervention to treat an ethnically diverse client population suffering from panic disorder. Thirty patients, 53% of whom were Hispanic, participated in 12 CBT sessions. From pre- to posttreatment, significant and clinically meaningful improvements were observed on a variety of outcome measures that were intended to assess panic, agoraphobia, generalized anxiety, and depression. The authors benchmarked their results to those of Barlow et al.'s (1989) efficacy study. Treatment effects were comparable in magnitude to those of the efficacy trial, and European American and Hispanic clients responded to treatment similarly. The effectiveness and efficacy studies did differ in regard to the percentage of clients who were panic-free at the end of treatment, with only 50% of the effectiveness sample satisfying this criterion as compared to 85% in the efficacy trial. However, this difference might be misleading, given that Sanderson et al.'s participants reported more panic attacks before treatment than Barlow et al.'s clients. Finally, although Carter et al.'s (2003) study was an efficacy trial with random assignment to treatment and research therapists, their findings pertain to the effectiveness question in an important regard: Their sample exclusively comprised African Americans with panic disorder. The positive effects of this treatment are apparent in the large effect sizes reported in Table 5.4.

In addition to the routine therapy provided in service clinics, CBT for panic disorder has been administered through the provision of self-help books. A number of studies by Gould, Clum, and their colleagues (Gould & Clum, 1995; Gould et al., 1993; Lidren et al., 1994) indicate that for clients with panic disorder, bibliotherapy represents a legitimate and useful mode of treatment delivery. Indeed, these authors found that clients who received bibliotherapy fared as well as those who received their version of face-to-face CBT. Recall, however, that Sharp et al. (2003) obtained discrepant results: In their study, face-to-face CBT was more effective than bibliotherapy, although both led to change. An Internet version of CBT has also shown promise as a treatment for panic disorder (Carlbring, Westling, Ljungstrand, Ekselius, & Andersson, 2001). Successes such as these should be interpreted cautiously, however. In the majority of studies that have explored the effectiveness of bibliotherapy for panic disorder, clients interacted with researchers in some capacity, often with checks on whether the clients were actually reading the manuals provided. Therefore, positive findings from these studies might be partially attributable to demand characteristics of the interventions (e.g., reporting change because investigators expected it) or to the motivational properties of contact with the research staff, and might not generalize to clients left entirely on their own with self-help books.

Clearly, additional research is needed to better clarify the full extent to which CBT for panic disorder can be effectively used in service clinics. For the most part, available studies support the intervention's generalizability. In the studies described above, treatment settings, client populations, or treatment providers were more heterogeneous than those from controlled efficacy trials. Despite these differences, CBT led to significant and often clinically meaningful improvement on a variety of treatment outcome measures. However, therapists were generally well trained in treatment procedures. How well CBT will fare with less carefully trained therapists (e.g., those who have only read a treatment manual and who do not receive supervision) is yet to be determined.

CONCLUSIONS

Our review of the second decade of research on CBT for GAD and panic disorder reveals a high level of activity in this field, especially in panic disorder, for which we found 19 efficacy studies published after our first (Chambless & Gillis, 1993) review. It is encouraging to see new researchers entering the GAD arena as well, although it still requires additional attention. We found 10 new efficacy studies for GAD. The success of CBT apparent in its first decade continues: CBT for panic disorder and GAD remains an efficacious treatment—superior to waiting-list, attention control, and pill placebo conditions; modestly superior to supportive psychotherapy; and equivalent to other behavioral treatments (largely applied relaxation and/or exposure) in outcome. Initial evidence of effectiveness research indicates that, at least when therapists are given training and supervision, CBT transfers well to practice settings and is beneficial to members of ethnic minority groups. All studies to date were conducted in the United States, Canada, or Western Europe. Whether CBT will generalize well to Third World countries remains to be seen.

The data reported in Tables 5.1–5.6 indicate that CBT has beneficial effects not only on core symptoms of anxiety, panic, and anxious thinking, but also on depression. A small set of studies provides evidence of positive effects on quality of life as well, although this is an area requiring additional documentation. The dropout rates reported in these tables, ranging from 8% to 27% for CBT, compare very favorably to an average rate (excluding those with alcohol and substance abuse/dependence problems) of 47% (SD = 24%) reported in a meta-analysis of 78 psychotherapy studies for adult clients (Wierzbicki & Pekarik, 1993).

The focus of our meta-analysis has been on treatment research with adults, including elderly adults. An important, relatively new frontier for CBT for GAD and panic disorder is the treatment of children and adolescents. Studies with this population are not yet sufficiently abundant to warrant meta-analysis. However, initial investigations indicate that with age-appropriate modifications, CBT is efficacious for older children and adolescents with GAD and panic disorder (e.g., Barrett, Dadds, & Rapee, 1996; Kendall, 1994; Ollendick, 1995).

These positive results cannot be taken to mean that CBT is a panacea. Examination of the percentage of clients who achieve clinically significant gains (i.e., who are not only improved but who score, after treatment, in the normal range on measures of their disorder) is sobering, particularly for GAD. The results for panic disorder are more encouraging in this regard, but better long-term follow-up, tracking fluctuations for individual clients, is needed before we can be confident that this is so (cf. Brown & Barlow, 1995). The present emphasis in funding for research in the United States is on effectiveness trials—taking treatments like CBT into the community, making them shorter, teaching them to less expert therapists, and using them with clients with a host of medical and psychological problems. Such research is clearly valuable, but also needed is additional research on achieving clinically significant change for a larger proportion of clients. Additional investigations targeting clients' comorbid disorders (typically depression and other anxiety disorders) may yield payoffs in this regard. In the meantime, the cognitive-behavioral therapist following one of the protocols used in these studies may be assured of offering clients a form of psychotherapy for GAD or panic disorder that is as good as or better than any other with which it has been contrasted.

ACKNOWLEDGMENTS

We thank the following individuals for their generosity in sharing unpublished data and manuscripts and for providing clarifications about their papers: Arnaud Arntz, Michele Carter, Michelle Craske, Michel Dugas, Jeffrey Hecker, Michael Linden, and Melinda Stanley.

REFERENCES

Arntz, A. (2002). Cognitive therapy versus interoceptive exposure as treatment of panic disorder without agoraphobia. *Behaviour Research and Therapy, 40*, 325–341.

Arntz, A., & van den Hout, M. (1996). Psychological treatments of panic disorder without agoraphobia: Cognitive therapy versus applied relaxation. *Behaviour Research and Therapy, 34*, 113–121.

Bakker, A., Spinhoven, P., van Balkom, A. J. L. M., Vleugel, L., & van Dyke, R. (2000). Cognitive therapy by allocation versus cognitive therapy by preference in the treatment of panic disorder. *Psychotherapy and Psychosomatics, 69*, 240–243.

Barlow, D. H., Craske, M. G., Cerny, J. A., & Klosko, J. (1989). Behavioral treatment of panic disorder. *Behavior Therapy, 20*, 261–282.

Barlow, D. H., Gorman, J. M., Shear, M. K., & Woods, S. W. (2000). Cognitive-behavioral therapy, imipramine, or their combination for panic disorder: A randomized controlled trial. *Journal of the American Medical Association, 283*, 2529–2536.

Barrett, P. M., Dadds, M. R., & Rapee, R. M. (1996). Family treatment of childhood anxiety: A controlled trial. *Journal of Consulting and Clinical Psychology, 64*, 333–342.

Beck, J. G., Stanley, M. A., Baldwin, L. E., Deagle, E. A., III, & Averill, P. M. (1994). Comparison of cognitive therapy and relaxation training for panic disorder. *Journal of Consulting and Clinical Psychology, 62*, 818–826.

Black, D. W., Wesner, R., Bowers, W., & Gabel, J. (1993). A comparison of fluvoxamine, cognitive therapy, and placebo in the treatment of panic disorder. *Archives of General Psychiatry, 50*, 44–50.

Borkovec, T. D., Abel, J. L., & Newman, H. (1995). Effects of psychotherapy on comorbid conditions in generalized anxiety disorder. *Journal of Consulting and Clinical Psychology, 63*, 479–483.

Borkovec, T. D., & Costello, E. (1993). Efficacy of applied relaxation and cognitive-behavioral therapy in the treatment of generalized anxiety disorder. *Journal of Consulting and Clinical Psychology, 61*, 611–619.

Borkovec, T. D., Newman, M. G., Pincus, A. L., & Lytle, R. (2002). A component analysis of cognitive behavioral therapy for generalized anxiety disorder and the role of interpersonal problems. *Journal of Consulting and Clinical Psychology, 70*, 288–298.

Bouchard, S., Gauthier, J., Laberge, B., French, D., Pelletier, M.-H., & Godbout, C. (1996). Exposure versus cognitive restructuring in the treatment of panic disorder with agoraphobia. *Behaviour Research and Therapy, 34*, 213–224.

Brown, T. A., Antony, M. M., & Barlow, D. H. (1995). Diagnostic comorbidity in panic disorder: Effect on treatment outcome and course of comorbid diagnoses following treatment. *Journal of Consulting and Clinical Psychology, 63*, 408–418.

Brown, T. A., & Barlow, D. H. (1995). Long-term outcome in cognitive-behavioral treatment of panic disorder: Clinical predictors and alternative strategies for assessment. *Journal of Consulting and Clinical Psychology, 63*, 754–765.

Burke, M., Drummond, L. M., & Johnston, D. W. (1997). Treatment choice for agoraphobic women: Exposure or cognitive-behaviour therapy? *British Journal of Clinical Psychology, 36*, 409–420.

Carlbring, P., Westling, B. E., Ljungstrand, P., Ekselius, L., & Andersson, G. (2001). Treatment of panic disorder via the Internet: A randomized trial of a self-help program. *Behavior Therapy, 32*, 751–764.

Carter, M. M., Sbrocco, T., Gore, K. L., Marin, N. W., & Lewis, E. L. (2003). Cognitive-behavioral therapy versus a wait-list control in the treatment of African American women with panic disorder. *Cognitive Therapy and Research, 27*, 505–518.

Chambless, D. L., & Gillis, M. M. (1993). Cognitive therapy of anxiety disorders. *Journal of Consulting and Clinical Psychology, 61*, 248–260.

Clark, D. M., Salkovskis, P. M., Hackmann, A., Wells, A., Ludgate, J., & Gelder, M. (1999). Brief cognitive therapy for panic disorder: A randomized controlled trial. *Journal of Consulting and Clinical Psychology, 67*, 583–589.

Cohen, J. (1988). *Statistical power analysis for the behavioral sciences* (2nd ed.). Hillsdale, NJ: Erlbaum.

Craske, M. G., Maidenberg, E., & Bystritsky, A. (1995). Brief cognitive-behavioral versus nondirective therapy for panic disorder. *Journal of Behavior Therapy and Experimental Psychiatry, 26*, 113–120.

Dobson, K. S. (1989). A meta-analysis of the efficacy of cognitive therapy for depression. *Journal of Consulting and Clinical Psychology, 57*, 414–419.

Dugas, M. J., Ladouceur, R., Leger, E., Freeston, M. H., Langlois, F., Provencher, M., et al. (2003). Group cognitive-behavior therapy for generalized anxiety disorders: Treatment outcome and long-term follow-up. *Journal of Consulting and Clinical Psychology, 71*, 821–825.

Durham, R. C., Murphy, T., Allan, T., Richard, K., Treliving, L. R., & Fenton, G. W. (1994). Cognitive therapy, analytic psychotherapy, and anxiety management training for generalized anxiety disorder. *British Journal of Psychiatry, 165*, 315–323.

Gould, R. A., & Clum, G. A. (1995). Self-help plus minimal therapist contact in the treatment of panic disorder: A replication and extension. *Behavior Therapy, 26*, 533–545.

Gould, R. A., Clum, G. A., & Shapiro, D. (1993). The use of bibliotherapy in the treatment of panic: A preliminary investigation. *Behavior Therapy, 24*, 241–252.

Gould, R. A., Otto, M. W., Pollack, M. H., & Yap, L. (1997). Cognitive behavioral and pharmacological treatment of generalized anxiety disorder: A preliminary meta-analysis. *Behavior Therapy, 28*, 285–305.

Hecker, J. E., Fink, C. M., Vogeltanz, N. E., Thorpe, G. L., & Sigmon, S. T. (1998). Cognitive restructuring and interoceptive exposure in the treatment of panic disorder: A crossover study. *Behavioural and Cognitive Psychotherapy, 26*, 115–131.

Hofmann, S. G., Barlow, D. H., Papp, L. A., Detweiler, M. F., Ray, S. E., Shear, K., et al. (1998). Pretreatment attrition in a comparative treatment outcome study on panic disorder. *American Journal of Psychiatry, 155*(1), 43–47.

Jacobson, N. S., & Truax, P. (1991). Clinical significance: A statistical approach to defining meaningful change in psychotherapy research. *Journal of Consulting and Clinical Psychology, 59*, 12–19.

Kendall, P. C. (1994). Treating anxiety disorders in children: Results of a randomized clinical trial. *Journal of Consulting and Clinical Psychology, 62,* 100–110.

Kovacs, A. L. (1996). "We have met the enemy and he is us!" *AAP Advance,* pp. 6, 19, 20, 22.

Ladouceur, R., Dugas, M. J., Freeston, M. H., Leger, E., Gagnon, F., & Thibodeau, N. (2000). Efficacy of a cognitive-behavioral treatment for generalized anxiety disorder: Evaluation in a controlled clinical trial. *Journal of Consulting and Clinical Psychology, 68,* 957–964.

Lidren, D. M., Watkins, P. L., Gould, R. A., Clum, G. A., Asterino, M., & Tulloch, H. L. (1994). A comparison of bibliotherapy and group therapy in the treatment of panic disorder. *Journal of Consulting and Clinical Psychology, 62,* 865–869.

Linden, M., Zubrägel, D., Bär, T., Wendt, U., & Schlattmann, P. (in press). Efficacy of cognitive behaviour therapy in generalized anxiety disorders: Results of a controlled clinical trial. *Psychotherapy and Psychomatics.*

Moras, K. (1998). Internal and external validity of intervention studies. In A. S. Bellack & M. Hersen (Eds.), *Comprehensive clinical psychology* (Vol. 3, pp. 201–224). Oxford: Elsevier.

Ollendick, T. H. (1995). Cognitive-behavioral treatment of panic disorder with agoraphobia in adolescents: A multiple baseline design analysis. *Behavior Therapy, 26,* 517–531.

Öst, L.-G., & Breitholtz, E. (2000). Applied relaxation vs. cognitive therapy in the treatment of generalized anxiety disorder. *Behaviour Research and Therapy, 38,* 777–790.

Rosenthal, R. (1991). *Meta-analytic procedures for social research* (rev. ed.). Newbury Park, CA: Sage.

Sanderson, W. C., Raue, P. J., & Wetzler, S. (1998). The generalizability of cognitive behavior therapy for panic disorder. *Journal of Cognitive Psychotherapy: An International Quarterly, 12,* 323–330.

Seligman, M. E. P. (1995). The effectiveness of psychotherapy: The *Consumer Reports* study. *American Psychologist, 50,* 965–974.

Sharp, D. M., Power, K. G., Simpson, R. J., Swanson, V., Moodie, E., Anstee, J. A., et al. (1996). Fluvoxamine, placebo, and cognitive behaviour therapy used alone and in combination in the treatment of panic disorder and agoraphobia. *Journal of Anxiety Disorders, 10,* 219–242.

Sharp, D. M., Power, K. G., & Swanson, V. (2003). Reducing therapist contact in cognitive behaviour therapy for panic disorder and agoraphobia in primary care: Global measures of outcome in a randomized controlled trial. *British Journal of General Practice, 50,* 963–968.

Shear, M. K., Houck, P., Greeno, C., & Masters, S. (2001). Emotion-focused psychotherapy for patients with panic disorder. *American Journal of Psychiatry, 158,* 1993–1998.

Shear, M. K., Pilkonis, P. A., Cloitre, M., & Leon, A. C. (1994). Cognitive behavioral treatment compared with nonprescriptive treatment of panic disorder. *Archives of General Psychiatry, 51,* 395–401.

Stanley, M. A., Beck, J. G., & Glassco, J. D. (1996). Treatment of generalized anxiety in older adults: A preliminary comparison of cognitive-behavioral and supportive approaches. *Behavior Therapy, 27,* 565–581.

Stanley, M. A., Beck, J. G., Novy, D. M., Averill, P. M., Swann, A. C., Diefenbach, G. J., et al. (2003). Cognitive behavior treatment of late-life generalized anxiety disorder. *Journal of Consulting and Clinical Psychology*, 309–319.

Stanley, M. A., Hopko, D. R., Diefenbach, G. J., Bourland, S. L., Rodriguez, H., & Wagener, P. (2003). Cognitive-behavior therapy for late-life generalized anxiety disorder in primary care. *American Journal of Geriatric Psychiatry*, 11(1), 1–5.

Stuart, G. L., Treat, T. A., & Wade, W. A. (2000). Effectiveness of an empirically based treatment for panic disorder delivered in a service clinic setting: One-year follow-up. *Journal of Consulting and Clinical Psychology*, 68, 506–512.

Telch, M. J., Lucas, J. A., Schmidt, N. B., Hanna, H. H., Jaimez, T. L., & Lucas, R. A. (1993). Group cognitive behavioral treatment of panic disorder. *Behaviour Research and Therapy*, 31, 279–287.

Telch, M. J., Schmidt, N. B., Jaimez, L., Jacquin, K. M., & Harrington, P. J. (1995). Impact of cognitive-behavioral treatment on quality of life in panic disorder patients. *Journal of Consulting and Clinical Psychology*, 63, 823–830.

Tsao, J. C., Mystkowski, J. L., Zucker, B. G., & Craske, M. G. (2002). Effects of cognitive-behavioral therapy for panic disorder on comorbid conditions: Replication and extension. *Behavior Therapy*, 33, 493–509.

van den Hout, M., Arntz, A., & Hoekstra, R. (1994). Exposure reduced agoraphobia but not panic, and cognitive therapy reduced panic but not agoraphobia. *Behaviour Research and Therapy*, 32, 447–451.

Wade, W. A., Treat, T. A., & Stuart, G. L. (1998). Transporting an empirically supported treatment for panic disorder to a service clinic setting: A benchmarking strategy. *Journal of Consulting and Clinical Psychology*, 66, 231–239.

Westen, D., & Morrison, K. (2001). A multidimensional meta-analysis of treatments for depression, panic, and generalized anxiety disorder: An empirical examination of the status of empirically supported therapies. *Journal of Consulting and Clinical Psychology*, 69, 875–899.

Wetherell, J. L., Gatz, M., & Craske, M. G. (2003). Treatment of generalized anxiety disorder in older adults. *Journal of Consulting and Clinical Psychology*, 71, 31–40.

White, J., Keenan, M., & Brooks, N. (1992). Stress control: A controlled comparative investigation of large group therapy for generalized anxiety disorder. *Behavioural Psychotherapy*, 20, 97–114.

Wierzbicki, M., & Pekarik, G. (1993). A meta-analysis of psychotherapy dropout. *Professional Psychology: Research and Practice*, 24, 190–195.

Williams, S. L., & Falbo, J. (1996). Cognitive and performance-based treatments for panic attacks in people with varying degrees of agoraphobic disability. *Behaviour Research and Therapy*, 34, 253–264.

Chapter 6

Decision Making and Psychopathology

ROBERT L. LEAHY

Cognitive theories of psychopathology have stressed the information-processing metaphor as a model. Specifically, they propose that individuals will differ as to their biased perception of loss and failure (depression); threat to safety or self (anxiety); vulnerability to humiliation or defeat (anger); or specific personal content of defectiveness, abandonment, special status, or autonomy (personality disorders) (Beck & Emery with Greenberg, 1985; Beck, Freeman, Davis, & Associates, 2004; Beck, Rush, Shaw, & Emery, 1979; Young, Klosko, & Weishaar, 2003). A second model within the cognitive tradition draws on explanatory style, distinguishing individuals as to their tendency to employ an "optimistic" or a "pessimistic" attribution style for behavior at which they have failed or succeeded (Abramson, Metalsky, & Alloy, 1989; Abramson, Seligman, & Teasdale, 1978). Derived from the attribution models of motivation developed by Weiner, Kelley, and others (Davis, 1965; Kelley, 1967, 1973; Weiner, Nierenberg, & Goldstein, 1976), this model suggests that individuals will differ in their vulnerability to depression contingent on their preexisting attribution style.

There is considerable empirical support for the schematic model as a vulnerability factor for depression (Clark & Beck with Alford, 1999; Ingram, Miranda, & Segal, 1998), for anxiety (Purdon & Clark, 1993; Stopa & Clark, 1993; Winton, Clark, & Edelmann, 1995), and for specific personality disorders (Beck et al., 2001, 2004; Butler, Brown, Beck, & Grisham, 2002). There is also considerable empirical support for a cogni-

116

tive diathesis model of vulnerability for depression based on explanatory style (Abramson et al., 1989; Alloy, Abramson, Metalsky, & Hartledge, 1988; Alloy, Reilly-Harrington, Fresco, Whitehouse, & Zechmeister, 1999).

However, as compelling as these models (and the empirical support that they have achieved) are, there has been little attention to processes of decision making in the cognitive approach to psychopathology. A cursory examination of the clinical problems presented by patients illustrates that many individuals are characterized by a history of procrastination, impulsive decisions, regret, and/or the inability to decide between alternatives. Indeed, the clinical import of decision making is reflected by the fact that the therapist is attempting to help the patient change thinking and behavior— that is, to make decisions about the nature of reality and about how to act differently.

In the current chapter, I briefly review classical models of decision making—which are referred to as "normative" models, reflecting their "ideal" or "rational" nature. I then turn to a discussion of consistencies in the errors of decision makers—consistencies resulting from heuristics (or rules of thumb) that lead to biased predilections. I next review three areas of biased decision making that are of specific relevance to psychopathology. The first area is the modern "portfolio theory" model of decision making that I have elaborated, which suggests that individuals differ as to their underlying assumptions about resources, strategies for dealing with uncertainty, and risk tolerance. Related to these individual differences in investment strategies in decision making are two distinct styles: those of the depressive and the manic decision maker. A second area I review is that of "myopic" decision making, in which the consistent focus on shorter-term gains over longer-term gains results in "contingency traps." The third area I discuss is the issue of "sunk costs," or the consequences of prior commitments to lost causes. I propose theoretical reasons why we all tend to honor sunk costs, and I indicate how these sunk costs are specifically related to particular areas of psychopathology. In connection with sunk costs, I review the evidence that decision makers do not utilize a "rational" model in decision making based on future utility; rather, they base their current decisions on their past decision-making outcomes.

NORMATIVE MODELS OF DECISION MAKING

A "normative" model is one that describes how decision makers should think if they are rational and utilize all of the information presented to them. Rationality is determined by what we would expect would work in decision making if individuals eventually obtained perfect information with infinite iterations of their decisions (see von Neumann & Morgenstern, 1944). Thus, if I had perfect information that a die is "honest" (with equal probability of an outcome between 1 and 6), and I throw the die, I should rationally wager based on the expected probabilities of each of the outcomes. I should not engage in gambling fallacies—such as believing that I am having a streak of luck; that my luck is running out; that I am particularly fond of the number 4 and always bet on that number; or that I have seen someone else winning on betting on 6, and so I am now forsaking my favored 4 for the new fetish of 6. Rational decision making is presumably based on an objective calculation of the probabilities of an outcome, as well as its future utility.

Exceptions to normative decision making are common—reflecting the "anomalies" that characterize mundane decision making and that make gamblers excited and miserable, while perplexing depressed and anxious people. Thus, manic individuals may believe that they are having a streak of luck (based on limited information); depressed people believe their luck has run out and will never return; obsessive–compulsive individuals will superstitiously favor specific behaviors because they provide a "felt sense" of satisfaction; and many of us are envious of other people and copy their behavior, even if it is self-destructive to us. The goal of this chapter is to describe some of these anomalies and the clinical implications that follow from them.

Cost–Benefit Analyses

An essential component of normative models of decision making is that individuals will focus entirely on future utility and ignore prior costs or outcomes. This model of the "ahistorical" decision maker is based on the metaphor of the human being as a computer, rather than as someone trying to save face and make sense of the past. A central component of this normative model is the calculation of costs and benefits for a decision.

As cognitive therapists, we engage our patients in discussions of "cost–benefit" analyses, as if we are asking our patients to do an objective "weighting" of outcomes—very much like someone comparing four oranges with six oranges. Cost–benefit analyses, however, are exceedingly complex; philosophers, economists, and legal scholars have all pondered the intricacies of this kind of analysis (see Becker, 1976, 1991; Becker, Grossman, & Murphy, 1991; Becker & Murphy, 1988; Breyer, 1993; Sunstein, 2000).

Consider a patient contemplating whether he should divorce his wife and pursue a new life independently of her. How does he go about making a cost–benefit analysis? Is this an entirely logical or rational endeavor? It is doubtful that it is. First, it is apparent that the patient does are not utilize a stable metric. How does one weigh a cost—what *units* of "cost" are implied? How does the patient weigh the costs of not seeing his daughter or the costs of losing much of his financial security? How does he weigh the benefit of reducing arguments or achieving opportunities for new relationships? These are not units of information measured in yards or meters. It is unclear how they are measured. Second, how does one translate or compare costs in one area with benefits in another area? How can this patient say that the costs of loss of a relationship are comparable to the benefits of achieving freedom to pursue new relationships? Third, costs that are calculated in the first phase of consideration may gain a "primacy" effect; that is, the individual may give greater weight to the costs simply because he is thinking of them first. For example, he may first think of the costs of seeing his daughter less and then ignore any other possible thoughts of any benefits. Or he may be utilizing a "satisfaction" principle—he is "satisfied" that there is too much cost to bear.

Fourth, cost–benefit calculations ignore whether individuals differ as to their desire to minimize all costs or to maximize all gains. It is common for a patient to acknowledge that the benefits of a change outweigh the costs, but the patient may also believe that *any* costs are intolerable. For this individual, ratios are less important than the existence of a cost. For example, in social policy Breyer (1993) has identified a tendency in litigation to eliminate any possible cost (or risk) of toxic contamination, regardless of the insurmountable costs. Since available resources for combating health risks are not limitless, overexpenditure in eliminating the "last 10%" often far outweighs the advantages of utilizing this money to decrease other risks. For example, far more lives are saved by money expended advocating auto safety than by money expended in trying to eliminate the last 10% of (very low) risks in toxic waste dumps (see Breyer, 1993). This is related to the reluctance of individuals to obtain "probabilistic insurance"—that is, insurance that would cover only part of the loss with a commensurate reduction in the premium (Kahneman, 1995; Kahneman & Tversky, 1979). Individuals will overpay to cover all risks, rather than take their chances with a reduced premium that covers only some risks. A similar overemphasis on attempting to eliminate any possible cost (or risk) is found among patients with obsessive–compulsive disorder and generalized anxiety disorder (GAD). For example, individuals with GAD seek perfect solutions that will eliminate any risk or uncertainty, thereby driving their worry toward rejection of plausible solutions (Dugas, Buhr, & Ladouceur, 2004). These individuals ignore base rates (Wells, 1995) and seek certainty, sometimes even preferring a *certain* negative outcome to an *uncertain* positive outcome (Dugas et al., 2004).

Fifth, cost–benefit ratios ignore the probability of an outcome—a central component of calculating subjective estimates of risk. Simply saying that the costs "outweigh" the benefits by a 3:2 ratio may ignore the probability that the costs have a higher probability. Risk is not necessarily reducible to the magnitude of an outcome; it includes the probability of the outcome. Sixth, individuals will be myopic about costs, since they may fear that they will face the costs first. Or, if they are impulsive, they may be myopic about the benefits, discounting the costs as a future factor to be ignored. In the former case, we see individuals who are avoidant and procrastinating, since they wish to avoid the discomfort of the costs. In the latter case, the individual places greater emphasis on immediate benefits that overshadow longer-term costs—a familiar pattern in the "contingency traps" of patients with addictions or certain other disorders (to be discussed in a later section).

An alternative to a "subjective" estimate of a cost–benefit ratio is a pragmatic estimate based on what a patient is willing to do when action is required. For example, the patient who claims that the costs of his marriage outweigh the benefits, but then decides to stay in the marriage, may later articulate that his decision to stay was based on his reluctance to change his relationship with his daughter. Thus the "true" cost–benefit ratio is determined by what he observes in his actions, not by what he says about what he might do "if I were rational." Similarly, examining outcomes or actions can help us evaluate whether a the patient uses a "satisfaction" or a "primacy/recency" decision rule. The "satisfaction" rule suggests that the patient will be satisfied if one criterion (or some criteria) are met. In the example above, the man has determined that he is satisfied to stay in his marriage, since he will not want to change his relationship with his daughter; the "daughter" criterion satisfies him and therefore overrules other criteria. Indeed, he may not even consider other criteria once he has examined the daughter issue. Another factor that arises in his action is that he may weigh more heavily primacy information (the information that he first thinks of—e.g., "Will I see my daughter less?"), or he may value recency information more (e.g., "My relationship with my wife was better today").

HEURISTICS

"Heuristics" are shorthand "rules of thumb" that allow individuals to make a decision rapidly, without having to calculate baselines, evaluate past performance, or conduct pairwise comparisons of future probabilities and utilities. For example, if I go to a diner for lunch, I am pressed for time, since I must return to my office shortly for an appointment. The menu arrives, presenting me with the opportunity to examine the possible pairwise comparisons of 100 entrees, appetizers, and salads. What decision strategy do I utilize? One rule of thumb might be "Choose something that I am familiar with that was really 'good enough to eat.'" Along with this "satisfaction" rule might be the "first one" rule—that is, "The first dish that meets this criterion is good enough." An alternative rule of thumb (which is not a short cut) would be to ask the waiter for the pros and cons of every dish and to ask for comparisons between these dishes. Since time is of the essence, I utilize the first one that satisfies (Simon, 1979). Choosing the tuna salad platter, however, may leave me open to regrets due to perfectionism if I should hear from a colleague that the beef stroganoff was "out of this world." However, if I utilize the "satisfaction" and "first one" rules, I can count on eating my lunch efficiently, never having to regret that the meal was less than satisfying.

Another heuristic that guides decision makers is "loss aversion": People tend to suffer from their losses more than they enjoy their gains. Thus a loss of $1,000 is experienced as more important than a gain of $1,000. Kahneman and Tversky's (1979) prospect theory proposes that the way in which alternatives are framed or considered—for example, as losses or gains—may lead to violations of expected utility theory. For example, when considering the following alternatives—"50% chance of losing $1,000 versus a sure loss of $500"—individuals choose the more "risky" 50% chance of losing, even though the expected utility of both alternatives is equivalent. The issue of loss aversion outlined by Kahneman and Tversky is a key element of my adaptation of portfolio theory to explain depressive decision making (Leahy, 1997). My view (as outlined below) is that depressed individuals are especially averse to further losses and will therefore avoid changing their behavior, because outcomes are disproportionately viewed as losses rather than as potential gains.

Related to this loss aversion is the "endowment effect," which reflects the tendency to attach a higher value to what one has already paid for and possesses. Thus investors who own a stock will require a higher payment for the stock than they would pay to buy the stock themselves if they never owned it (Thaler, 1992). The endowment effect is conceptually related to the concept of "sunk costs" that I describe later in this chapter. Because people overvalue the possessions (or decisions) to which they have committed themselves, they are more likely to "ride a loser"—whether it is a stock investment, a relationship, or an opinion.

Other heuristics described by Kahneman and Tversky include recency and salience effects. Thus information that is recent and conceptually salient is far more likely to determine decisions than information that is abstract, such as baseline information (Kahneman, 1995; Kahneman & Tversky, 1979; Tversky & Kahneman, 1974). This has implications for individuals with GAD who worry excessively when they hear of a recent and widely publicized accident ("I don't think flying an airplane is safe, because there was an accident yesterday"). Estimates of "risk" or "danger" are often based on the accessibility of information rather than on a survey of base rates over time. When an individual with hypochondriasis scans the Internet and reviews information about all the "symptoms" of cancer, this information and the disease are more accessible than the abstract and rather unconvincing base rates, which this person seldom examines.

Finally, emotional arousal affects the perception of risk, such that increasing anxiety (by mood induction) can increase the estimates of risks in other areas of life (Finucane, Alhakami, Slovic, & Johnson, 2000; Slovic, 2000). Once the anxiety is activated, it serves as a priming catalyst for perceptions of possible danger. Cognitive therapists (who will consider this an example of "emotional reasoning") are correct in noting that one can use one's own emotions to estimate the external threat. This emotional heuristic—and the consequent perception of risk or scarcity of resources—is a major component of decision making and the perception of alternatives in depression and the various anxiety disorders.

PORTFOLIO THEORY

Modern Portfolio Theory

Decision making has long been of interest both to cognitive psychologists and to economic theorists. Kahneman and Tversky (Kahneman, 1995; Kahneman & Tversky, 1979; Tversky & Kahneman, 1974), as well as other cognitive psychologists (Finucane et al., 2000), have focused on heuristics that guide decision making, reflecting the "bounded rationality"—or the limits to rationality—in everyday decisions (see Simon, 1979, 1983). Similarly, behavioral finance theory is guided by the view that the cognitive processes that underlie irrational decision making in investments are not random, but rather reflect a consistent bias in thinking (Thaler, 1992). Many years prior to the integration of cognitive psychology and behavioral finance theory, Harry Markowitz (1952) advanced a model of "portfolio selection" in finance theory, which suggested that individuals differ as to their assumptions, goals, and conditions in contemplating their investments in the market.

Risk is measured in modern portfolio theory by the standard deviation of an investment. Thus investments that reflect greater variability confer greater risk, but may also confer greater reward potential. Markowitz proposed that individuals differ as to their risk tolerance: Some prefer more aggressive or risky strategies in order to maximize gains, while others seek to avoid risk while valuing minimization of loss over maximization of gain. Investors may reduce their risk—or the standard deviation effects noted here—by diversifying their investments (in a manner where these separate investments are either negatively correlated with or orthogonal to each other) and by increasing the time horizon of the investment. For example, overexposure to the potential disadvantages of one investment can be offset or hedged by taking a position in another investment that may rise when the first one falls (a negatively correlated investment) or that is unrelated to the initial investment. Repeated investment over a long period of time reduces the standard deviation of any specific position, as Markowitz and others have demonstrated.

Of relevance to our discussion of individual decision makers facing mundane decisions, the portfolio theory model suggests that individuals differ in their psychological tolerance of risk and in their duration and replication of investment. Specifically, some individuals will believe that they have significant resources and that they can face a longer time horizon (i.e., stay in the market longer), whereas others have fewer resources or a shorter time horizon. Other individuals will hedge against risk by diversifying their investments, since a loss in one area may not affect another area of investments. These factors, according to Markowitz, will affect the degree to which individuals will tolerate risks.

I have expanded on these themes first identified by Markowitz in developing a model of how individuals make mundane decisions—not simply decisions focused on financial investments (Leahy, 1997, 1999, 2001a, 2003). According to this model, individuals consider a number of factors both in contemplating a decision and in taking a risk. These include the following: perception of current resources; anticipation of future earnings or gains (independent of the current decision); ability to predict and control outcomes; generalizability of negative and positive outcomes; criteria for defining a gain or a loss; disposition to blame self or other; tendency to take credit for gains; acceleration of loss or gain; replication of "investment" or behavior directed toward a goal; time horizon; need for information; and risk aversion or toleration. I shall develop these themes in the following section in discussing pessimistic and optimistic models of decision making.

Pessimistic and Optimistic Decision Makers

The underlying premise guiding modern portfolio theory is that decision makers differ as to their assumptions and perceived realities. Thus individuals have different portfolio theories, or models of decision making and investment. I have proposed that the realities of these different portfolio theories are best captured by comparing how depressed, nondepressed, and manic individuals approach a decision. This contrast is reflected in Table 6.1.

As we examine this table, we note that the decision-making assumptions guiding depressed or pessimistic investors are the "flip side" of those guiding manic investors. Specifically, as depressed individuals con-

TABLE 6.1. Portfolio Theories of Depressed, Nondepressed, and Manic Individuals

Portfolio concern	Depressed	Nondepressed	Manic
Assets available	Few	Some/many	Unlimited
Future earning potential	Low	Moderate	Unlimited
Market variation	Volatile	Low/predictable	Certain predictability
Investment goal	Minimal loss	Minimal loss with maximum gain	Maximum gain, indifference to loss
Risk orientation	Risk-averse	Risk-neutral	Risk-loving
Functional utility of gain	Low	Moderate	Very high
Replications of investment	None/few	Many	Unlimited
Duration of investment	Short-term	Long-term	Short-term
Portfolio diversification	Low	Moderate	Very high

template a change, they view themselves as having few current resources or assets and their future earning potential as quite low. Thus they may believe that any future loss will drive them into oblivion. In contrast, manic individuals perceive themselves as having substantial current and future resources, and thus believe that a loss will not affect their substantial "holdings." Pessimistic individuals view the market as quite unpredictable or variable, thus making any change risky from the perspective of control or information needs. Optimistic individuals may believe that the market is predictable and that they can go with their hunches. The highest goal for depressed individuals is to avoid loss (reflecting their minimizing strategy), while manic individuals may be indifferent to loss and may focus exclusively on potential gains. Depressed individuals believe that they have few replications and a short time horizon, and thus that they cannot continue to persist in their efforts to achieve their goals; manic individuals may believe that they can persist in their investments or behavior indefinitely, thereby making it more likely (they believe) that they will eventually succeed. Depressed individuals are anhedonic and do not enjoy things anyway (this makes any "gains" not particularly "beneficial" to them), whereas manic individuals may overestimate how much they enjoy an outcome. All of these assumptions and perceptions guide depressed and manic individuals to consider decisions in distinctive, but predictable, ways.

In Table 6.2, I present aspects of loss orientation for depressed individuals. As inspection of this table reveals, depressed individuals view any slight change in loss as a major change. Given that the goal is to minimize further loss, early detection of loss, coupled with a pessimism about the "market" (or available resources), would suggest that early loss detection would be helpful—especially if there is a perception that losses will "cascade" like a waterfall or will follow a chain reaction. The decision to "quit early," after experiencing a loss, is based on these individuals' view that they have few resources to utilize and that outcomes are hopeless. This is similar to the findings by Dweck and her colleagues that individuals marked by "learned helplessness" will give up early, thereby confirming their low self-esteem and their belief that they do not have the ability to perform (Dweck, 1975, 1986; Dweck, Davidson, Nelson, & Enna, 1978). Furthermore, depressed individuals operate both with scarcity assumptions ("There are few rewards out there anyway") and with depletion views of behavior ("The more effort I utilize, the more exhausted and defeated I will feel"). Thus they believe that persistence in behavior is not likely to pay off

TABLE 6.2. Aspects of Loss Orientation for Depressed Individuals

Aspect of loss orientation	Definition
Low threshold	The slightest decrease is viewed as a loss of significant proportions.
High "stop-loss" criteria	A small loss leads to termination of behavior. Consequently, depressive individuals get "stopped out" early.
Scarcity assumptions	The world is viewed as having few opportunities for success. This is generalized to a zero-sum model of rewards for self and other.
Depletion assumptions	Losses are not seen as simple inconveniences or temporary setbacks. They are viewed as permanently drawing down resources.
Cost cascades	Losses are viewed as linked to an accelerating linear trend of further losses.
Short-term temporal focus	Depressive individuals take a short-term focus, viewing their investments only in terms of how they will pay off or lose in the short term.
Reversibility and revocability	Losses are viewed as irreversible and not compensated or offset by gains. Negative investments are irrevocable; depressive individuals cannot see themselves as able to "pull out" easily.
Regret orientation	Depressive individuals' losses are followed by regret that they should have known better. Their hindsight bias is focused on the assumption that they should have been able to make perfect decisions with limited information.

TABLE 6.3. Risk Management Concerns of Depressive Individuals

Risk management concern	Definition
Low diversification	Depressive individuals believe that they have only a single investment—the one at hand—and therefore that they are highly exposed to loss.
Short duration	Because depressive individuals believe that they are in the game for the short term, they are highly exposed to volatility.
Low or no replication	They believe that they will not have additional chances to succeed in this situation. Therefore, they must be sure that the first attempt will work.
Need to wait	They believe that they need to wait for a more opportune moment to act, and they forgo opportunity costs because no alternative seems attractive.
High information	They require near-absolute certainty before they decide.
High disappointment aversion	They are less concerned with the ongoing lack of reinforcement than with the possibility of a negative *change*. They avoid *negative delta* at all costs.
Manipulation of expectations	They attempt either to lower expectations that they will succeed, or to raise expectations excessively in order to avoid disappointment and to avoid direct assessment of their "true" ability.
Rejection of hope	They view hope ambivalently, believing that getting their hopes up leaves them open to greater exposure and disappointment.
Straddling	They exert a minimal effort as a probe to determine whether their behavior can have some effect. Holding themselves back, they pull out at the first sign of a negative.
Hedging	They bet against themselves by keeping other options open that, ironically, may undermine their current choice.
Hiding	They attempt to maintain a low profile in order to avoid being exposed to evaluation.
Obscuring self-evaluation	They create conditions that prevent a direct assessment of their competence under optimal conditions. This provides them with the face-saving option of misattributing their failure to lack of effort, illness, poor attendance, and/or lack of preparation, rather than to a fixed trait.

in a sinking market of rewards, and that they will become exhausted in their efforts. This is to be contrasted with the optimistic and resilient expectations of individuals characterized by "learned resourcefulness"—that is, by the belief that effort is a point of pride and a necessary aspect of self-efficacy (Eisenberger, 1992).

Finally, the portfolio theory of decision making proposes that depressed individuals will utilize self-protective strategies to avoid further losses. These are reflected in Table 6.3. Individuals who are depressed are risk-averse (Leahy, 2001a, 2001b). Since they believe that they are not diversified (i.e., that they do not have a range of sources of rewards—they may be exceptionally sensitive to any loss. However, there are strategies that depressed individuals can utilize to offset their "exposure." These include waiting for the "right time," collecting more information to reduce uncertainty, lowering their expectations (and the expectations that others have of them), rejecting hope (since hope may lead to risky behavior), straddling across two alternatives, and hedging, hiding, and obscuring self-evaluation. Ironically, in the longer term, these risk-management strategies may actually perpetuate further depression and the elimination of opportunities for change. The essential point here is that depressed individuals seek to avoid *further loss*.

There is empirical support for the portfolio theory model. In a study of 153 adult psychiatric patients (Leahy, 2001a), the participants completed a 25-item Decision Questionnaire that assessed 25 dimensions of decision making, and these responses were correlated with scores on the Beck Depression Inventory. The results substantially supported the assumptions of a general portfolio theory of risk. Risk aversion and depression were related to most of the dimensions, and depression was related to risk aversion. Less depression was related to maximizing positives as a goal, but was unrelated to minimizing negatives. Four factors accounted for most of the variance: general efficacy, discouragement, unpredictability, and risk aversion. Thus individuals who were more depressed were more likely to view themselves as having lower general efficacy, being more discouraged, being less able to predict, and having higher risk aversion. Moreover, predicted risk aversion was related to the factors of general efficacy, discouragement, and predictability.

In a second study, 101 adult psychiatric patients completed the Millon Clinical Multiaxial Inventory and the Decision Questionnaire. Dimensional scores (rather than categorical comparisons) were employed for the various personality disorders. The pessimistic portfolio style was utilized by individuals scoring higher on avoidant, dependent, and borderline personality disorders. The results for these diagnostic groups reflected perceptions of low current and future access to rewards; high information demands; quick stop-loss or quitting rules; and a greater likelihood of suffering negatives and having less enjoyment of gains.

The data on obsessive–compulsive personality disorder were revealing, in that they supported the view of individuals with this disorder as inhibited and cautious, but not as lacking in self-esteem. Especially interesting were the data on paranoid personality disorder, which suggested an underlying negative portfolio view of the self, low self-efficacy, greater discouragement, and caution about change. Persons with histrionic personality disorder reported a *preference* for risk, low frustration tolerance, and a tendency to quit early. Finally, the findings relevant to those with narcissistic personality disorder did not support the commonly held view that such individuals are masking low self-esteem, but rather indicated that they are afraid of making mistakes.

A CLOSER LOOK AT MYOPIA

Normative models of decision-making assume that individuals will consider longer-term utility in a hedonic calculus: "What are the longer-term costs and benefits?" As we have seen, calculation of utility ratios is confounded by the idiosyncratic meanings of psychological value for outcomes. There is considerable empirical and clinical evidence that individuals highly value shorter-term gains over longer-term gains, especially when the decision makers have experienced deprivation of rewards or are under considerable stress. Clinical manifestations of this "myopic" decision-making process include inability to delay gratification (Metcalfe & Mischel, 1999; Mischel, Shoda, & Rodriguez, 1989), binge-eating disorder, substance abuse, and excessive financial spending (Leahy, 2003; Orford, 2001). Indeed, one can view the overvaluation of shorter-term gains as marking a "contingency trap," such that these individuals consistently choose a short-term intense reward that has longer-term high costs, even when they know that the longer-term costs can be devastating. In these cases, the individuals get "trapped" by a contingency such as the following: "I feel bad → I can feel better immediately by using this substance → I choose this substance → I become addicted → I need more of this substance."

In my analysis of the contingency traps inherent in these self-defeating myopic choices, I have suggested that several factors maintain this vicious cycle (Leahy, 2003). Consider the model of a contingency trap presented in Figure 6.1. The earlier biological precursors are the evolutionary adapted strategies of seeking immediate gratification in a primitive environment: Primitive humans necessarily sought immediate rewards in an environment of scarcity, unpredictability, and danger. A strategy of seeking rewards involves cognitive assumptions such as "Get it now while the getting is good," or "Better to consume a reward now than to hope for a better day." An emotional diathesis toward myopia is that an individual feels deprived

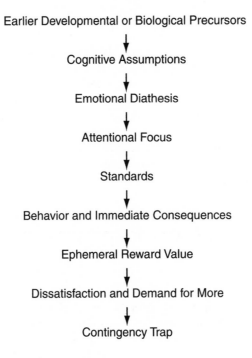

Earlier Developmental or Biological Precursors

Cognitive Assumptions

Emotional Diathesis

Attentional Focus

Standards

Behavior and Immediate Consequences

Ephemeral Reward Value

Dissatisfaction and Demand for More

Contingency Trap

FIGURE 6.1. A model of a contingency trap.

and desperate, and therefore seeks immediate reduction in distress or immediate gratification for a reward. The more exhilarating the reward—such as the use of food, alcohol, or drugs—the greater the tendency toward myopic choice. Attentional focus on myopic options is enhanced by an individual's prepotent drive level and arousal, as well as the relevance of the reward to immediate gratification (while alternative rewards, especially those that are not immediately present or that require waiting, are obscured). The standards that are used—for gratification or for reward value—may undermine the longer-term "satisfaction" of the reward; the reward does not measure up. Although, the reward provides immediate positive consequences (reduction of anxiety, distraction from psychic pain, pleasure), the "lasting" effect of this reward is ephemeral—it does not persist. Consequently, further attempts must be made to seek out more of the immediate gratification. This continued vicious cycle is a "contingency trap."

A contingency trap may be illustrated by the decision to use alcohol to reduce anxiety or to seek pleasure. A person with alcoholism may be genetically predisposed toward this problem and may be more responsive to the effects of alcohol on the brain. Assumptions about drinking and emotional states may include "I need to get rid of this bad feeling immediately," "It would be terrific to get high," and "My drinking doesn't harm anyone" (see Beck, Wright, Newman, & Liese, 1993). These facilitative and discounting assumptions, along with the emotional diathesis of anxiety and depression, then lead to attentional focus on alcohol as the sole source of reward, obscuring examination of the longer-term consequences and the alternative rewards available. The standard is to feel better immediately, leading to immediate positive rewards of drinking; however, drinking has only short-term effects, leading to greater demands for more alcohol, and thus resulting in a contingency trap.

BACKWARD-LOOKING DECISIONS

Sunk-Cost Effects

Normative models of decision making propose that individuals will only consider the future utility and costs of a particular decision, compared to those of the available alternatives. According to this model, individuals should ignore their past investments in a behavior or alternative, and should focus only on future payoffs. However, considerable research illustrates that people are seldom neutral about their past investments, and that they will utilize this past cost (or disutility) in determining their future course of action (Arkes & Ayton, 1999; Garland, 1990; Staw, 1976; Staw, Barsade, & Koput, 1997; Staw & Fox, 1977; Staw & Ross, 1978, 1987; Staw, Sandelands, & Dutton, 1981; Thaler, 1980, 1992). The "sunk-cost" effect is sometimes referred to as the "Concorde effect" in celebration of the supersonic jet that could never recover its costs, was operated as a deficit proposition, and recently took its last commercial flight. In "honoring" a sunk cost, the decision maker takes into consideration the prior costs as an *added reason* to continue in an endeavor that has already proven to be a failure. Thus real-life decisions are often "backward-looking" rather than prospective or "forward-looking."

Consider the following. You have purchased a jacket, paying "good money," and return home only to seclude the jacket in your closet of "lost clothes." You take the jacket out periodically but never actually wear it, since it does not seem right to you. Your partner disdainfully notices this garment that hangs in your closet for years, but you resist discarding it. You argue, "I paid good money for this, and eventually I will wear it." This jacket is a sunk cost—a past decision that has proven to be a failure, but a decision that you cannot finalize. You hope some day to find utility for this jacket, although years go by.

Another example of a sunk cost is reflected in the woman who has been involved with a married man named Roger for 5 years. She acknowledges that she is miserable in this relationship, and she tells her therapist that she knows that it is irrational to stay. However, she just can't bring herself to break away: She claims it would prove that she has wasted all that time, and that she has been a jerk to stay. Unlike a good decision maker, who will look for the first sign of a mistake to take action to escape from a trap, she looks at her mistake as a decision that she must redeem. Consequently, she uses the experience of 5 years in a no-win relationship as a rationale to stay even longer.

Sunk costs often involve an escalation of commitment to a failed pattern of decisions. Rather than thinking that "I don't want to throw good money after bad," the individual may claim, "I've invested too much to give up on this now." Ideally, in making a decision, people consider the future benefits that may be achieved by a course of action; that is, they consider the expected utility. For example, a woman who has already committed substantial behavior, at high cost, to a relationship that seems to be going nowhere might be expected to consider these costs as a "learning experience" and to anticipate further trouble ahead. Classical learning theories, guided by a reinforcement or extinction model, would imply that she will abandon the relationship, even if no other rewarding relationship is available. From the perspective of reinforcement theory, the reinforcements would be seen as diminishing as the costs increase. The woman's longer learning history in the relationship would predict even greater impetus to abandon the relationship. However, she resists abandoning the high-cost, long-history relationship. Individuals are not always guided by reinforcement history, nor are they easily convinced by cost–benefit analysis. Her current decision point—whether to continue or quit—is determined by her prior investment in the relationship.

Sunk-cost effects can be explained by commitment theory (Kiesler, Nisbett, & Zanna, 1969), cognitive dissonance theory (Festinger, 1957, 1961), prospect theory and loss frames (Kahneman & Tversky, 1979), fear-of-wasting theory (Arkes, 1996; Arkes & Blumer, 1985), attribution processes (e.g., (Davis, 1965; Kelley, 1967, 1973), and inaction inertia (Gilovich & Medvec, 1994; Gilovich, Medvec, & Chen, 1995). For example, commitment theory suggests that individuals will persist with a commitment to past actions, sometimes ignoring future utility ratios. Once a commitment is made, the reason for going forth is the commitment rather than the expected utility. Festinger's (1957, 1961) cognitive dissonance model suggests that prior losses precipitate a cognitive conflict, which can be resolved either by overvaluing the prior behavior or by increasing the hope that the sunk cost will be redeemed, and thereby will justify the past behavior. Thus the woman in the no-win relationship may view her prior commitments and costs as dissonant with her view of herself as someone who makes good decisions. She can reduce this dissonance by arguing that her beloved Roger possesses qualities only she can know and appreciate—or she may devalue other alternatives (e.g., all other available men).

Kahneman and Tversky's (1979) prospect theory suggests that individuals suffer losses more than they enjoy their gains and that changing from a sunk cost may be experienced as a loss. If the woman in our example views the change—that is, breaking off with Roger—as a loss (of Roger) rather than a gain (of freedom to pursue other relationships), then she will forgo other alternatives in order to maintain the commitment to Roger.

Fear-of-wasting theory suggests a strong, perhaps innate, motive to avoid wasting resources or behavior (Arkes, 1996; Arkes & Blumer, 1985). Thus, in our example, commitment to the sunk cost (Roger) avoids the recognition that this has been a waste of time, since the woman can take an "option" on hoping at some time to redeem the relationship and finally separate Roger from his wife. Attribution processes (or self-perception processes) may be reflected in how this woman perceives her own behavior. Viewing herself as paying a high cost for the relationship, she may conclude that a high investment must be due to a worthwhile cause. Finally, inaction inertia is based on the fact that there is asymmetrical regret for inaction and action; thus, in the short run, individuals regret taking new actions more than they do continuing in a course of inaction (Gilovich & Medvec, 1994). By continuing in the sunk cost, the woman avoids an increase of regret in the short run.

Individuals are more likely to continue in a course of behavior if the prior cost incurred has been greater (Arkes & Blumer, 1985; Garland, 1990). Thus, if the woman involved with Roger has suffered a great deal, she may utilize this suffering as a justification that the relationship is better than others believe it to be, in order to reduce the greater dissonance that she experiences. Making a change is based partly on the costs to be incurred relative to current "assets" or rewards available. If she views a change as having high cost relative to her existing "assets," she will continue longer in the behavior (Garland & Newport, 1991; Kahneman & Tversky, 1979). Thus as she stays in the bad relationship longer, and her self-esteem and access to alternative relationships decrease, she will expect that the cost of leaving will be high—and will be relatively higher in relationship to her diminishing resources. As a result of this, the sense of feeling demeaned reduces her current "assets" or resources, meaning that the costs of leaving are measured against a sinking position. Therefore, she will be more likely to stay, since she has little left to offset her losses if she should leave the relationship—a common pattern in abusive relationships (Dutton, 1999).

Ironically (but as expected from the foregoing models), research indicates that increasing the individual's sense of personal responsibility for the original action also increases the sunk-cost effect (Staw, 1976; Whyte, 1993), but that making the individual accountable to others for a decision decreases the sunk-cost effect (Simonson & Nye, 1992). As the woman in our example views herself as personally responsible for staying in the sunk-cost commitment, she experiences greater fear of wasting and greater dissonance; these motivate her to try harder to redeem the prior commitment, rather than to finally acknowledge failure. Diversion of responsibility to someone else—through modifying accountability and disattribution—can reverse the sunk-cost effect.

Modifying Sunk-Cost Effects

A clinician can effectively reverse the sunk-cost effect by doing the following (see Leahy, 2000, 2001b, 2003):

1. Explain the sunk-cost effect to the patient (the example of the purchased garment that hangs in the closet for years is completely understandable to almost everyone).
2. Help the patient examine the costs and benefits—for the immediate and distant future, separately—of continuing in the sunk cost.
3. Help the patient examine the opportunity costs of continuing in the sunk cost (what opportunities elsewhere are foreclosed?).
4. Separate the current decision to change from the past commitment to the sunk cost: "If you had not made the prior decision to commit to this behavior—and it was a new option now—would you commit to it? Why or why not?"
5. Ask, "What advice would you give someone else in this situation?"
6. Ask, "Are you concerned that abandoning the sunk cost means it was a total waste?" Perhaps the benefits outweighed the costs earlier, even though the costs outweigh the benefits now.

Individuals contemplating making a change from a sunk-cost commitment also often worry how other people will see this change: "My friends will think I was an idiot for staying, and now it's like saying that they are right and I was wrong." The patient can collect information on how his or her friends would view the new decision by canvassing them and asking them what their response will be. In addition, even if friends say, "I told you so," there is a benefit in taking good advice—even if it is late in being utilized. Indeed, what is so bad about friends' saying, "I told you so"? If the patient is now making the right decision, he or she can feel comfortable that the future is more likely to be better than the past.

Of particular interest in the sunk-cost effect is that the prior commitment may be related to the patient's personal schemas. For example, it is useful to ask patients whether there are certain sunk costs that are easier to abandon. In one case, an executive was quite adept at abandoning a sunk cost in his investments, but had greater difficulty abandoning a sunk cost in his relationship with his wife. On closer examination, it became apparent that recognizing that the relationship was not going to work activated his personal schema that he was unlovable and would never find a suitable partner. By utilizing the sunk-cost approach, he was also able to see that staying in a loveless relationship was "confirming" his belief that he was unlovable, thereby trapping him in a Catch-22: "If I leave, it means I'm unlovable, but if I stay, it means that I can't get the love that I want."

CONCLUSIONS

Cognitive models of psychopathology can be elaborated by drawing upon the vast literature on decision-making, choice, or investment strategies in order to better understand how mundane decision making can be affected by heuristics, biases, emotional arousal, and underlying assumptions of scarcity. Logical or rational models of normative decision making—first advanced by von Neuman and Morgenstern (1944)—assume that decision makers are sampling all of the data over long periods of time and are indifferent toward their past experiences or outcomes. However, the models I have examined here contend that few people make decisions in such a rational and dispassionate manner, and that understanding the "regularity" of the "anomalies" in decision making—that is, the consistent "pattern of errors"—can help us comprehend how depressed, anxious, manic, or otherwise distressed individuals make decisions.

If we therapists are able to discern these patterns of anomalies for such individuals, then we can intervene by identifying—with our patients—the heuristics or limits to rationality that guide them. For example, helping patients understand their commitment to sunk costs can help them extricate themselves from the limitations that have trapped them in the past. Or assisting bipolar individuals to understand their overly optimistic, manic theories of choice may help them avoid unnecessary risks. This integration of cognitive models of choice and schematic models of psychopathology can help guide us as therapists in counseling patients whose choices often seem "irrational"—but are guided by an internal and consistent logic of bounded rationality.

REFERENCES

Abramson, L. Y., Metalsky, G. I., & Alloy, L. B. (1989). Hopelessness depression: A theory-based subtype of depression. *Psychological Review, 96,* 358–372.

Abramson, L. Y., Seligman, M. E. P., & Teasdale, J. (1978). Learned helplessness in humans: Critique and reformulation. *Journal of Abnormal Psychology, 87,* 49–74.

Alloy, L. B., Abramson, L. Y., Metalsky, G. I., & Hartledge, S. (1988). The hopelessness theory of depression. *British Journal of Clinical Psychology, 27,* 5–12.

Alloy, L. B., Reilly-Harrington, N., Fresco, D. M., Whitehouse, W. G., & Zechmeister, J. S. (1999). Cognitive styles and life events in subsyndromal unipolar and bipolar disorders: Stability and prospective prediction of depressive and hypomanic mood swings. *Journal of Cognitive Psychotherapy, 13,* 21–40.

Arkes, H. R. (1996). The psychology of waste. *Journal of Behavioral Decision Making, 9*(3), 213–224.

Arkes, H. R., & Ayton, P. (1999). The sunk cost and Concorde effects: Are humans less rational than lower animals? *Psychological Bulletin, 125*(5), 591–600.

Arkes, H. R., & Blumer, C. (1985). The psychology of sunk cost. *Organizational Behavior and Human Decision Processes, 35,* 124–140.

Beck, A. T., Butler, A. C., Brown, G. K., Dahlsgaard, K. K., Newman, C. F., & Beck, J. S. (2001). Dysfunctional beliefs discriminate personality disorders. *Behaviour Research and Therapy, 39,* 1213–1225.

Beck, A. T., & Emery, G., with Greenberg, R. L. (1985). *Anxiety disorders and phobias: A cognitive perspective.* New York: Basic Books.

Beck, A. T., Freeman, A., Davis, D. D., & Associates. (2004). *Cognitive therapy of personality disorders* (2nd ed.). New York: Guilford Press.

Beck, A. T., Rush, A. J., Shaw, B. F., & Emery, G. (1979). *Cognitive therapy of depression.* New York: Guilford Press.

Beck, A. T., Wright, F. D., Newman, C. F., & Liese, B. S. (1993). *Cognitive therapy of substance abuse.* New York: Guilford Press.

Becker, G. S. (1976). *The economic approach to human behavior.* Chicago: University of Chicago Press.

Becker, G. S. (1991). *A treatise on the family.* Cambridge, MA: Harvard University Press.

Becker, G. S., Grossman, M., & Murphy, K. M. (1991). Rational addiction and the effect of price on consumption. *American Economic Review, 81,* 237–241.

Becker, G. S., & Murphy, K. M. (1988). A theory of rational addiction. *Journal of Political Economy, 96,* 675–700.

Breyer, S. (1993). *Breaking the vicious cycle: Toward effective risk calculations.* Cambridge, MA: Harvard University Press.

Butler, A. C., Brown, G. K., Beck, A. T., & Grisham, J. R. (2002). Assessment of dysfunctional beliefs in borderline personality disorder. *Behavioural Research and Therapy, 40*(10), 1231–1240.

Clark, D. A., & Beck, A. T., with Alford, B. A. (1999). *Scientific foundations of cognitive theory and therapy of depression.* New York: Wiley.

Davis, K. E. (1965). From acts to dispositions: The attribution process in person perception. In L. Berkowitz (Ed.), *Advances in experimental social psychology* (Vol. 2, pp. 219–266). New York: Academic Press.

Dugas, M. J., Buhr, K., & Ladouceur, R. (2004). The role of intolerance of uncertainty in the etiology and maintenance of generalized anxiety disorder. In R. G. Heimberg, C. L. Turk, & D. S. Mennin (Eds.), *Generalized anxiety disorder: Advances in research and practice* (pp. 143–163). New York: Guilford Press.

Dutton, D. G. (1999). Limitations of social learning models in explaining intimate aggression. In X. B. Arriaga & S. Oskamp (Eds.), *Violence in intimate relationships* (pp. 73–87). Thousand Oaks, CA: Sage.

Dweck, C. S. (1975). The role of expectations and attributions in the alleviation of learned helplessness. *Journal of Personality and Social Psychology, 31,* 674–685.

Dweck, C. S. (1986). Motivational processes affecting learning. *American Psychologist, 41,* 1040–1048.

Dweck, C. S., Davidson, W., Nelson, S., & Enna, B. (1978). Sex differences in learned helplessness: II. The contingencies of evaluative feedback in the classroom. III. An experimental analysis. *Developmental Psychology, 14,* 268–276.

Eisenberger, R. (1992). Learned industriousness. *Psychological Review, 99*(2), 248–267.

Festinger, L. (1957). *A theory of cognitive dissonance.* Stanford, CA: Stanford University Press.

Festinger, L. (1961). The psychological effects of insufficient rewards. *American Psychologist, 16,* 1–11.

Finucane, M., Alhakami, A., Slovic, P., & Johnson, S. (2000). The affect heuristic in judgments of risks and benefits. *Journal of Behavioral Decision Making, 13,* 1–13.

Garland, H. (1990). Throwing good money after bad: The effect of sunk costs on the decision to esculate commitment to an ongoing project. *Journal of Applied Psychology, 75*(6), 728–731.

Garland, H., & Newport, S. (1991). Effects of absolute and relative sunk costs on the decision to persist with a course of action. *Organizational Behavior and Human Decision Processes, 48*(1), 55–69.

Gilovich, T., & Medvec, V. H. (1994). The temporal pattern to the experience of regret. *Journal of Personality and Social Psychology, 67*(3), 357–365.

Gilovich, T., Medvec, V. H., & Chen, S. (1995). Commission, omission, and dissonance reduction: Coping with regret in the "Monty Hall" problem. *Personality and Social Psychology Bulletin, 21*(2), 182–190.

Ingram, R. E., Miranda, J., & Segal, Z. V. (1998). *Cognitive vulnerability to depression.* New York: Guilford Press.

Kahneman, D. (1995). Varieties of counterfactual thinking. In N. J. Roese & J. J. Olson (Eds.), *What might have been: The social psychology of counterfactual thinking* (pp. 375–396). Mahwah, NJ: Erlbaum.

Kahneman, D., & Tversky, A. (1979). Prospect theory: An analysis of decision under risk. *Econometrica, 47,* 263–291.

Kelley, H. H. (1967). Attribution theory in social psychology. *Nebraska Symposium on Motivation, 15,* 192–238.

Kelley, H. H. (1973). The processes of causal attribution. *American Psychologist, 28*(2), 107–128.

Kiesler, C. A., Nisbett, R. E., & Zanna, M. P. (1969). On inferring one's beliefs from one's behavior. *Journal of Personality and Social Psychology, 11*(4), 321–327.

Leahy, R. L. (1997). An investment model of depressive resistance. *Journal of Cognitive Psychotherapy: An International Quarterly, 11*, 3–19.

Leahy, R. L. (1999). Decision making and mania. *Journal of Cognitive Psychotherapy: An International Quarterly, 13*, 83–105.

Leahy, R. L. (2000). Sunk costs and resistance to change. *Journal of Cognitive Psychotherapy: An International Quarterly, 14*(4), 355–371.

Leahy, R. L. (2001a). Depressive decision making: Validation of the portfolio theory model. *Journal of Cognitive Psychotherapy: An International Quarterly, 15*, 341–362.

Leahy, R. L. (2001b). *Overcoming resistance in cognitive therapy.* New York: Guilford Press.

Leahy, R. L. (2003). *Psychology and the economic mind: Cognitive processes and conceptualization.* New York: Springer.

Markowitz, H. (1952). Portfolio selection. *Journal of Finance, 7*, 77–91.

Metcalfe, J., & Mischel, W. (1999). A hot/cool-system analysis of delay of gratification dynamics of willpower. *Psychological Review, 106*(1), 3–19.

Mischel, W., Shoda, Y., & Rodriguez, M. L. (1989). Delay of gratification in children. *Science, 244*, 933–988.

Orford, J. (2001). *Excessive appetites: A psychological view of addictions.* Chichester, UK: Wiley.

Purdon, C., & Clark, D. A. (1993). Obsessive intrusive thoughts in nonclinical subjects: I. Content and relation with depressive, anxious and obsessional symptoms. *Behaviour Research and Therapy, 31*(8), 713–720.

Simon, H. A. (1979). Rational decision making in business organizations. *American Economic Review, 69*, 493–513.

Simon, H. A. (1983). *Reason in human affairs.* Stanford, CA: Stanford University Press.

Simonson, I., & Nye, P. (1992). The effect of accountability on susceptibility to decision errors. *Organizational Behavior and Human Decision Processes, 51*(3), 416–446.

Slovic, P. (Ed.). (2000). *The perception of risk.* Sterling, VA: Earthscan.

Staw, B. M. (1976). Knee-deep in the Big Muddy: A study of escalating commitment to a chosen course of action. *Organizational Behavior and Human Decision Processes, 16*(1), 27–44.

Staw, B. M., Barsade, S. G., & Koput, K. W. (1997). Escalation at the credit window: A longitudinal study of bank executives' recognition and write-off of problem loans. *Journal of Applied Psychology, 82*(1), 130–142.

Staw, B. M., & Fox, F. V. (1977). Escalation: The determinants of commitment to a chosen course of action. *Human Relations, 30*(5), 431–450.

Staw, B. M., & Ross, J. (1978). Commitment to a policy decision: A multi-theoretical perspective. *Administrative Science Quarterly, 23*(1), 40–64.

Staw, B. M., & Ross, J. (1987). Behavior in escalation situations: Antecedents, prototypes, and solutions. *Research in Organizational Behavior, 9*, 39–78.

Staw, B. M., Sandelands, L. E., & Dutton, J. E. (1981). Threat-rigidity effects in organizational behavior: A multilevel analysis. *Administrative Science Quarterly*, 26(4), 501–524.

Stopa, L., & Clark, D. M. (1993). Cognitive processes in social phobia. *Behaviour Research and Therapy*, 31(3), 255–267.

Sunstein, C. R. (Ed.). (2000). *Behavioural law and economics*. Cambridge, UK: Cambridge University Press.

Thaler, R. (1980). Toward a positive theory of consumer choice. *Journal of Economic Behavior and Organization*, 1, 39–60.

Thaler, R. (1992). *The winner's curse: Paradoxes and anomalies of economic life*. Princeton, NJ: Princeton University Press.

Tversky, A., & Kahneman, D. (1974). Judgment under uncertainty: Heuristics and biases. *Science*, 185(4157), 1124–1131.

von Neumann, J., & Morgenstern, O. (1944). *Theory of games and economic behavior*. Princeton, NJ: Princeton University Press.

Weiner, B., Nierenberg, R., & Goldstein, M. (1976). Social learning (locus of control) versus attributional (causal stability) interpretations of expectancy of success. *Journal of Personality*, 44(1), 52–68.

Wells, A. (1995). Meta-cognition and worry: A cognitive model of generalized anxiety disorder. *Behavioural and Cognitive Psychotherapy*, 23, 301–320.

Whyte, G. (1993). Escalating commitment in individual and group decision making: A prospect theory approach. *Organizational Behavior and Human Decision Processes*, 54(3), 430–455.

Winton, E. C., Clark, D. M., & Edelmann, R. J. (1995). Social anxiety, fear of negative evaluation and the detection of negative emotion in others. *Behaviour Research and Therapy*, 33, 193–196.

Young, J. E., Klosko, J. S., & Weishaar, M. E. (2003). *Schema therapy: A practitioner's guide*. New York: Guilford Press.

Part III

ANXIETY, MOOD, AND OTHER AXIS I DISORDERS

Chapter 7

Posttraumatic Stress Disorder

From Cognitive Theory to Therapy

DAVID M. CLARK
ANKE EHLERS

Posttraumatic stress disorder (PTSD) is a well recognized reaction to traumatic events, such as assault, disasters, and severe accidents. The symptoms include involuntary reexperiencing of aspects of the event, hyperarousal, emotional numbing, and avoidance of stimuli that could serve as reminders of the event. Many people experience at least some of these symptoms in the immediate aftermath of a traumatic event. A large proportion recover in the ensuing months or years, but in a significant subgroup the symptoms persist, often for many years (Ehlers, Mayou, & Bryant, 1998; Rothbaum, Foa, Riggs, Murdock, & Walsh, 1992; Kessler, Sonnega, Bromet, Hughes, & Nelson, 1995). This raises the question of why PTSD persists in some individuals and how the condition can be treated. The present chapter overviews our group's cognitive approach to these questions.

AARON T. BECK

It is fitting that the overview appears in a volume honoring the enormous achievements of Aaron T. Beck, the founder of cognitive therapy and an unparalleled exponent of cognitive approaches to psychopathology. In his early writing on depression, Beck developed a particular approach to the psychological understanding and treatment of emotional disorders. Following astute clinical observation, he proposed a theory of the maintenance of depression in which cognitive processes play a central role, in interaction with behavioral responses that are driven by the cognitive abnormalities. An elegant set of studies substantiated and refined the theory. A cognitive therapy program that specifically focused on the therapeutic targets specified in the theory was developed and rigorously evaluated in randomized controlled trials. As the reader will see, we have adopted the same general approach as that pioneered by Beck. However, our debt extends much further. Aaron T. Beck has been a close friend and mentor for many years. We have greatly benefited from his innovative thinking, incisive criticism, endless enthusiasm, and generosity of spirit.

A COGNITIVE MODEL OF PERSISTENT PTSD

Elsewhere, we (Ehlers & Clark, 2000) have suggested that persistent PTSD occurs only if individuals process the traumatic experience in a way that produces a sense of a serious current threat. Once activated, the perception of current threat is accompanied by intrusions and other reexperiencing symptoms; symptoms of arousal; and strong emotions, such as anxiety, anger, shame or sadness. The model, which is illustrated in Figure 7.1, proposes that two key processes lead to a sense of current threat.

First, it is suggested that individual differences in the personal meaning (appraisal) of the trauma *and/or* its sequelae determine whether persistent PTSD develops. Some people are able to see the trauma as a time-limited terrible experience that does not necessarily have threatening implications for their future. These people are likely to recover quickly. Individuals with persistent PTSD are characterized by excessively negative appraisals of the event and/or its sequelae. (See Table 7.1 for examples of such appraisals.)

Second, it is suggested that the trauma memory in people with PTSD differs from other autobiographical memories in a problematic manner. Autobiographical memories are normally organized and elaborated in a way that facilitates intentional retrieval and inhibits cue-driven[1] reexperiencing of an event. The intentional recall of an autobiographical event contains both specific information about the event itself and context information, and is characterized by "autonoetic awareness" (the sense or experience of the self in the past) (Conway, 1997; Tulving, 2002). We (Ehlers & Clark, 2000) propose that trauma memories do not have this

---

[1] "Cue-driven" reexperiencing is the triggering of an aspect of a trauma memory by a stimulus that matches a stimulus that was present at the time of the trauma. Triggering stimuli include low-level physical aspects, such as color, sound, movement, shape, and proprioceptive information.

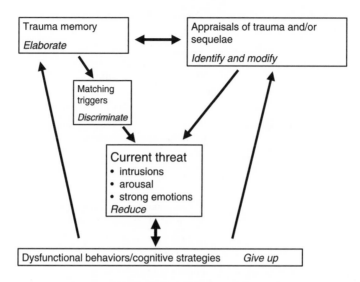

FIGURE 7.1. A cognitive model of PTSD and the treatment goals (in *italics*) that follow from the model. Adapted from Ehlers and Clark (2000, p. 321). Copyright 2000 by Elsevier. Adapted by permission.

level of organization and elaboration (see also Ehlers, Hackmann, & Michael, in press, for details). The series of experiences during a traumatic event are inadequately integrated into their context (both within the event, and within the context of previous and subsequent experiences/information). This has the effect that the resulting intentional recall is disjointed; for example, some elements of the event may be recalled out of sequence, and when distressing elements are recalled, it may be difficult for the individual to access later information that corrected impressions the person had or predictions he or she made at the time. For example, a man who thought during an assault that he would never see his children again was not able (while recalling this particularly distressing moment) to access the fact that he still lived with his children.

Furthermore, the poor organization and elaboration leads to poor inhibition of cue-driven retrieval of elements of the trauma memory. In addition, perceptual priming (reduced threshold for perception) for stimuli that occurred at the time of the traumatic event, and strong associative links between these stimuli, further enhance the probability of cue-driven retrieval. By classical conditioning, the stimuli are also associated with strong affective responses. Thus, when the traumatized person encounters cues that bear resemblance to those occurring shortly before or during the particularly distressing moments of the traumatic event, cue-driven retrieval leads to distressing reexperiencing of elements of the event. The reexperiencing

TABLE 7.1. Examples of Idiosyncratic Negative Appraisals Leading to Sense of Current Threat in Persistent PTSD

What is appraised?	Negative appraisals
Fact that trauma happened	"Nowhere is safe," "The next disaster will strike soon."
Trauma happened to me	"I attract disaster," "Others can see that I am a victim."
Behavior/emotions during trauma	"I deserve that bad things happen to me," "I cannot cope with stress."
Initial PTSD symptoms	
Irritability, anger outbursts	"My personality has changed for the worse," "My marriage will break up."
Emotional numbing	"I'm dead inside," "I'll never be able to relate to people again."
Flashbacks, intrusive recollections, and nightmares	"I'm going mad," "I'll never get over this."
Difficulty concentrating	"My brain has been damaged," "I'll lose my job."
Other people's reactions after trauma	
Positive responses	"They think I am too weak to cope on my own," "I am unable to feel close to anyone."
Negative responses	"Nobody is there for me," "I cannot rely on other people."
Other consequences of trauma	
Physical consequences	"My body is ruined," "I will never be able to lead a normal life again."
Loss of job, money, etc.	"I will lose my children," "I will be homeless."

Note. Adapted from Ehlers and Clark (2000, p. 322). Copyright 2000 by Elsevier. Adapted by permission.

lacks autonoetic awareness, and the threat that the person experienced during these moments is reexperienced as if it was happening right now rather than being a memory from the past. This includes a phenomenon that we have termed "affect without recollection" (Ehlers & Clark, 2000). For example, a patient with PTSD who had experienced a severe car accident reported that he became extremely anxious and felt something terrible was going to happen during a train journey. At the time, he was not able to put his finger on what triggered the anxiety. Only afterwards, he realized that he had heard a baby cry shortly before he became anxious. The pitch of the baby's voice was the same as that of the sound of the impact during his accident. At the time he became anxious on the train, he was not aware of this link and did not recall the accident.

Why do the negative appraisals and the problematic nature of trauma memory persist? It is proposed that the negative appraisals and emotions prompt a series of dysfunctional cognitive and behavioral responses that have the short-term aim of reducing distress, but have the long-term consequence of preventing cognitive change and therefore maintain the disorder. We (Ehlers & Clark, 2000) propose that these behaviors and cognitive strategies maintain PTSD in three ways. First, some behaviors directly lead to increases in symptoms; for example, thought suppression leads to paradoxical increases in intrusion frequency. Second, other behaviors prevent changes in the problematic appraisals; for instance, constantly checking one's rear-view mirror (a safety behavior) after a car accident prevents change in the appraisal that another accident will happen if one does not check the mirror. Third, other behaviors prevent elaboration of the trauma memory and its link to other experiences. For example, avoiding thinking about the event prevents people from incorporating the fact that they did not die into the trauma memory, and they thus continue to reexperience the fear of dying they originally experienced during the event.

EMPIRICAL STATUS OF THE
EHLERS AND CLARK MODEL

Studies that are relevant to the evaluation of components of our (Ehlers & Clark, 2000) cognitive model of PTSD are summarized below.

Negative Appraisals of the Traumatic Event and/or Its Sequelae

Effect of Trauma on Beliefs about the Self and the World

A traumatic event threatens the persons' view of themselves and their world. Several theorists have proposed that change in basic beliefs about self and world is at the core of PTSD, or of responses to trauma in general (e.g., Ehlers & Clark, 2000; Foa & Riggs, 1993; Janoff-Bulman, 1992; Horowitz, 1976; Resick & Schnicke, 1993). For example, Janoff-Bulman (1992) has proposed that traumatic events "shatter" previously held beliefs (e.g., "The world is a safe place"), and that posttrauma adjustment requires rebuilding of basic beliefs about the self and the world. Foa and Riggs (1993) and Resick and Schnicke (1993) have pointed out that PTSD is quite often associated with a *confirmation* of previously held negative beliefs rather than a shattering of positive beliefs (e.g., "Bad things always happen to me"), and that recovery requires the modification of these beliefs. Several studies have found empirical evidence for a relationship between PTSD and negative beliefs concerning the self and the world (Ali, Dunmore, Clark, & Ehlers, 2002; Dunmore, Clark, & Ehlers, 1997, 1999; Foa, Ehlers, Clark, Tolin, & Orsillo, 1999; Resick, Schnicke, & Markway, 1991; Wenninger & Ehlers, 1998). In addition, in a prospective study of assault survivors, negative beliefs about the self and one's world predicted the subsequent persistence of PTSD (Dunmore, Clark, & Ehlers, 2001).

Appraisals of Trauma Sequelae

Appraisals of trauma sequelae have been a particular research interest of our group. We have assumed that the power of appraisal processes in predicting persistent PTSD can be enhanced if trauma sequelae are included.

Appraisal of PTSD Symptoms. Ehlers and Steil (1995) have observed that people differ widely in the meaning they assign to the occurrence and content of intrusive recollections of traumatic events. Whereas many individuals see them as a normal part of recovery from an upsetting event, others interpret them in a more negative way—for example, as an indication that they are going crazy. Ehlers and Steil (1995) proposed that such negative interpretations are important in explaining the maintenance of intrusive recollections and PTSD in general, because they determine (1) how distressing the intrusions are; and (2) the extent to which a patient engages in strategies to control the intrusions, which then prevent change in the meaning of the trauma and posttraumatic intrusions. They provided evidence for these hypotheses in correlational studies of road traffic accident (RTA) survivors (Steil & Ehlers, 2000) and of ambulance workers (Clohessy & Ehlers, 1999), and in a large-scale prospective longitudinal study of 967 RTA survivors (Ehlers, Mayou, & Bryant, 1998). The latter study found that negative interpretations of intrusive memories 3 months after the accident predicted PTSD severity at 1 year, even after PTSD severity at 3 months was controlled for. Overall, early negative interpretation of symptoms was one of the most important predictors of PTSD at 1 year. Similar findings were obtained in a prospective study of children involved in RTAs (Ehlers, Mayou, & Bryant, 2003).

People with persistent PTSD interpret not only intrusive memories in a negative way, but also other PTSD symptoms such as irritability (e.g., "I will lose control and harm somebody"), poor concentration (e.g., "I must have a brain injury"), or emotional numbing (e.g., "Feeling numb means that I will never have normal emotions again"). In a concurrent correlation study that we conducted in collaboration with Foa's group in Philadelphia, negative interpretation of PTSD symptoms distinguished between trauma survivors (many of whom had experienced accidents) with and without PTSD (Foa et al., 1999). In a series of prospective studies, we have found that negative interpretation of a range of initial PTSD symptoms predicts subsequent PTSD severity in adults after physical and sexual assaults (Dunmore et al., 2001; Halligan, Michael, Clark, & Ehlers, 2003).

Appraisal of Other People's Responses. Many people with persistent PTSD consider that other people responded to them in a negative way after the traumatic event or were less supportive than expected. For example, an assault survivor was very distressed because she had felt that the hospital staff had been uncaring and had left her alone for long periods while she was in the hospital. She interpreted her hospital experience as meaning that "Nobody is there for me." Sometimes, well-meant or otherwise positive behaviors can also be interpreted by the traumatized individual in a negative way. For example, another trauma survivor interpreted her friend's offer to help her after the accident as meaning that the friend thought she was unable to cope on her own. Several studies have shown that negative appraisals of others' responses are related to PTSD and predict its persistence (Andrews, Brewin, & Rose, 2003; Dunmore et al., 1997, 1999, 2001).

Perceived negative responses of other people or a perceived inability to relate to others after trauma can give rise to an overall feeling of alienation from others. We have found that an overall feeling of alienation impedes recovery in survivors of rape and of torture (Ehlers, Clark, Dunmore, et al., 1998; Ehlers, Maercker, & Boos, 2000). Furthermore, alienation is related to PTSD in survivors of different traumas (Foa et al., 1999).

Perceived Permanent Change. Traumatic events can have long-term negative consequences. For example, many trauma survivors suffer long-term physical problems, such as pain and financial hardship. Persistent health problems were among the most important predictors of persistent PTSD after RTAs (Blanchard et al., 1996; Ehlers, Mayou, & Bryant, 1998; Mayou, Bryant, & Duthie, 1993; Mayou, Tindel, & Bryant, 1997), and were more important in predicting persistent PTSD than injury severity was.

Some traumatized individuals interpret such long-standing physical problems as meaning that their lives have permanently changed for the worse. Others interpret their initial reactions to the trauma, including the initial PTSD symptoms, as indicating a permanent negative change in their personality. Several studies have shown that perceived permanent change predicts PTSD severity in survivors of RTA, assault, rape, and torture (Dunmore et al., 1997, 1999, 2001; Foa et al., 1999; Ehlers et al., 2000).

Nature of the Trauma Memory

Poor Organization and Elaboration

In line with the proposed deficit in organization and elaboration of trauma memories in PTSD (Ehlers & Clark, 2000), preliminary studies have found that the *intentional* recall of traumatic events in PTSD is relatively poorly organized and lacks coherence (e.g., Amir, Stafford, Freshman, & Foa, 1998; Halligan et al., 2003; Harvey & Bryant, 1999; Koss, Figueredo, Bell, Tharan, & Tromp, 1996). With treatment, trauma narratives become more organized (Foa, Molnar, & Cashman, 1995; van der Minnen, 2002). In two naturalistic prospective studies, initial disorganization of trauma narratives predicted subsequent PTSD in survivors of RTAs (Murray, Ehlers, & Mayou, 2002) and assaults (Halligan et al., 2003). Further systematic observations suggest that patients with PTSD may have difficulty in accessing details that are important for the interpretation of the event (although the overall number of details recalled may not be different from other autobiographical memories), and that patients often have difficulty recollecting the exact temporal order of events during the trauma (Ehlers, Hackmann, & Michael, in press).

Lack of Context and Time Perspective

In line with the features of unintentional trauma memories highlighted in the Ehlers and Clark (2000) model, a prospective study of assault survivors found that the lack of time perspective (operationalized by the degree to which the intrusion was experienced as something happening "now") and lack of context of intrusive memories (operationalized by the degree to which the intrusive memory was experienced as isolated and disconnected to what happened before and afterward) predicted more variance of subsequent PTSD severity than initial intrusion frequency did (Michael, 2000).

Perceptual Priming

In a preliminary test of the proposed role of perceptual priming in the triggering of unwanted trauma memories (Ehlers & Clark, 2000), Ehlers, Michael, and Chen (2004) presented volunteers with a sequence of three pictures that made up a story. The initial pictures were neutral, and the last picture showed either a traumatic or a neutral outcome of the story. In a trauma sequence, the first picture showed a woman standing by a table with a drinking glass and a table lamp. The next picture showed a man's hands holding a bathrobe cord, and the final picture showed the woman strangled. In a parallel neutral sequence, the first picture was rather similar, but the final picture showed a woman looking thoughtful after making a telephone call. Following presentation of the "picture stories," memory for objects shown in the initial pictures was assessed in two different ways. First, in order to assess perceptual priming, participants were presented with blurred objects and asked to identify them. Some of the objects had been presented in the "stories," and others had not. Perceptual priming would be evidenced by better identification of the objects that had been presented. Second, explicit memory was assessed by asking participants to recognize nonblurred objects from the story pictures within a set of similar distractor objects. There were no differences in recognition memory between objects from the traumatic and nontraumatic stories. However, as predicted, perceptual priming was better for the objects shown in the trauma stories. To assess whether enhanced perceptual priming might be linked to subsequent PTSD-like intrusions, participants in the experiment were followed up after 4 months and asked whether they had any unwanted intrusive memories of the material that had been presented within the experiment. As predicted, there was a significant positive association between perceptual priming for objects from traumatic stories and the presence of subsequent intrusions.

The promising preliminary results obtained in this analogue experiment study have recently been extended in a clinical study (Michael, Ehlers, & Halligan, 2003). Priming for trauma-related material distinguished between assault survivors with and without PTSD, and predicted subsequent PTSD symptoms.

Encoding during Trauma

A series of studies addressed the question of what aspects of cognitive processing during the trauma contribute to subsequent reexperiencing symptoms. Several authors have suggested that dissociation during the trauma affects the way the trauma is laid down in memory, and therefore predicts subsequent reexperiencing symptoms (Brewin, Dalgleish, & Joseph, 1996; Ehlers & Clark, 2000; Foa & Hearst-Ikeda, 1996; van der Kolk & Fisler, 1995). Several prospective longitudinal studies of RTA and assault survivors have found that dissociation during and shortly after a traumatic event predicts subsequent PTSD (Ehlers, Mayou, & Bryant, 1998; Halligan et al., 2003; Rosario, Ehlers, Williams, & Glucksman, 2004; Murray et al., 2002; Shalev, Peri, Canetti, & Schreiber, 1996). Dissociation is defined as a "disruption of the usually integrated functions of consciousness, memory, identity, or perception of the environment" (American Psychiatric Association, 1994, p. 477). As the definition suggests, dissociation is a complex process that has several components—for instance, feelings of derealization and depersonalization, emotional numbing, and distorted time perception. We (Ehlers & Clark, 2000) have linked the concept of dissociation to findings from experimental psychology and suggested that dissociation partly overlaps with two aspects of cognitive processing that have been shown to influence memory: lack of self-referent processing and data-driven (as opposed to conceptual) processing. The studies of Halligan et al. (2003) and Rosario et al. (2004) have supported this hypothesis.

Behaviors and Cognitive Responses That Maintain PTSD

It is well known from research on phobias that *avoidance behavior* maintains anxiety disorders. Several studies have demonstrated that avoidance also plays a crucial role in maintaining PTSD (e.g., Bryant & Harvey, 1995; Dunmore et al., 1998, 2001). Avoidance includes both situational avoidance (e.g., of places, people, conversations, and other stimuli that remind the individual of the trauma) and cognitive avoidance (i.e., efforts not to think about the trauma). Situational avoidance is not restricted to avoidance of reminders of the traumatic event. People who have perceived negative responses from others in the aftermath of the event, or those who feel that other people will not understand their response to the trauma, often withdraw from a wide range of social situations. This has several negative effects: They are less likely to receive social support, to correct negative beliefs about themselves and others, and to benefit from the therapeutic effects of talking about their emotions with others (e.g., Pennebaker, 1989), and thus contributes to the maintenance of PTSD.

Even if there is no obvious situational avoidance, people with PTSD commonly show subtle avoidance behaviors ("safety behaviors") that prevent change of problematic appraisals and maintain anxiety. For example, a survivor of an RTA, who had been trapped in her car after the accident because her seat belt could not be opened, kept checking whether her seat belts were still functioning. This prevented her from testing the appraisal "If I do not check my seat belt, I will be trapped again." Other common safety behaviors in RTA survivors include driving very slowly, stepping on the brakes repeatedly, checking the mirrors repeatedly, or holding onto the seat. In assault survivors, typical examples include checking whether all doors and windows are locked, sleeping with the lights on, or carrying a weapon. In line with their hypothesized role in maintaining PTSD, safety behaviors predicted persistent PTSD in a prospective longitudinal study of assault survivors (Dunmore et al., 2001).

Several authors have pointed that maintenance of PTSD cannot be solely explained by avoidance, and have suggested that cognitive responses play a crucial role (e.g., Ehlers & Steil, 1995; Foa & Riggs, 1993; Horowitz, 1976).

Research on the effects of *thought suppression* (e.g., Wegner, 1989) suggests that efforts to suppress memories of the traumatic event may increase their frequency (Ehlers & Steil, 1995). Two retrospective studies of RTA survivors and a retrospective study of ambulance workers (Steil & Ehlers, 2000; Clohessy & Ehlers, 1999) found that suppression of memories of the traumatic event was related to PTSD. This finding was subsequently confirmed in prospective longitudinal studies with RTA survivors. Early suppression of memories predicted later PTSD severity in adults (Ehlers, Mayou, & Bryant, 1998) and in children (Ehlers, Mayou, & Bryant, 2003). Furthermore, recent experimental studies have demonstrated that thought suppression increases the frequency of trauma-related intrusions in RTA and rape survivors (Harvey & Bryant, 1998; Shepherd & Beck, 1999), and in volunteers who had seen a traumatic film (Davies & Clark, 1998).

People with PTSD commonly *ruminate* about aspects of the traumatic event and its sequelae (e.g., "If *only* the accident had not happened or I had done something differently," or "Why did it happen to me?"). Rumination appears to play a role in maintaining PTSD. Steil and Ehlers (2000) and Clohessy and Ehlers (1999) showed that rumination about intrusive memories was correlated with PTSD severity in RTA survivors and ambulance workers. Warda and Bryant (1998) showed that rumination distinguished between RTA survivors with and without acute stress disorder, a precursor of PTSD. In several prospective studies of RTA survivors, rumination was one of the most important predictors of PTSD, and of delayed onset of PTSD (Ehlers, Mayou, & Bryant, 1998, 2003; Murray et al., 2002). At this stage, the mechanism by which rumination maintains PTSD is unclear. Rumination probably strengthens problematic appraisals of the trauma (e.g., "The trauma has ruined my life"); it is also probably similar to cognitive avoidance in interfering with the formation of a more organized and elaborated trauma memory, because it focuses on "What if ... " questions rather than on the experience of the trauma itself. Finally, rumination is likely to directly increase feelings of nervous tension, dysphoria, or hopelessness, and cue the retrieval of intrusive memories of the traumatic event.

Attentional deployment is likely to contribute to the maintenance of PTSD. Patients with PTSD have an attentional bias to stimuli that are reminiscent of the traumatic event (see McNally, 1999, for a review). Selective attention to reminders is likely to enhance the frequency of reexperiencing symptoms.

Dissociation is another, and as yet poorly understood, cognitive process that interferes with recovery in PTSD. Most studies of dissociation have focused on dissociation during and immediately after the trauma. However, persistent dissociation may actually be more predictive of chronic PTSD. Continuing dissociation in response to intrusive memories was a predictor of persistence of PTSD in prospective studies of RTA and assault survivors (Halligan et al., 2003; Murray et al., 2002).

A THEORY-DERIVED COGNITIVE THERAPY

The studies reviewed in the preceding section have provided encouraging initial support for the Ehlers and Clark (2000) model. In this section, we focus on the therapeutic implications of the model and describe the cognitive therapy program that our group has developed on the basis of the model. The Ehlers and Clark (2000) model specifies three therapy goals, which are identified by italics in Figure 7.1.

Goal 1: Reduce Reexperiencing by Elaboration of the Trauma Memory and Discrimination of Triggers

The aim in elaborating the trauma memory is to help the patient develop a coherent narrative account—one that starts before the trauma begins; ends after the patient is safe again; and places the series of events during the trauma in between in context, in sequence, and in the past. Three main techniques are used: writing out a detailed account of the event, imaginal reliving of the event, and revisiting the scene. Each has advantages. Writing is particularly useful when aspects of what happened and how it happened are unclear. Reconstructing the event with diagrams and models can be of further assistance in such instances. Imaginal reliving, in which the patient vividly images the event while simultaneously describing what is happening and what he or she is feeling and thinking, is particularly good at eliciting all aspects of the memory (including emotions and sensory components) and can therefore be very helpful in linking elements together and placing them in context. Revisiting the scene is a particularly helpful way of putting a time code into the memory (and hence reducing the sense of "nowness" that characterizes intrusions), because, with the therapist's guidance, the patient can clearly see that the event is no longer happening; it is in the past and the scene has moved on/changed. Revisiting the scene can also provide new information that helps explain why or how an event occurred.

Discrimination of triggers usually involves two stages. First, careful analysis of where and when intrusions occur is used to identify triggers. Second, the link between the triggers and the trauma memory is intentionally broken. For example, a man who had been involved in an RTA at night experienced frequent intrusions; these sometimes consisted of just reexperiencing the terror he had felt as he saw that a van was about to plow into the back of his vehicle, and sometimes also included images from the crash. He was under the impression that the intrusions came on "out of the blue." A prominent aspect of the trauma memory was the headlights of the van, and it soon became clear that the intrusions were often triggered by patches of bright light (such as a patch of sunlight on a lawn or an overhead projector at work). Once this became clear, the patient discriminated between "then" and "now" when the intrusion occurred by telling himself that he was reacting to a past meaning of the light. This point was strengthening by intentionally provoking the memory with bright lights and then behaving in ways that he could not have done at the time (e.g., standing up and moving about).

Goal 2: Modify Excessively Negative Appraisals

Excessively negative appraisals of the traumatic event are identified by careful questioning, particularly about the meaning of "hot spots" (moments of greatest distress in the memory). Hot spots are often identified by examining the content of intrusions and by a probe reliving. Standard verbal cognitive therapy techniques are then used to modify the negative appraisals. Once an alternative appraisal that the patient finds compelling has been identified, the new appraisal is incorporated into the trauma memory, either by adding it to the written account or by inserting it into a subsequent imaginal reliving. For example, a woman who had been raped identified the moment when her assailant said, "I can't do this looking at your ugly face," as the worst hot spot. The moment was her most common intrusion. In addition, since the rape she had felt unattractive and had engaged in casual sex in an apparent attempt to convince herself that she was attractive. Socratic questioning was used to identify an alternative appraisal, which was that the rapist had identified her because she was attractive, and had made his comment because he was unable to become aroused without abusing and humiliating women. During a subsequent reliving, she introduced the new appraisal into the hot spot by saying it to the rapist at the moment that he verbally abused her.

Imagery transformation techniques can be a useful way of getting new, less threatening information to stick. For example, a woman whose car had crashed into a brick pillar was haunted by intrusions in which the pillar flew to within a few inches of her face. Discussion and measuring the distance between her seat and the crumpled front of her vehicle established that in reality the pillar came no closer than 5 feet. This information alone did not stop the intrusion. However, vividly demonstrating to herself that the intrusion was misleading/not real by transforming it into the Microsoft "flying windows" logo did.

Excessively negative appraisals of trauma sequelae, such as the initial PTSD symptoms and other people's responses after the event, are modified by Socratic questioning and behavioral experiments. For example, a bystander when a bomb exploded interpreted the fact that friends didn't ask him about his experience as a sign that they viewed his attempt to help dying victims of the bomb as inadequate and pathetic. After Socratic questioning had identified the alternative explanation that they might not want to distress him by making him think about the bombing, he made a point of discussing the event and found that, contrary to his belief, others were full of admiration for his actions. Similarly, a woman who had always been a "coper" in her family was greatly distressed by the sudden mood swings, periods of tearfulness, and intrusive memories she experienced after a severe RTA. All these symptoms meant to her that she was becoming like her sister, who was generally acknowledged as the "neurotic" of the family. She tried very hard to suppress her intrusions and emotions when reminded of the accident; she believed that if she didn't, she would become a nervous wreck. The alternative view that her symptoms were the normal sequelae of a severe trauma, and were perhaps being maintained by her attempts to suppress them, was discussed. To test her belief that she would become like her sister if she allowed herself to become upset about the trauma, she intentionally entered a situation that would provoke strong flashbacks (sitting with the therapist in a vehicle in a car wash). She was delighted to discover that although she became very anxious and briefly dissociated, she was still herself afterward.

Goal 3: Drop Dysfunctional Behavioral and Cognitive Strategies

Strategies that have the immediate aim of reducing one's sense of current threat, but have the long-term effect of maintaining the disorder, are common in PTSD. The strategies maintain the disorder by preventing elaboration of the trauma memory (e.g., avoidance of talking about the event) or by preventing reappraisal (e.g., excessive use of the rear-view mirror after a rear-end crash, maintaining overestimation of the likelihood of a further crash because the absence of a new accident is attributed to the excessive vigilance). Treatment usually starts by discussing the problematic consequences of the strategy. The strategy is then dropped/reversed in the context of a behavioral experiment. For example, a young man who believed that he would go mad if he did not try hard to suppress the trauma memory and intrusions was encouraged to test the idea by intentionally allowing intrusions to enter and leave his head without trying to control them. To his surprise, this led to a subsequent decline in intrusion frequency.

EFFECTIVENESS OF THE COGNITIVE THERAPY

To date, four studies have investigated the effectiveness of the cognitive therapy program described here. In the first (Ehlers, Clark, Hackmann, McManus, & Fennell, in press, Study 1), a consecutive series of patients with PTSD from a variety of traumas received between 4 and 20 sessions (mean =8.3) of cognitive therapy. The treatment showed high acceptability. Only one patient (5%) dropped out, and that was for reasons unrelated to therapy. Significant improvements in PTSD symptoms, disability, and depression were observed and maintained at 6-month follow-up. The overall pretreatment-to-posttreatment effect size for PTSD symptoms was very large (ES = 2.7 for the intention-to-treat sample). Ninety percent of patients no longer met diagnostic criteria for PTSD at the end of treatment, and 80% achieved high end-state functioning.

The highly promising results obtained in our initial case series were replicated in a subsequent controlled trial (Ehlers, Clark, et al., in press, Study 2), in which patients with chronic PTSD (lasting longer than 6 months) were randomly assigned to either immediate cognitive therapy (up to 12 weekly sessions) or a 13-week waiting period, followed by cognitive therapy. The immediate-treatment group were significantly better than the waiting-list group at 13 weeks. Immediate cognitive therapy was associated with significant improvement on all measures. There were no significant changes during the waiting period, but patients from the waiting-list group improved as much as the immediate-treatment group when they subsequently received cognitive therapy. The pretreatment-to-posttreatment PTSD effect size was again very large (ES = 2.82 for the intention-to-treat sample).

The studies described above indicate that cognitive therapy is an effective treatment for chronic PTSD. Clearly, it would be preferable if treatment could be successfully provided earlier. Our third study (Ehlers, Clark, Hackmann, et al., 2003) investigated this possibility in patients who developed PTSD shortly after an RTA. Early intervention research (see Ehlers & Clark, 2003) had recently provided a surprise finding. Psychological debriefing has long been advocated as an effective early intervention; however, a series of controlled trials investigating individual debriefing found that it was ineffective (Rose, Bisson, & Wessely, 2002) and in some cases might even retard natural recovery (Bisson, Jenkins, Alexander, & Bannister, 1997; Mayou, Ehlers, & Hobbs, 2000). To determine whether cognitive therapy might be effective when delivered relatively early, patients who had PTSD 3 months after an RTA were randomly assigned to cognitive therapy (up to 12 weekly sessions), an assessment interview and a self-help booklet, or no treatment. At the end of treatment and 9 months later, cognitive therapy was associated with significantly greater improvements in PTSD than the self-help and no-treatment conditions, which did not differ from each other. The pretreatment-to-posttreatment effect size for cognitive therapy was again high (ES = 2.5 at posttreatment and 2.7 at follow-up).

Most controlled trials have a number of patient exclusion criteria. This raises important questions about the extent to which the positive results obtained in trials can be generalized to routine clinical practice. To address this issue, our fourth study (Gillespie, Duffy, Hackmann, & Clark, 2002) was an audit of a consecutive series of 91 patients who developed PTSD following a car bomb that exploded in the center of Omagh, Northern Ireland, in August 1998. There were no major patient exclusion criteria, and 53% of participants had one or more additional Axis I disorders (comorbidity). Treatment was conducted by National Health Service staff who had modest prior training in the treatment of trauma. A brief specialist training in cognitive therapy for PTSD was provided. Therapists were allowed flexibility in the number of treatment sessions they offered a patient. Significant and substantial improvements in PTSD were observed in the pretreatment-to-posttreatment effect size (ES = 2.5), which was comparable to those obtained in our two controlled trials (Ehlers, Clark, et al., 2003, in press). Comorbidity was not associated with poorer outcome, perhaps because comorbid patients were given more sessions of treatment (an average of 10 vs. 5 sessions). Although all patients showed some degree of improvement, those who were physically injured improved less than those who were not physically injured. This suggests that further development of treatment modules for patients who have continuing physical injury may be useful.

Overall, the results of the evaluations that have so far been conducted suggest that cognitive therapy is an acceptable and effective treatment for PTSD. Encouragingly, the substantial improvements that occur during treatment are well maintained at follow-up, and it appears that the treatment can be successfully transported from specialist research centers to front-line, nonselective clinical services.

SUMMARY AND CONCLUSIONS

In recent years, we have applied the general approach to psychopathology that Beck has used in many disorders to the understanding and treatment of PTSD. A cognitive model of PTSD that is consistent with the main clinical features of the disorder has been developed. Experimental and prospective longitudinal investigations have provided support for key aspects of the model, including the role of excessively negative appraisals of the trauma and/or its sequelae; the proposed disturbance in autobiographical memory; and the role of dysfunctional behavioral and cognitive strategies.

A specialized form of cognitive therapy that targets the key processes in the model has been developed. Controlled trials indicate that the cognitive therapy has high acceptability with patients, is effective, and can be successfully disseminated into routine clinical services.

ACKNOWLEDGMENTS

The research of David M. Clark and Anke Ehlers is supported by the Wellcome Trust.

REFERENCES

Ali, T., Dunmore, E., Clark, D. M., & Ehlers, A. (2002) The role of negative beliefs in posttraumatic stress disorder: A comparison of assault victims and non-victims. *Behavioural and Cognitive Psychotherapy, 30*, 249–257.

American Psychiatric Association. (1994). *Diagnostic and statistical manual of mental disorders* (4th ed.). Washington, DC: Author.

Amir, N., Stafford, J., Freshman, M. S., & Foa, E. B. (1998). Relationship between trauma narratives and trauma pathology. *Journal of Traumatic Stress, 11*, 385–392.

Andrews, B., Brewin, C. R., & Rose, S. (2003). Gender, social support, and PTSD in victims of violent crime. *Journal of Traumatic Stress, 16*, 421–427.

Bisson, J. L., Jenkins, P. L., Alexander, J., & Bannister, C. (1997). Randomized controlled trial of psychological debriefing for victims of acute burn trauma. *British Journal of Psychiatry, 171*, 78–81.

Blanchard, E. B., Hickling, E. J., Barton, K. A., Taylor, A. E., Loos, W. R., & Jones-Alexander, J. (1996). One-year prospective follow-up of motor vehicle accident victims. *Behaviour Research and Therapy, 34*, 775–786.

Brewin, C. R., Dalgleish, T., & Joseph, S. (1996). A dual representation theory of posttraumatic stress disorder. *Psychological Review, 103*, 670–686.

Bryant, R. B., & Harvey, A. G. (1995). Avoidant coping style and post-traumatic stress disorder following motor vehicle accidents. *Behaviour Research and Therapy, 33*, 631–635.

Clohessy, S., & Ehlers, A. (1999). PTSD symptoms, response to intrusive memories, and coping in ambulance service workers. *British Journal of Clinical Psychology, 38*, 251–265.

Conway, M. A. (1997). Introduction: What are memories? In M. A. Conway (Ed.), *Recovered memories and false memories* (pp. 1–22). Oxford: Oxford University Press.

Davies, M. I., & Clark, D. M. (1998). Thought suppression produces a rebound effect with analogue post-traumatic intrusions. *Behaviour Research and Therapy, 36*, 571–582.

Dunmore, E., Clark, D. M., & Ehlers, A. (1997). Cognitive factors in persistent versus recovered post-traumatic stress disorder after physical or sexual assault: A pilot study. *Behavioural and Cognitive Psychotherapy, 25,* 147–159.

Dunmore, E., Clark, D. M., & Ehlers, A. (1999). Cognitive factors involved in the onset and maintenance of posttraumatic stress disorder (PTSD) after physical or sexual assault. *Behaviour Research and Therapy, 37,* 809–830.

Dunmore, E., Clark, D. M., & Ehlers, A. (2001). A prospective investigation of the role of cognitive factors in persistent posttraumatic stress disorder (PTSD) after physical or sexual assault. *Behaviour Research and Therapy, 39,* 1063–1084.

Ehlers, A., & Clark, D. M. (2000). A cognitive model of persistent posttraumatic stress disorder. *Behaviour Research and Therapy, 38,* 319–345.

Ehlers, A., & Clark, D. M. (2003). Early psychological interventions for adult survivors of trauma. *Biological Psychiatry, 53,* 817–826.

Ehlers, A., Clark, D. M., Dunmore, E. B., Jaycox, L., Meadows, E., & Foa, E. B. (1998). Predicting response to exposure in PTSD: The role of mental defeat and alienation. *Journal of Traumatic Stress, 11,* 457–471.

Ehlers, A., Clark, D. M., Hackmann, A., McManus, F., & Fennell, M. J. V. (in press). Cognitive therapy for posttraumatic stress disorder: Development and evaluation. *Behaviour Research and Therapy.*

Ehlers, A., Clark, D. M., Hackmann, A., McManus, F., Fennell, M. J. V., Herbert, C., et al. (2003). A randomized controlled trial of cognitive therapy, a self-help booklet, and repeated assessment as early interventions for PTSD. *Archives of General Psychiatry, 60,* 1024–1032.

Ehlers, A., Hackmann, A., & Michael, T. (in press). Intrusive reexperiencing in posttraumatic stress disorder: Phenomenology, theory, and therapy. *Memory.*

Ehlers, A., Maercker, A., & Boos, A. (2000). PTSD following political imprisonment: The role of mental defeat, alienation, and perceived permanent change. *Journal of Abnormal Psychology, 109,* 45–55.

Ehlers, A., Mayou, R. A., & Bryant, B. (1998). Psychological predictors of chronic posttraumatic stress disorder after motor vehicle accidents. *Journal of Abnormal Psychology, 107,* 508–519.

Ehlers, A., Mayou, R. A., & Bryant, B. (2003). Cognitive predictors of posttraumatic stress disorder in children: Results of a prospective longitudinal study. *Behaviour Research and Therapy, 41,* 1–10.

Ehlers, A., Michael, T., & Chen, Y. P. (2004). *Perceptual priming for stimuli that occur in a traumatic context.* Manuscript in preparation.

Ehlers, A., & Steil, R. (1995). Maintenance of intrusive memories in posttraumatic stress disorder: A cognitive approach. *Behavioural and Cognitive Psychotherapy, 23,* 217–249.

Foa, E. B, Ehlers, A., Clark, D. M., Tolin, D. F., & Orsillo S. M. (1999). The Post-traumatic Cognitions Inventory (PCTI): Development, reliability and validity. *Psychological Assessment, 11,* 303–314.

Foa, E. B., & Hearst-Ikeda, D. (1996). Emotional dissociation in response to trauma: An information-processing approach. In L. K. Michelson & W. J. Ray (Eds.), *Handbook of dissociation: Theoretical, empirical, and clinical perspectives.* New York: Plenum Press.

Foa, E. B., Molnar, C., & Cashman, L. (1995). Change in rape narratives during exposure therapy for posttraumatic stress disorder. *Journal of Traumatic Stress, 8,* 675–690.

Foa, E. B., & Riggs, D. S. (1993). Post-traumatic stress disorder in rape victims. In J. Oldham, M. B. Riba & A. Tasman (Eds.), *Annual review of psychiatry* (Vol. 12, pp. 273–303). Washington, DC: American Psychiatric Association.

Gillespie, K., Duffy, M., Hackmann, A., & Clark, D. M. (2002). Community based cognitive therapy in the treatment of posttraumatic stress disorder following the Omagh bomb. *Behaviour Research and Therapy, 40,* 345–357.

Halligan, S. L., Michael, T., Clark, D. M., & Ehlers, A. (2003). Posttraumatic stress disorder following assault: The role of cognitive processing, trauma memory and appraisals. *Journal of Consulting and Clinical Psychology, 71,* 419–431.

Harvey, A. G., & Bryant, R. A. (1998). The effect of attempted thought suppression in acute stress disorder. *Behaviour Research and Therapy, 36,* 583–590.

Harvey, A. G. & Bryant, R. A. (1999). A qualitative investigation of the organization of traumatic memories. *British Journal of Clinical Psychology, 38,* 401–405.

Horowitz, M. J. (1976). *Stress response syndromes.* New York: Aronson.

Janoff-Bulman, R. (1992). *Shattered assumptions: Towards a new psychology of trauma.* New York: Free Press.

Kessler, R. C., Sonnega, A., Bromet, E., Hughes, M., & Nelson, C. B. (1995). Posttraumatic stress disorder in the National Comorbidity Survey. *Archives of General Psychiatry, 52,* 1048–1060.

Koss, M. P., Figueredo, A. J., Bell, I., Tharan, M., & Tromp, S. (1996). Traumatic memory characteristics: A cross-validated mediational mode of response to rape among employed women. *Journal of Abnormal Psychology, 105,* 421–432.

Mayou, R. A., Bryant, B., & Duthie, R. (1993). Psychiatric consequences of road traffic accidents. *British Medical Journal, 307,* 647–651.

Mayou, R. A., Ehlers, A., & Hobbs, M. (2000). Psychological debriefing for road traffic accident victims: 3 year follow-up of a randomized controlled trial. *British Journal of Psychiatry, 176,* 589–593.

Mayou, R. A., Tyndel, S., & Bryant, B. (1997). Long term outcome of motor vehicle accident injury. *Psychosomatic Medicine, 59,* 578–584.

McNally, R. J. (1999). Posttraumatic stress disorder. In T. Millon, P. H. Blaney, & R. D. Davis (Eds.), *Oxford textbook of psychopathology* (pp. 144–165). Oxford: Oxford University Press.

Michael, T. (2000). *The nature of trauma memory and intrusive cognitions in posttraumatic stress disorder.* Unpublished doctoral dissertation, University of Oxford, UK.

Michael, T., Ehlers, A., & Halligan, S. L. (2003). *Perceptual bias for trauma-related material predicts posttraumatic stress disorder.* Manuscript submitted for publication.

Murray, J., Ehlers, A., & Mayou, R. M. (2002). Dissociation and posttraumatic stress disorder: Two prospective studies of road traffic accident victims. *British Journal of Psychiatry, 180,* 363–368.

Pennebaker, J. (1989), Confession, inhibition, and disease. In L. Berkowitz (Ed.), *Advances in experimental social psychology* (Vol. 22, pp. 211–244). New York: Academic Press.

Resick, P. A., & Schnicke, M. K. (1993). *Cognitive processing therapy for rape victims: A treatment manual.* Newbury Park, CA: Sage.

Resick, P. A., Schnicke, M. K., & Markway, B. G. (1991, November). *The relationship between cognitive content and posttraumatic stress disorder.* Paper presented at the annual meeting of the Association for Advancement of Behavior Therapy, New York.

Rosario, M., Ehlers, A., Williams, R., & Glucksman, E. (2004). *Peri-traumatic predictors of posttraumatic stress disorder following road traffic accidents.* Manuscript in preparation.

Rose, S., Bisson, J., & Wessely, S. (2002). Psychological debriefing for preventing posttraumatic stress disorder (PTSD). In *The Cochrane Library, Issue 2.* Oxford, UK: Update Software.

Rothbaum, B. O., Foa, E. B., Riggs, D. S., Murdock, T. B., & Walsh, W. (1992). A prospective examination of posttraumatic stress disorder in rape victims. *Journal of Traumatic Stress, 5,* 455–475.

Shalev, A., Peri, T., Canetti, L., & Schreiber, S. (1996). Predictors of PTSD and injured trauma survivors: A prospective study. *American Journal of Psychiatry, 153,* 219–225.

Shepherd, J. C., & Beck, J. G. (1999). The effects of suppressing trauma-related thoughts on women with rape-related post-traumatic stress disorder. *Behaviour Research and Therapy, 37,* 99–112.

Steil, R., & Ehlers, A. (2000). Cognitive correlates of intrusive memories after road traffic accidents. *Behaviour Research and Therapy, 38,* 537–558.

Tulving, E. (2002). Episodic memory. *Annual Review of Psychology, 53,* 1–25.

van der Kolk, B. A., & Fisler, R. (1995). Dissociation and the fragmentary nature of traumatic memories: Overview and exploratory study. *Journal of Traumatic Stress, 8,* 505–525.

Van der Minnen, A. (2002). Changes in trauma narratives with exposure treatment *Journal of Traumatic Stress, 15,* 255–258.

Warda, G., & Bryant, R. A. (1998). Thought control strategies in acute stress disorder. *Behaviour Research and Therapy, 36,* 1171–1175.

Wegner, D. M. (1989). *White bears and other unwanted thoughts: Suppression, obsession, and the psychology of mental control.* New York: Viking.

Wenninger, K., & Ehlers, A. (1998). Dysfunctional cognitions and adult psychological functioning in child sexual abuse survivors. *Journal of Traumatic Stress, 11,* 281–300.

Chapter 8

Cognitive-Behavioral Theory and Treatment of Obsessive–Compulsive Disorder

Past Contributions and Current Developments

DAVID A. CLARK

According to the fourth edition of the *Diagnostic and Statistical Manual of Mental Disorders* (DSM-IV; American Psychiatric Association, 1994), obsessive–compulsive disorder (OCD) is characterized by the presence of obsessions and/or compulsions that are recognized at some point during the disorder as excessive or unreasonable, and that cause marked distress, are time-consuming, or significantly interfere in daily functioning. "Obsessions" are intrusive, recurrent, and persistent thoughts, images, or impulses that are personally unacceptable, unwanted, and most often subjectively resisted by the sufferer (Rachman & Hodgson, 1980). The obsessional content most often deals with imagined or highly improbable threats involving dirt or contamination; causing harm or injury to self or others; pathological doubt over one's actions; religious or sexual impropriety; or violations of orderliness, exactness, or symmetry (Foa & Kozak, 1995; Rasmussen & Eisen, 1992).

"Compulsions" are repetitive, stereotypic, and intentional behavioral or mental responses that are subjectively experienced as an urge or pressure to act (American Psychiatric Association, 1994; Rachman & Hodgson, 1980). A compulsion is usually triggered by an obsession, and even though there is a sense of reduced volitional control over the ritual, it most often persists because of its anxiolytic properties or because it is thought to prevent a dreaded outcome associated with the obsession (Rachman & Shafran, 1998). The main types of compulsions are washing, checking, ordering, reassurance seeking, and hoarding (Rachman & Shafran, 1998).

OCD has a lifetime prevalence of 1–2% (see Antony, Downie, & Swinson, 1998), although estimates vary. It most typically takes a chronic, fluctuating course, with little evidence of spontaneous remission of symptoms (Rasmussen & Eisen, 1992). Onset is gradual and most often occurs in early adolescence to young adulthood (Rasmussen & Tsuang, 1986). OCD can occur in children, though this is uncommon(see March & Mulle, 1998). The gender distribution is approximately equal, with a chronic waxing and waning of symptoms, often in response to stressors or other critical incidents in a person's life. OCD has a high comorbidity rate for major depression, panic disorder, social phobia, and generalized anxiety disorder (see Antony et al., 1998; Crino & Andrews, 1996). Given the chronicity and severity of this disorder, OCD can have a substantial negative impact on individuals' quality of life, family and couple relationships, occupational functioning, and even general health (Antony et al., 1998). Despite the seriousness of obsessional states, first treatment is often sought many years after the emergence of initial symptoms.

This chapter will explore the contribution of the cognitive perspective to theory, research, and treatment of obsessional states, tracing its development from the earlier behavioral perspective. Particular emphasis is placed on the influence of Aaron T. Beck's cognitive theory and therapy of depression on present-day cognitive-behavioral (CB) models and treatment (CBT) of OCD. The chapter concludes with a summary of the current status and future direction of CBT for obsessions and compulsions.

COGNITIVE AND BEHAVIORAL
ANTECEDENTS TO CBT

Behavioral Theory and Treatment of OCD

According to the behavioral model, obsessions are noxious *conditioned* stimuli that cause pain and distress for patients, and so persist because of an increased responsiveness (i.e., sensitization) to obsessional stimuli. This responsiveness leads to failure in habituation, despite repeated occurrences of the obsession (Rachman, 1971, 1976, 1978). Compulsions, on the other hand, develop through an avoidance learning paradigm. Because the performance of a compulsive ritual temporarily reduces the anxiety or distress caused by the obsession, it becomes strengthened by operant conditioning (i.e., reinforcement), and thus becomes a persistent response to the obsession (Emmelkamp, 1982). At the same time, the performance of the compulsive ritual will increase the salience of the obsession, thereby ensuring that the individual becomes even more sensitized to this type of mental intrusion. More extensive discussions of the behavioral theory of OCD can be found in Emmelkamp (1982), Foa and Steketee (1979), and Rachman and Hodgson (1980).

The behavioral account of obsessions and compulsions seemed at first intuitively appealing. Obsessions evidence certain phobic-like qualities, and the anxiety reduction hypothesis for compulsions has fairly strong empirical support (for reviews, see Clark, 2004; Foa & Steketee, 1979; Rachman & Hodgson, 1980). More importantly, a new behavioral treatment—"exposure and response prevention" (ERP), which was based on learning theory—proved to be a highly effective treatment for most types of OCD, but especially compulsive washing and checking. ERP, first introduced by Victor Meyer (1966), involves controlled, repeated exposure to an anxiety-eliciting stimulus (i.e., the obsession) and prevention of any neutralization or other avoidance response (i.e., the compulsive ritual). The rationale is that anxiety should be allowed to dissipate naturally, without performance of the anxiety-reducing compulsion. In this way the patient learns to habituate to the fear-eliciting obsession, while the urge to perform the compulsive ritual is reduced through an absence of reinforcement (Rachman, Hodgson, & Marzillier, 1970). The reader is directed to Steketee (1993), Kozak and Foa (1997), and Rachman and Hodgson (1980) for a detailed description of the ERP treatment protocol.

ERP is considered the psychological treatment of choice for OCD. The American Psychological Association's Division 12 Task Force on Promotion and Dissemination of Psychological Procedures has categorized ERP as a well-established, empirically validated treatment for OCD (Chambless et al., 1998; see also the recommendations from the Expert Consensus Survey by March, Frances, Carpenter, & Kahn, 1997). A number of controlled outcome studies have shown that (1) from 70% to 80% of treatment completers exhibit significant improvement at posttreatment, (2) most patients maintain their improvement over the long term, and (3) ERP is often more effective than pharmacotherapy at posttreatment (see reviews by Abramowitz, 1998; Foa & Kozak, 1996; Stanley & Turner, 1995; Steketee & Shapiro, 1995; van Balkom, van Oppen, Vermeulen, Nauta, & Vorst, 1994). Currently ERP is considered a necessary component in any psychological treatment of OCD.

Dissatisfaction with the Behavioral Approach to OCD

The effectiveness of ERP for the treatment of obsessions and compulsions might lead one to assume that cognitive clinical theory and therapy have little to offer for this disorder. Given that individuals with OCD already recognize the unreasonableness of their obsessions and compulsions, any attempt to utilize the verbal disputation techniques of cognitive therapy to refute the "truth" or improbability of obsessional fears will be futile or perhaps even counterproductive (Salkovskis, 1985, 1999; Steketee, Frost, Rhéaume, & Wilhelm, 1998). For this reason, Reed (1985) concluded that standard cognitive interventions used to treat depression and other anxiety disorders will have limited application to obsessional complaints. Even Hollon and Beck (1986), in their review of cognitive therapy, concluded that *in vivo* ERP was the treatment of choice for OCD, and that "it also remains possible that explicit cognitive interventions have little to offer in this disorder" (p. 467). And yet all was not well with a "purely" behavioral approach to OCD.

By the mid-1980s, serious problems became apparent with the conditioning theory of obsessions and compulsions. Despite the effectiveness of ERP, limitations were becoming increasingly evident in various treatment trials. Detailed discussions of the weaknesses of the learning theory of obsessions and compulsions can be found elsewhere (Carr, 1974; Emmelkamp, 1982; Foa & Steketee, 1979; Rachman & Hodgson, 1980; Steketee, 1993). The most significant shortcoming of the behavioral account was its difficulty in explaining the onset of obsessions. There is little empirical evidence that traumatic learning is involved in the genesis of obsessions. In fact, without the introduction of cognitive, developmental, and even personality variables, the behavioral account cannot mount a credible explanation of the etiology or specificity of obsessional fears (e.g., Rachman, 1978). To deal with the complexities of obsessional phenomena, behavioral researchers like Rachman (1978) introduced such cognitive concepts as "appraisals of unacceptability," "inadequate mental control," and "perceived uncontrollability" (see also Rachman & Hodgson, 1980).

Criticism of a strictly behavioral perspective on OCD has focused more intently on treatment limitations. Salkovskis (1989b), for example, noted that a significant number of patients do not respond to exposure treatment. Rates of refusal, premature termination, and noncompliance with exposure tasks reduce the overall effectiveness of ERP (see Stanley & Turner, 1995). Direct behavioral treatment of obsessions, whether based on thought stopping, habituation training, or thought satiation, is less than adequate (Beech & Vaughan, 1978; Freeston & Ladouceur, 1997; Rachman, 1983). Rachman (1985) concluded that ERP is not well suited for treating "pure" obsessions without overt compulsions. Other subtypes of OCD, such as compulsive hoarding (Frost & Steketee, 1998) or primary obsessional slowness (Rachman, 1985), may be less responsive to ERP. It is also known that the average treated patient still exhibits higher levels of obsessive–compulsive (OC) symptoms at posttreatment than nonclinical controls do (Abramowitz, 1998). Together, these factors argue for a broader theoretical perspective and intervention protocol for the treatment of OCD.

Contributions from Beck's Cognitive Therapy

Given the prodigious rate of scholarly and scientific writing on the cognitive basis and treatment of depression and anxiety, it is interesting that Beck was relatively silent on the application of cognitive therapy to the treatment of OCD. In their detailed account of the cognitive model of anxiety disorders, Beck and Emery with Greenberg (1985) did not extend this model to treatment of obsessions and compulsions. As noted previously, Hollon and Beck (1986) concluded that cognitive interventions may not be effective in the treatment of obsessional complaints.

A number of early contributions suggested that cognitive constructs may be important in OCD. Carr (1974), for example, argued that obsessional states are characterized by abnormally high subjective estimates of the probability that unfavorable outcomes will occur (e.g., "I might become contaminated if I touch this water faucet"). McFall and Wollersheim (1979) proposed a more detailed cognitive model of OCD—one that involves a faulty primary threat appraisal in which the probability of threat and its negative consequences are overestimated, and an erroneous secondary appraisal in which patients underestimate their ability to cope with the perceived threat. Both the primary and secondary appraisals are based on certain preconscious maladaptive beliefs about perfectionism, responsibility, control of thoughts, and uncertainty. Rachman and Hodgson (1980) also proposed that specific cognitive features of intrusive thoughts are involved in the genesis and maintenance of obsessions.

The catalyst for a more cognitive approach to OCD came in a seminal article published by Paul Salkovskis (1985) in *Behaviour Research and Therapy*. Salkovskis proposed that a comprehensive CB account of obsessions could be developed by merging Rachman's (1978) formulation of obsessions with Beck's views on the role of negative automatic thoughts in emotional disorders. Salkovskis argued that a distinction can be made between obsessions and automatic thoughts. He suggested that obsessions function as stimuli that trigger adverse evaluations or automatic thoughts. Thus the occurrence of an obsession may activate certain preexisting dysfunctional schemas, which in turn lead to faulty appraisals about the unacceptability, personal significance, and possible threatening nature of the unwanted intrusive thought. Salkovskis argued that the faulty appraisal of the importance of the obsession is a form of "negative automatic thought." Appraisals indicating that one is personally responsible to prevent anticipated harm to self or others were considered a particularly potent type of negative automatic thought involved in the pathogenesis of obsessions. Borrowing from the behavioral account of OCD, Salkovskis added that neutralization attempts, by either compulsive rituals or other control strategies, are attempts to put things right and so to avert the possibility of being blamed for harm to self or others.

Current CB models of OCD owe a substantial debt to Beck's cognitive theory of depression, and yet this link to the cognitive model has gone unrecognized. In large part, this oversight is due to the use of different labels to refer to the negative automatic thoughts in OCD. Later Salkovskis (1989a) dropped the label of "automatic thoughts" in favor of the term "appraisal" when referring to how obsession-prone individuals evaluate or cognitively respond to particular unwanted intrusive thoughts. Thus contemporary CB researchers routinely focus on faulty appraisals as the core cognitive process leading to the persistence of obsessions, without realizing that these appraisals fit closely with Beck's notion of negative automatic thoughts. In depression, these thoughts refer to negative evaluations about one's self, world, or future (Beck, 1967/1972), whereas in OCD the automatic thoughts or appraisals focus on negative evaluations about the personal importance and threatening nature of obsessions. Thus the cognitive theory of depression has contributed a very critical concept to our understanding of the cognitive basis of obsessions.

There are other features of contemporary CB theories and treatment of OCD that owe considerably to Beck's cognitive theory of depression. The idea that certain schemas or enduring beliefs act as an underlying cognitive vulnerability to OCD (see Clark, 2004; Freeston, Rhéaume & Ladouceur, 1996; Obsessive Compulsive Cognitions Working Group [OCCWG], 1997), is reminiscent of Beck's cognitive diathesis–stress model of depression (Beck, 1987; Clark & Beck with Alford, 1999). As well, activation of these underlying schemas is considered responsible for producing faulty appraisals of the obsession, in a manner similar to the activation of hypervalent schemas and negative self-referent thinking in depression. Finally, as discussed below, many features of cognitive therapy of depression have been adapted to the treatment of obsessions. These include (1) the emphasis placed on Socratic questioning and guided discovery; (2) the importance of identifying faulty appraisals and differentiating appraisals (negative automatic thoughts) from the obsessions; (3) the use of cognitive restructuring to challenge dysfunctional appraisals and beliefs of responsibility, importance, and control; and (4) the development of behavioral experiments to test the validity of specific dysfunctional beliefs central to the obsession.

CB APPRAISAL THEORIES OF OCD

Figure 8.1 illustrates the general theoretical framework adopted in most current CB theories of OCD. Although the formulations proposed by Salkovskis, Rachman, the OCCWG, myself, and others may emphasize different beliefs and appraisals, nevertheless all accept the importance of faulty appraisals and neutralization in the persistence of obsessions. As can be seen from Figure 8.1, CB theories trace the source of obsessions to the natural occurrence of unwanted intrusive thoughts, images or impulses. Questionnaire and interview studies indicate that 80–90% of nonclinical samples have occasional unwanted and unacceptable thoughts that are similar in content to the obsessions seen in OCD (e.g., Parkinson & Rachman, 1981; Purdon & Clark, 1993; Rachman & de Silva, 1978). If the intrusive thought is appraised as benign or irrelevant, then the thought will quickly fade from conscious awareness. However, if vulnerable persons interpret their mental intrusions as personally significant because they are viewed as indicating responsibility for some anticipated negative consequence or threat, then the thought will become a highly salient cognitive event. The faulty appraisals of importance will lead to some action intended to alleviate the distress caused by the intrusive thought, to avert the anticipated negative consequence, or simply to "put matters right." The response to the intrusion may be a compulsive ritual, some other form of neutralization, avoidance, or intentional mental control (i.e., distraction). The production of faulty appraisals of significance and the execution of a compulsion or other neutralization response are the two main processes responsible for an escalation of normal unwanted

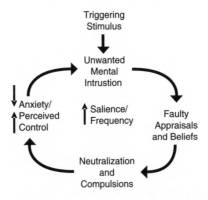

FIGURE 8.1. General framework of CB appraisal theories of OCD. From Clark (2004, p. 90). Copyright 2004 by The Guilford Press. Reprinted by permission.

intrusive thoughts into obsessions. Together, these processes lead to a temporary reduction in anxiety and an increase in the perceived control over the obsession. Unfortunately, these effects are temporary, because a serious by-product of the faulty appraisals and neutralization is an increase in the salience of the unwanted, obsessive-like intrusive thoughts (for further discussion of the CB model of obsessions, see Clark, 2004; Rachman, 2003; Salkovskis, 1989a, 1999).

Salkovskis's Model

Salkovskis (1985, 1989a, 1999) argues that *appraisals and beliefs involving inflated responsibility* for the occurrence or prevention of threat to self or others are the central cognitive processes involved in the pathogenesis of obsessions. Salkovskis and colleagues define responsibility as "the belief that one has power which is pivotal to bring about or prevent subjectively crucial negative outcomes. These outcomes may be actual, that is, having consequences in the real world, and/or at a moral level" (Salkovskis, 1998, p. 40). According to Salkovskis, once an intrusive thought, image, or impulse is misinterpreted as signifying increased personal responsibility for the occurrence or prevention of harm, it will then lead to an increase in the distressing qualities of the intrusion; the intrusion will attain greater accessibility or salience; there will be increased attention to the intrusive thought; and neutralization responses will be initiated in order to escape or avoid responsibility (Salkovskis & Wahl, 2004).

What is the empirical evidence that heightened appraisals of responsibility are a necessary causal element in the pathogenesis of obsessions? A number of studies found that responsibility appraisals and beliefs are elevated in OCD and correlate with OC symptom measures (e.g., OCCWG, 2001, 2003; Salkovskis et al., 2000; Steketee, Frost, & Cohen, 1998). Furthermore, there is some experimental evidence that manipulations leading to heightened subjective estimates of personal responsibility result in more discomfort and a greater urge to neutralize (Bouchard, Rhéaume, & Ladouceur, 1999; Ladouceur et al., 1995; Lopatka & Rachman, 1995; Shafran, 1997). Although these findings are supportive of Salkovskis's model, other studies have been less encouraging. For example, heightened appraisals and beliefs of personal responsibility for threat (1) may not be specific or unique to OCD (Foa, Amir, Bogert, Molnar, & Przeworski, 2001); (2) may account for less variance in OC symptoms than originally expected (Emmelkamp & Aardema, 1999; Wilson & Chambless, 1999); (3) may be more transient and situationally influenced than predicted by Salkovskis's model (Rachman, Thordarson, Shafran, & Woody, 1995); and (4) may be less relevant to certain subtypes of OCD, such as compulsive washing (Menzies, Harris, Cumming, & Einstein, 2000). In addition, it is unclear whether inflated responsibility is a cause or a consequence of frequent disturbing obsessions.

Rachman's Model

Rachman (1997, 1998, 2003) has proposed that obsessions are caused by the *catastrophic misinterpretation of the significance* of unwanted mental intrusions. Obsessions will persist as long as the misinterpretations of significance continue, but will decrease when the misinterpretation is weakened (Rachman, 1997). The key process in the escalation of unwanted intrusive thoughts into abnormal obsessions is the misinterpretation that an intrusion indicates something highly important, personally significant, and threatening or even catastrophic (Rachman, 2003). Rachman argues that his proposal is based on three findings: "that cognitions can cause anxiety, anxiety provoking interpretations of cognitions can lead to obsessions, and particular cognitive biases are associated with vulnerability to obsessions" (Rachman, 2003, p. 14).

There is, of course, considerable evidence that negative cognitions can cause anxiety, and Rachman (2003) cites D. M. Clark's research on the catastrophic misinterpretation of bodily sensations in panic disorder as a prime example of the functional relation between cognition and subjective anxiety. There is also substantial empirical evidence that the production of unwanted intrusive thoughts or obsessions leads to an increase in subjective distress and possibly also in psychophysiological arousal (for reviews, see Clark, 2004; Rachman & Hodgson, 1980). However, the model does have more difficulty accounting for the persistence of obsessions that do not give rise to subjective anxiety, such as the repetition of nonsensical images or meaninglessness phrases, or obsessional thinking associated with order, exactness, and symmetry compulsions (Rachman, 1997).

The second prediction of Rachman's model—the misinterpretation of an intrusion as indicating significant threat—again has some empirical support in the research literature. Individuals with OCD are significantly more likely to rate their unwanted intrusive thoughts or obsessions as important, unacceptable, threatening, and personally meaningful (e.g., OCCWG, 2001, 2003; Rachman & de Silva, 1978). Moreover, the frequency of unwanted intrusive thoughts is positively associated with increased ratings of significance, importance, and threat or unacceptability (Freeston, Ladouceur, Thibodeau, & Gagnon, 1991; Freeston, & Ladouceur, 1993; Parkinson & Rachman, 1981; Purdon, 2001).

Finally, there is evidence that certain cognitive biases, such as inflated responsibility (see above) and "thought–action fusion" (TAF), are salient cognitive features of obsessional states and may lead to misinterpretations of the significance of unwanted intrusive thoughts. Rachman (1993;

Rachman & Shafran, 1999) described "TAF–Likelihood" as the belief that having an unacceptable thought increases the likelihood that a negative outcome will occur (e.g., "If I think that my daughter will have an accident, it is more likely that she will have an accident"), and "TAF–Moral" as the belief that having a "bad thought" is morally equivalent to committing the deed (e.g., "Having thoughts of sexually abusing a child is as evil as actually doing it"). There is emerging empirical evidence that TAF may be a cognitive bias specific to obsessional states, and that it may even play a causal role in the pathogenesis of obsessions (see reviews by Clark, 2004; Rachman, 2003; Thordarson & Shafran, 2002). However, questions remain about which aspect of TAF is most relevant to OCD, and whether TAF and other cognitive biases are true predisposing vulnerability factors for obsessionality. As well, the functional relationships among misinterpretations of significance, cognitive biases like TAF, and neutralization are not well understood.

Cognitive Control Theory

Recently, a number of researchers have proposed that beliefs and appraisals about the control of unwanted intrusive thoughts may play an important role in the pathogenesis of obsessions (Clark & Purdon, 1993; OCCWG, 1997; Purdon & Clark, 2002; Salkovskis, Richards, & Forrester, 1995). The importance of appraisals and beliefs about the control of obsessions is discussed extensively elsewhere (Clark, 2004). Briefly, it is well known that individuals with OCD try too hard to control their obsessional thinking (Salkovskis et al., 1995). It is also known that even under the best of circumstances, people's ability to suppress unwanted thoughts intentionally is less than perfect; in fact, thought suppression may even result in a paradoxical increase in the intrusive thought, once suppression efforts cease (Wegner, 1994; Wenzlaff & Wegner, 2000). Thus active attempts to suppress obsessions may account in part for their increased frequency, although the empirical evidence is quite inconsistent that thought suppression plays a significant role in the persistence of obsessions (see Abramowitz, Tolin, & Street, 2001; Clark, 2004; Purdon, 1999).

It is proposed that beliefs and appraisals concerning the importance of thought control and the exaggerated misinterpreted consequences of failure to control one's unwanted cognitions may have a more adverse impact on the salience and frequency of the obsession than the presence of active thought suppression. For example, if vulnerable individuals conclude that they can and must control an unwanted thought, because failure to do so would lead to dire consequences, then this belief will increase the amount of attention devoted to the persistent mental intrusion. These primary appraisals will lead to attempts to prevent or suppress the obsession. Such efforts are bound to be less than perfect, leaving these individuals with repeated occurrences of failed thought control. If the individuals now interpret their failed thought control efforts in a catastrophic fashion (i.e., secondary appraisals of control), this will lead to even more distress and increased efforts to control the obsession. In sum, primary appraisals of the importance of obsessions, coupled with faulty secondary appraisals of the significance of failed thought control, lead to a spiraling increase in the frequency and intensity of the obsessions.

Investigations into the role of appraisals and beliefs of control in OCD have just begun. There is emerging evidence that dysfunctional control appraisals and beliefs are elevated in OCD (OCCWG, 2001, 2003) and that these beliefs are related to OC symptoms (Clark, Purdon, & Wang, 2003). More recently, Tolin, Abramowitz, Hamlin, and Synodi (2002) found that patients with OCD reported stronger internal attributions for thought control failure in a thought suppression experiment than did other anxious patients or nonclinical controls. Although these findings suggest that maladaptive thought control appraisals and beliefs, as well as misinterpretations about the consequences of failed thought control, may be significant in understanding the maintenance of obsessions, it is far too early to judge the relevance of a cognitive control perspective on obsessional states.

COGNITIVE-BEHAVIORAL TREATMENT OF OCD: ELEMENTS AND EMPIRICAL STATUS

Basic Elements of CBT

Contemporary CBT protocols for obsessions and compulsions are clear examples of the theory-driven approach to the development of a psychotherapeutic intervention for a specific disorder. If the persistence of obsessions depends on faulty appraisals of significance and accompanying neutralization responses, then a reduction in the frequency and intensity of the obsessions will occur if the faulty appraisals are modified and if counterproductive compulsions and other neutralization efforts are prevented (Rachman, 2003). The eight features of CBT for obsessions and compulsions listed in Table 8.1 are briefly discussed below. The reader can find more extensive accounts of this treatment approach in Clark (2004), Freeston and Ladouceur (1997), Rachman (2003), Salkovskis (1999), Salkovskis and Wahl (2004), and Whittal and McLean (1999, 2002).

The CB therapist places considerable emphasis on educating the patient into the CB model of OCD. Individuals with OCD enter therapy believing that their problem centers on poor self-control over distressing obsessions and powerful compulsive urges. They interpret these symptoms as a sign of their personal abnormality and weakness, and so believe that treatment should focus on elimination of their obsessions. The CB therapist, however, must first educate patients that their faulty appraisal of the significance of the obsessions is the primary cause of the repeated occurrence of the unwanted thought. The educational component focuses on normalizing the experience of unwanted intrusive thoughts by demonstrating to patients that most individuals experience unwanted thoughts of similar content to their obsessions. Whether an unwanted intrusive thought remains a low-frequency occurrence or develops into a frequent, distressing cognition depends on whether a person considers the thought personally significant or not. In order to obtain an adequate level of treatment compliance, the educational phase must present a convincing rationale. The essence of the treatment rationale is that a focus on the modification of faulty appraisals and the prevention of neutralization responses is necessary to achieve improvement in OC symptoms. As well, patients must learn how to distinguish between their faulty appraisals or evaluations of their obsessions and the obsessions themselves. This will include helping patients learn the difference between appraisals ("the importance you give to your thoughts") and the obsessional thoughts, as well as how they use different types of faulty appraisals, neutralization, mental control strategies, compulsive rituals, and avoidance to deal with their obsessional state. This phase of treatment will involve considerable exploration of the patients' OC cognitive and behavioral responses within sessions, as well as the assignment of self-monitoring homework tasks.

Once patients understand their reaction to their obsessions, cognitive restructuring strategies are introduced to challenge the "interpretations of importance" associated with the obsessions. Cognitive restructuring is used to help patients realize that their faulty appraisals of importance are only one of several possible ways to interpret unwanted intrusive thoughts; that their in-

TABLE 8.1. Therapeutic Elements of CBT for OCD

· Education about the appraisal model

· Identification and differentiation of appraisals and intrusions

· Cognitive restructuring strategies

· Alternative appraisals of the obsession

· Exposure and response prevention (ERP)

· Behavioral experimentation

· Modifying self-referent and metacognitive beliefs

· Relapse prevention

Note. Adapted from Clark (2004). Copyright 2004 by The Guilford Press. Adapted by permission.

terpretations are based on "what could happen" and not on "what will happen" (O'Connor & Robillard, 1999); and that the faulty appraisals are a highly selective approach taken to a certain type of unwanted thought. A variety of cognitive intervention strategies—such as the downward-arrow technique, double-column evidence gathering, the continuum-reframing task, and probability reestimations—are employed to challenge faulty appraisals of overestimated threat, TAF bias, inflated responsibility, overimportance of thoughts, need to control thoughts, neutralization, intolerance of uncertainty, perfectionism, and intolerance of anxiety/distress (for further details, see Clark, 2004; OCCWG, 1997; Rachman, 2003; Whittal & McLean, 2002).

It is important early in the treatment process to present patients with an alternative explanation for why they suffer from distressing and recurring obsessions and compulsions. Cognitive and behavioral restructuring exercises should lead patients to view their obsessions in a less threatening manner. The therapist uses guided discovery to assist patients in realizing that their appraisals of importance and efforts to control their obsessions are what lead to a paradoxical increase in the obsessions' frequency and intensity. The alternative explanation that the CB therapist wishes to reinforce is that unwanted intrusive thoughts, even obsessions, are harmless, irrelevant by-products of a creative mind; as such, they require no particular response (i.e., doing nothing; Salkovskis, 1999). In fact, only by letting the obsessions ebb and flow naturally through conscious awareness, without any attempt to control their occurrence or respond to their content, will there be significant improvement in obsessional symptoms.

Although cognitive interventions are important in CBT for obsessions, the most potent therapeutic ingredient is still ERP. Faulty appraisals and beliefs about threat, importance, responsibility, control, and the like are most effectively modified when patients experience repeated, sustained exposure to their obsessional fears and cease trying to "put matters right" through compulsive rituals or other neutralization strategies. In CBT, ERP is used to directly challenge and modify faulty appraisals and beliefs. Thus it is important that the CB therapist structure ERP as a hypothesis-testing experiment. For example, rather than viewing repeated exposure to "contaminated objects" as a process of habituation, the CB therapist treats these exposure tasks as a means of testing beliefs about the threatening nature of touching certain objects, the intolerance of anxiety/distress, the responsibility to avoid becoming "contaminated," or the best way to control upsetting thoughts about disease and germs. Depending on the OCD subtype, a large proportion of CBT is devoted to ERP.

Another very effective type of intervention for challenging OC appraisals and beliefs is direct behavioral experimentation. Beck, Rush, Shaw, and

Emery (1979) indicated that behavioral techniques can take the form of "miniexperiments" that test the validity of dysfunctional thoughts and beliefs in order to bring about cognitive change. A number of different behavioral experiments have been described for challenging OC appraisal and beliefs (for examples of specific interventions, see Clark, 2004; Freeston et al., 1996; Rachman, 2003; Whittal & McLean, 2002).

The final two elements of CBT for obsessions are the modification of core self-referent or metacognitive schemas and the emphasis on relapse prevention in the final sessions of therapy. Certain recurring cognitive themes will emerge in the treatment of obsessional patients' faulty appraisals and beliefs. These themes represent more generalized, enduring ideas and assumptions about the self and the significance of unwanted intrusive thoughts. Some of these underlying core schemas are self-referent, dealing with basic beliefs about the self, world, and future (Beck et al., 1979). Other schemas reflect metacognitive beliefs, or beliefs about one's thought processes, such as the importance and significance of thoughts and their control. As in cognitive therapy for other disorders, it is important that these core beliefs are targeted for change in the course of therapy in order to improve treatment maintenance. Other steps that can be taken to build in relapse prevention include (1) providing written instructions on positive self-help strategies for the recurrence of obsessions; (2) teaching a problem-solving approach to episodes of unwanted thoughts or obsessions; (3) ensuring that patients practice ERP when OC symptoms reemerge; (4) teaching coping skills for stress and other life difficulties; and (5) gradually fading out the final therapy sessions, followed by occasional booster sessions.

Empirical Status of CBT

The new theory-derived CBT for obsessions and compulsions is such a recent development that only a few outcome studies have been published and others are still in progress. A number of controlled group outcome studies indicate that a focus on cognitive modification can be effective in reducing the frequency and severity of obsessional symptoms (Emmelkamp & Beens, 1991; Emmelkamp, Visser, & Hoekstra, 1988; Jones & Menzies, 1998). van Oppen et al. (1995) reported the first controlled outcome study of cognitive therapy for OCD, based on the treatment approach of Beck et al. (1985) and Salkovskis (1985). Cognitive therapy resulted in significant improvement on all outcome measures, showing even a slight superiority over the ERP-only condition. Freeston et al. (1997) found that CBT was significantly more effective than a waiting-list control in treating obsessional ruminations without overt compulsions. O'Connor, Todorov, Robillard, Borgeat, and Brault (1999) reported that 20 sessions of individual CBT alone over a 5-month period produced treatment effects equivalent to those of medication alone or CBT plus medication. Finally, McLean et al. (2001) found that 12 weeks of group CBT was more effective than a waiting-list control, but it was marginally less effective than ERP alone in achieving symptomatic improvement. Because of the complex and idiosyncratic nature of OC cognitive appraisals, the authors suggested that CBT might produce stronger effect sizes when offered individually than when provided in a group format. Overall, these findings indicate that CBT can be effective in treating obsessive and compulsive symptoms.

Given that ERP is an empirically supported treatment for OCD, a more critical question is whether the shift to a more cognitive perspective improves treatment effectiveness over that of ERP alone. In studies that tested the individual contributions of CBT versus ERP, the cognitive interventions proved to be as effective as ERP (Emmelkamp & Beens, 1991; Emmelkamp et al., 1988; de Haan et al., 1997; van Oppen et al., 1995), although McLean et al. (2001) found CBT to be less effective. However, at this time there is no evidence that adding a cognitive component to ERP produces significantly more symptomatic improvement than ERP alone, at least in a heterogeneous sample of patients with OCD. Although there is some preliminary indication that CBT may be more effective for certain subtypes of OCD (e.g., obsessional rumination), the necessary comparative treatment studies have not been conducted. Furthermore, one might expect cognitive interventions to improve treatment compliance and lower refusal or dropout rates, but there is insufficient evidence to support this assertion. Clearly, we are only beginning to explore the utility of this new approach to the treatment of obsessions and compulsions.

CONCLUSION AND FUTURE DIRECTIONS

OCD is one of the most perplexing and challenging of the anxiety disorders to understand and treat. Behavioral accounts based on the two-stage learning model at first provided a promising explanation for the persistence of obsessions and compulsions. More importantly, the behavioral perspective led to the development of a treatment for OCD based on repeated and prolonged exposure to fear-eliciting obsessions, accompanied by prevention of compulsive rituals or other forms of neutralization. ERP has proven to be a highly effective treatment for OCD, with averaged posttreatment response rates of over 80% (Foa & Kozak, 1996; Kozak, Liebowitz, & Foa, 2000).

Despite the success of ERP, a number of problems emerged with a strictly behavioral approach to OCD. The behavioral account could not provide an adequate explanation for the critical psychological processes involved in the etiology and persistence of OCD. Limitations also emerged in the use of ERP, such as fairly high treatment refuser and dropout rates; less effectiveness with certain OCD subtypes (e.g., hoarding or obsessional rumination without overt compulsions); and the presence of residual OC symptoms after a successful trial of ERP.

In response to deficiencies in the behavioral account, a more cognitive perspective on OCD has been advocated to explain the onset and maintenance of obsessional states. It is proposed that the normal occurrence of unwanted intrusive thoughts will escalate into clinical obsessions when individuals misinterpret these intrusions as highly significant personal threats, which are then dealt with by generating a compulsive ritual or some other neutralization response. These two processes—faulty appraisals and beliefs about intrusive thoughts, and active attempts to neutralize obsessional fears via compulsive rituals, avoidance, reassurance seeking, or the like—are considered responsible for the persistence of the obsessional state. As discussed in this chapter, a number of faulty beliefs and appraisals have been proposed as critical in the pathogenesis of obsessions. These include appraisals of inflated responsibility, personal significance, importance and control of thoughts, overestimated threat, TAF bias, intolerance of uncertainty, perfectionism, and intolerance of anxiety/distress (see Clark, 2004; OCCWG, 1997, 2001). Although research on these new cognitive appraisal concepts is still in its infancy, there is already evidence that some of them (e.g., inflated responsibility, overestimated threat, TAF, and control of thoughts) are implicated in OCD.

The current CB models of obsessional states proposed by Salkovskis, Rachman, the OCCWG, and others represent some of the best examples of theory-driven treatment in contemporary psychotherapy. In recent years a number of CBT protocols have been proposed, especially for the treatment of obsessions (e.g., Clark, 2004; Freeston & Ladouceur, 1997; Rachman, 2003; Salkovskis, 1999). As summarized in Table 8.1, the therapeutic elements of CBT for OCD represent a merger of behavior therapy (i.e., ERP) with the standard cognitive therapy of depression proposed by Beck et al. (1979). Initial trials indicate that the CBT approach is effective in treating OC symptoms.

No conclusion can be reached about the contribution of CB theory and CBT to our understanding of obsessional phenomena, because a number of critical questions remain unresolved. For example, it is unclear whether such cognitive concepts as inflated responsibility, TAF, or intolerance of uncertainty are specific to OCD, or whether these psychological dysfunctions are also evident in other disorders. As well, it is not known whether faulty appraisals and beliefs are causes or consequences of frequent intrusive thoughts or obsessions. Empirical research on vulnerability to obsessional states is largely nonexistent. In terms of treatment, it is uncertain whether the addition of cognitive intervention strategies has significant incremental value over ERP alone. More research is also needed to determine the short- and long-term effectiveness of CBT relative to other treatments for OCD, such as pharmacotherapy. Even though cognitive therapy was introduced to improve treatment compliance and lower refusal rates, there is practically no research on this issue. Finally, little is known about the mechanisms of change in CBT for obsessions. Are cognitive interventions in OCD effective because of the modification of faulty appraisals and beliefs, or is cognitive change a consequence of changes in compulsive behavior (Emmelkamp, van Oppen, & van Balkom, 2002)?

Theory, research, and treatment of the cognitive concomitants of OCD have shown noteworthy progress, innovation, and creativity in the last few years. Although many fundamental questions remain for CB theories and CBT of OCD, nevertheless this domain of psychological inquiry represents one of the finest examples of theory-driven research and treatment. The current advances seen in CBT for obsessional states owe a huge debt to Beck's pioneering work on the cognitive basis of anxiety and depression. Such constructs as negative automatic thoughts, cognitive biases, and vulnerability schemas have been adapted and elaborated to explain the cognitive basis of OCD. Cognitive therapy innovations such as guided discovery, cognitive restructuring, and behavioral experimentation (i.e., empirical hypothesis testing) have become critical therapeutic ingredients in CBT protocols for obsessions and compulsions. No doubt in the future we will continue to see new adaptations of Beck's cognitive therapy for the treatment of obsessional phenomena. As seen by the scale of their contribution to obsessional states, the cognitive theory and therapy of Aaron T. Beck are clearly among the most robust theoretical and psychotherapeutic formulations currently available to mental health researchers and practitioners.

REFERENCES

Abramowitz, J. S. (1998). Does cognitive-behavioral therapy cure obsessive–compulsive disorder?: A meta-analytic evaluation of clinical significance. *Behavior Therapy, 29*, 339–355.

Abramowitz, J. S., Tolin, D. F., & Street, G. P. (2001). Paradoxical effects of thought suppression: A meta-analysis of controlled studies. *Clinical Psychology Review, 21*, 683–703.

American Psychiatric Association. (1994). *Diagnostic and statistical manual of mental disorders* (4th ed.). Washington, DC: Author.

Antony, M. M., Downie, F., & Swinson, R. P. (1998). Diagnostic issues and epidemiology in obsessive–compulsive disorder. In R. P. Swinson, M. M. Antony, S. Rachman, & M. A. Richter (Eds.), *Obsessive–compulsive disorder: Theory, research, and treatment* (pp. 3–32). New York: Guilford Press.

Beech, H. R., & Vaughan, M. (1978). *Behavioural treatment of obsessional states.* Chichester, UK: Wiley.

Beck, A. T. (1972). *Depression: Causes and treatment.* Philadelphia: University of Pennsylvania Press. (Original work published 1967)

Beck, A. T. (1987). Cognitive models of depression. *Journal of Cognitive Psychotherapy: An International Quarterly, 1,* 5–37.

Beck, A. T., & Emery, G., with Greenberg, R. L. (1985). *Anxiety disorders and phobias: A cognitive perspective.* New York: Basic Books.

Beck, A. T., Rush, A. J., Shaw, B. F., & Emery, G. (1979). *Cognitive therapy of depression.* New York: Guilford Press.

Bouchard, C., Rhéaume, J., & Ladouceur, R. (1999). Responsibility and perfectionism in OCD: An experimental study. *Behaviour Research and Therapy, 37,* 239–248.

Carr, A. T. (1974). Compulsive neurosis: A review of the literature. *Psychological Bulletin, 81,* 311–318.

Chambless, D. L., Baker, M. J., Baucom, D. H., Beutler, L. E., Calhoun, K. S., Crits-Christoph, P., et al. (1998). Update on empirically validated therapies: II. *The Clinical Psychologist, 51,* 3–16.

Clark, D. A. (2004). *Cognitive-behavioral therapy for OCD.* New York: Guilford Press.

Clark, D. A., & Beck, A. T., with Alford, B. (1999). *Scientific foundations of cognitive theory and therapy of depression.* New York: Wiley.

Clark, D. A., & Purdon, C. L. (1993). New perspectives for a cognitive theory of obsessions. *Australian Psychologist, 28,* 161–167.

Clark, D. A., Purdon, C., & Wang, A. (2004). The Meta-Cognitive Beliefs Questionnaire: Development of a measure of obsessional beliefs. *Behaviour Research and Therapy, 41,* 655–669.

Crino, R. D., & Andrews, G. (1996). Obsessive–compulsive disorder and Axis I comorbidity. *Journal of Anxiety Disorders, 10,* 37–46.

de Haan, E., van Oppen, P., van Balkom, A. J. L. M., Spinhoven, P., Hoogduin, K. A. L., & van Dyck, R. (1997). Prediction of outcome and early vs. late improvement in OCD patients treated with cognitive behaviour therapy and pharmacotherapy. *Acta Psychiatrica Scandinavica, 96,* 354–361.

Emmelkamp, P. M. G. (1982). *Phobic and obsessive–compulsive disorders: Theory, research and practice.* New York: Plenum Press.

Emmelkamp, P. M. G., & Aardema, A. (1999). Metacognition, specific obsessive–compulsive beliefs and obsessive–compulsive behaviour. *Clinical Psychology and Psychotherapy, 6,* 139–145.

Emmelkamp, P. M. G., & Beens, H. (1991). Cognitive therapy with obsessive–compulsive disorder: A comparative evaluation. *Behaviour Research and Therapy, 29,* 293–300.

Emmelkamp, P. M. G., van Oppen, P., & van Balkom, A. J. L. M. (2002). Cognitive changes in patients with obsessive–compulsive rituals treated with exposure *in vivo* and response prevention. In R. O. Frost & G. Steketee (Eds.), *Cognitive approaches to obsessions and compulsions: Theory, assessment, and treatment* (pp. 392–401). Amsterdam: Elsevier.

Emmelkamp, P. M. G., Visser, S., & Hoekstra, R. J. (1988). Cognitive therapy vs. exposure *in vivo* in the treatment of obsessive–compulsives. *Cognitive Therapy and Research, 12,* 103–114.

Foa, E. B., Amir, N., Bogert, K. V. A., Molnar, C., & Przeworski, A. (2001). Inflated perception of responsibility for harm in obsessive–compulsive disorder. *Journal of Anxiety Disorders, 15,* 259–275.

Foa, E. B., & Kozak, M. J. (1995). DSM-IV field trial: Obsessive–compulsive disorder. *American Journal of Psychiatry, 152,* 90–96.

Foa, E. B., & Kozak, M. J. (1996). Psychological treatment for obsessive–compulsive disorder. In M. R. Mavissakalian & R. F. Prien (Eds.), *Long-term treatments of anxiety disorders* (pp. 285–309). Washington, DC: American Psychiatric Press.

Foa, E. B., & Steketee, G. (1979). Obsessive-compulsives: Conceptual issues and treatment interventions. In M. Hersen, R. M. Eisler, & P. M. Miller (Eds.), *Progress in behavior modification* (Vol. 8, pp. 1–53). New York: Academic Press.

Freeston, M. H., & Ladouceur, R. (1993). Appraisal of cognitive intrusions and response style: Replication and extension. *Behaviour Research and Therapy, 31,* 185–191.

Freeston, M. H., & Ladouceur, R. (1997). *The cognitive behavioral treatment of obsessions: A treatment manual.* Unpublished manuscript, École de Psychologie, Université Laval, Québec, Québec, Canada.

Freeston, M. H., Ladouceur, R., Gagnon, F., Thibodeau, N., Rhéaume, J., Letarte, H., & et al. (1997). Cognitive-behavioral treatment of obsessive thoughts: A controlled study. *Journal of Consulting and Clinical Psychology, 65,* 405–413.

Freeston, M. H., Ladouceur, R., Thibodeau, N., & Gagnon, F. (1991). Cognitive intrusions in a non-clinical population: I. Response style, subjective experience, and appraisal. *Behaviour Research and Therapy, 29,* 585–597.

Freeston, M. H., Rhéaume, J., & Ladouceur, R. (1996). Correcting faulty appraisals of obsessional thoughts. *Behaviour Research and Therapy, 34,* 433–446.

Frost, R. O., & Steketee, G. (1998). Hoarding: Clinical aspects and treatment strategies. In M. A. Jenike, L. Baer, & W. E. Minichiello (Eds.), *Obsessive–compulsive disorder: Practical management* (3rd ed., pp. 533–554). St. Louis, MO: Mosby.

Hollon, S. D., & Beck, A. T. (1986). Cognitive and cognitive-behavioral therapies. In S. L. Garfield & A. E. Bergin (Eds.), *Handbook of psychotherapy and behavior change* (3rd ed., pp. 443–482). New York: Wiley.

Jones, M. K., & Menzies, R. G. (1998). Danger ideation reduction therapy (DIRT) for obsessive–compulsive washers: A controlled trial. *Behavior Research and Therapy, 36,* 959–970.

Kozak, M. J., & Foa, E. B. (1997). *Mastery of obsessive–compulsive disorder: A cognitive-behavioral approach: Therapist guide.* Albany, NY: Graywind.

Kozak, M. J., Liebowitz, M. R., & Foa, E. B. (2000). Cognitive behavior therapy and pharmacotherapy for obsessive–compulsive disorder: The NIMH-sponsored collaborative study. In W. K. Goodman, M. V. Rudorfor, & J. D. Maser (Eds.), *Obsessive–compulsive disorder: Contemporary issues in treatment* (pp. 501–530). Mahwah, NJ: Erlbaum.

Ladouceur, R., Rhéaume, J., Freeston, M. H., Aublet, F., Jean, K., Lachange, S., et al. (1995). Experimental manipulations of responsibility: An analogue test for models of obsessive–compulsive disorder. *Behaviour Research and Therapy, 33*, 937–946.

Lopatka, C., & Rachman, S. (1995). Perceived responsibility and compulsive checking: An experimental analysis. *Behaviour Research and Therapy, 33*, 673–684.

March, J. S., Frances, A., Carpenter, D., & Kahn, D. A. (1997). Expert consensus guideline for treatment of obsessive–compulsive disorder. *Journal of Clinical Psychiatry, 58*(Suppl. 4), 5–72.

March, J. S., & Mulle, K. (1998). *OCD in children and adolescents: A cognitive-behavioral treatment manual*. New York: Guilford Press.

McFall, M. E., & Wollersheim, J. P. (1979). Obsessive–compulsive neurosis: A cognitive-behavioral formulation and approach to treatment. *Cognitive Therapy and Research, 3*, 333–348.

McLean, P. D., Whittal, M. L., Sochting, I., Koch, W. J., Paterson, R., Thordarson, D. S., et al. (2001). Cognitive versus behavior therapy in the group treatment of obsessive–compulsive disorder. *Journal of Consulting and Clinical Psychology, 69*, 205–214.

Menzies, R. G., Harris, L. M., Cumming, S. R., & Einstein, D. A. (2000). The relationship between inflated personal responsibility and exaggerated danger expectancies in obsessive–compulsive concerns. *Behaviour Research and Therapy, 38*, 1029–1037.

Meyer, V. (1966). Modifications of expectations in cases with obsessional rituals. *Behaviour Research and Therapy, 4*, 273–280.

Obsessive Compulsive Cognitions Working Group (OCCWG). (1997). Cognitive assessment of obsessive–compulsive disorder. *Behaviour Research and Therapy, 35*, 667–681.

Obsessive Compulsive Cognitions Working Group (OCCWG). (2001). Development and initial validation of the Obsessive Beliefs Questionnaire and the Interpretation of Intrusions Inventory. *Behaviour Research and Therapy, 39*, 987–1006.

Obsessive Compulsive Cognitions Working Group (OCCWG). (2003). Psychometric validation of the Obsessive Beliefs Questionnaire and the Interpretation of Intrusions Inventory: Part I. *Behaviour Research and Therapy, 41*, 863–878.

O'Connor, K., & Robillard, S. (1999). A cognitive approach to the treatment of primary inferences in obsessive–compulsive disorder. *Journal of Cognitive Psychotherapy: An International Quarterly, 13*, 359–375.

O'Connor, K., Todorov, C., Robillard, S., Borgeat, F., & Brault, M. (1999). Cognitive-behaviour therapy and medication in the treatment of obsessive–compulsive disorder: A controlled study. *Canadian Journal of Psychiatry, 44*, 64–71.

Parkinson, L., & Rachman, S. (1981). Part II. The nature of intrusive thoughts. *Advances in Behaviour Research and Therapy, 3*, 101–110.

Purdon, C. (1999). Thought suppression and psychopathology. *Behaviour Research and Therapy, 37*, 1029–1054.

Purdon, C. (2001). Appraisal of obsessional thought recurrences: Impact on anxiety and mood state. *Behavior Therapy, 32*, 47–64.

Purdon, C., & Clark, D. A. (1993). Obsessive intrusive thoughts in nonclinical subjects: Part I. Content and relation with depressive, anxious and obsessional symptoms. *Behaviour Research and Therapy, 31*, 713–720.

Purdon, C., & Clark, D. A. (2002). The need to control thoughts. In R. O. Frost & G. Steketee (Eds.), *Cognitive approaches to obsessions and compulsions: Theory, assessment and treatment* (pp. 29–43). Amsterdam: Elsevier.

Rachman, S. J. (1971). Obsessional ruminations. *Behaviour Research and Therapy, 9,* 229–235.

Rachman, S. J. (1976). The modification of obsessions: A new formulation. *Behaviour Research and Therapy, 14,* 437–443.

Rachman, S. J. (1978). An anatomy of obsessions. *Behaviour Analysis and Modification, 2,* 253–278.

Rachman, S. J. (1983). Obstacles to the successful treatment of obsessions. In E. B. Foa & P. M. G. Emmelkamp (Ed.), *Failures in behavior therapy* (pp. 35–57). New York: Wiley.

Rachman, S. J. (1985). An overview of clinical and research issues in obsessional–compulsive disorders. In M. Mavissakalian, S. M. Turner, & L. Michelson (Eds.), *Obsessive–compulsive disorder: Psychological and pharmacological treatment* (pp. 1–47). New York: Plenum Press.

Rachman, S. J. (1993). Obsessions, responsibility and guilt. *Behaviour Research and Therapy, 31,* 149–154.

Rachman, S. J. (1997). A cognitive theory of obsessions. *Behaviour Research and Therapy, 35,* 793–802.

Rachman, S. J. (1998). A cognitive theory of obsessions: Elaborations. *Behaviour Research and Therapy, 36,* 385–401.

Rachman, S. J. (2003). *The treatment of obsessions.* Oxford: Oxford University Press.

Rachman, S. J., & de Silva, P. (1978). Abnormal and normal obsessions. *Behaviour Research and Therapy, 16,* 233–248.

Rachman, S. J., & Hodgson, R. J. (1980). *Obsessions and compulsions.* Englewood Cliffs, NJ: Prentice-Hall.

Rachman, S. J., Hodgson, R., & Marzillier, J. (1970). Treatment of an obsessional–compulsive disorder by modeling. *Behaviour Research and Therapy, 8,* 385–392.

Rachman, S. J., & Shafran, R. (1998). Cognitive and behavioral features of obsessive–compulsive disorder. In R. P. Swinson, M. M. Antony, S. Rachman, & M. A. Richter (Eds.), *Obsessive–compulsive disorder: Theory, research, and treatment* (pp. 51–78). New York: Guilford Press.

Rachman, S., & Shafran, R. (1999). Cognitive distortions: Thought–action fusion. *Clinical Psychology and Psychotherapy, 6,* 80–85.

Rachman, S., Thordarson, D. S., Shafran, R., & Woody, S. R. (1995). Perceived responsibility: Structure and significance. *Behaviour Research and Therapy, 33,* 779–784.

Rasmussen, S. A., & Eisen, J. L. (1992). The epidemiology and clinical features of obsessive compulsive disorder. *Psychiatric Clinics of North America, 15,* 743–758.

Rasmussen, S. A., & Tsuang, M. T. (1986). Clinical characteristics and family history in DSM-III obsessive–compulsive disorder. *American Journal of Psychiatry, 143,* 317–322.

Reed, G. F. (1985). *Obsessional experience and compulsive behavior: A cognitive-structural approach.* Orlando, FL: Academic Press.

Salkovskis, P. M. (1985). Obsessional–compulsive problems: A cognitive-behavioural analysis. *Behaviour Research and Therapy, 23,* 571–583.

Salkovskis, P. M. (1989a). Cognitive-behavioural factors and the persistence of intrusive thoughts in obsessional problems. *Behaviour Research and Therapy, 27,* 677–682.

Salkovskis, P. M. (1989b). Obsessions and compulsions. In J. Scott, J. Mark, G. Williams & A. T. Beck (Eds.), *Cognitive therapy in clinical practice: An illustrative casebook* (pp. 50–77). New York: Routledge.

Salkovskis, P. M. (1998). Psychological approaches to the understanding of obsessional problems. In R. P. Swinson, M. M. Antony, S. Rachman, & M. A. Richter (Eds.), *Obsessive–compulsive disorder: Theory, research, and treatment* (pp. 33–50). New York: Guilford Press.

Salkovskis, P. M. (1999). Understanding and treating obsessive–compulsive disorder. *Behaviour Research and Therapy, 37,* S29–S52.

Salkovskis, P. M., Richards, H. C., & Forrester, E. (1995). The relationship between obsessional problems and intrusive thoughts. *Behavioural and Cognitive Psychotherapy, 23,* 281–299.

Salkovskis, P. M., & Wahl, K. (2004). Treating obsessional problems using cognitive-behavioural therapy. In M. Reinecke & D. A. Clark (Eds.), *Cognitive therapy across the lifespan: Theory, research and practice* (pp. 138–171). Cambridge, UK: Cambridge University Press.

Salkovskis, P. M., Wroe, A. L., Gledhill, A., Morrison, N., Forrester, E., Richards, C., et al. (2000). Responsibility attitudes and interpretations are characteristic of obsessive compulsive disorder. *Behaviour Research and Therapy, 38,* 347–372.

Shafran, R. (1997). The manipulation of responsibility in obsessive–compulsive disorder. *British Journal of Clinical Psychology, 36,* 397–407.

Stanley, M. A., & Turner, S. M. (1995). Current status of pharmacological and behavioral treatment of obsessive–compulsive disorder. *Behavior Therapy, 26,* 163–186.

Steketee, G. S. (1993). *Treatment of obsessive compulsive disorder.* New York: Guilford Press.

Steketee, G. S., Frost, R. O., & Cohen, I. (1998). Beliefs in obsessive–compulsive disorder. *Journal of Anxiety Disorders, 12,* 525–537.

Steketee, G., Frost, R. O., Rhéaume, J., & Wilhelm, S. (1998). Cognitive theory and treatment of obsessive–compulsive disorder. In M. A. Jenike, L. Baer, & W. E. Minichiello (Eds.), *Obsessive–compulsive disorders: Practical management* (3rd ed., pp. 368–399). St. Louis, MO: Mosby.

Steketee, G., & Shapiro, L. J. (1995). Predicting behavioral treatment outcome for agoraphobia and obsessive compulsive disorder. *Clinical Psychology, 15,* 317–346.

Thordarson, D. S., & Shafran, R. (2002). Importance of thoughts. In R. O. Frost & G. Steketee (Eds.), *Cognitive approaches to obsessions and compulsions: Theory, assessment and treatment* (pp. 15–28). Amsterdam: Elsevier.

Tolin, D. F., Abramowitz, J. S., Hamlin, C., & Synodi, D. S. (2002). Attributions for thought suppression failure in obsessive–compulsive disorder. *Cognitive Therapy and Research, 26,* 505–517.

van Balkom, A. J. L. M., van Oppen, P., Vermeulen, A. W. A., Nauta, M. C. E., & Vorst, H. C. M. (1994). A meta-analysis on the treatment of obsessive compulsive disorder: A comparison of antidepressants, behavior, and cognitive therapy. *Clinical Psychology Review, 14,* 359–381.

van Oppen, P., de Haan, E., van Balkom, A. J. L. M., Spinhoven, P., Hoogduin, K., & van Dyck, R. (1995). Cognitive therapy and exposure *in vivo* in the treatment of obsessive compulsive disorder. *Behaviour Research and Therapy, 33*, 379–390.

Wilson, K. A., & Chambless, D. L. (1999). Inflated perceptions of responsibility and obsessive–compulsive symptoms. *Behaviour Research and Therapy, 37*, 325–335.

Wegner, D. M. (1994). Ironic processes of mental control. *Psychological Review, 101*, 34–52.

Wenzlaff, R. M., & Wegner, D. M. (2000). Thought suppression. *Annual Review of Psychology, 51*, 59–91.

Whittal, M. L., & McLean, P. D. (1999). CBT for OCD: The rationale, protocol, and challenges. *Cognitive and Behavioral Practice, 6*, 383–396.

Whittal, M. L., & McLean, P. D. (2002). Group cognitive behavioral therapy for obsessive compulsive disorder. In R. O. Frost & G. Steketee (Eds.), *Cognitive approaches to obsessions and compulsions: Theory, assessment, and treatment* (pp. 417–433). Amsterdam: Elsevier.

Chapter 9

Metacognitive Therapy

Elements of Mental Control
in Understanding and Treating
Generalized Anxiety Disorder
and Posttraumatic Stress Disorder

ADRIAN WELLS

Emotionally disordered thinking has a particular style that is repetitive, brooding, and apparently difficult to control. Generalized anxiety disorder (GAD) is dominated by excessive and uncontrollable worrying. In posttraumatic stress disorder (PTSD), a significant symptom cluster comprises recurrent intrusive recollections of the traumatic event. Obsessive–compulsive disorder is marked by a preoccupation with intrusive thoughts of a repugnant quality, and depression is dominated by repetitive negative ruminations about the self, world, and future.

Cognitive theory and therapy (Beck, 1967/1972, 1976) have focused on examining the content of negative thoughts and beliefs, but analyzing the causes and effects of the repetitive and out-of-control thinking style that is characteristic of pathology provides a platform for advancing theory and treatment. In this chapter, I briefly outline features of the metacognitive theory and therapy of emotional disorders, with the aim of delineating the elements important for conceptualizing the regulation of thinking processes. The roles of these elements in the development and persistence of two disorders, GAD and PTSD, are described in detail. Finally, the nature of metacognitive therapy for GAD and PTSD is described. This chapter is dedicated to Aaron T. Beck in gratitude for his continued support, and in recognition of his seminal contributions to theory and treatment.

ELEMENTS OF MENTAL CONTROL

Conceptualizing the regulation of thinking requires a cognitive architecture that explains the relative roles of "bottom-up" and "top-down" processing. Top-down (strategic) processing is that guided by the individual's beliefs and is typically amenable to consciousness, whereas bottom-up processing is reflexively driven by interconnected networks of processing units and does not require significant attentional resources. Evidence suggests that many cognitive processes, such as biased attention and the continued execution of rumination or worry thinking styles, is controlled in nature and influenced by strategies under top-down control (for reviews, see Wells & Matthews, 1994; Matthews & Wells, 2000).

A model of mental control crucially requires a distinction between two qualitatively separable subtypes of cognition, in which cognitive activity itself is distinguished from the cognitions that lead to the regulation and appraisal of cognitive activity (i.e., metacognitions). The term "metacognitions" refers to knowledge or beliefs about thinking, the monitoring and control of cognition, and appraisals and subjective feelings that signal the meaning and status of cognitive processes (Flavell, 1979; Nelson & Narens, 1990; Wells, 2000). A classic example of a metacognition is the metacognitive experience of the "tip-of-the-tongue" state, in which an individual knows that an item of information is stored in memory even though it is not currently accessible. Such a state is associated with persistent efforts to retrieve the memory and escape the mildly unpleasant feelings associated with the "tip-of-the-tongue" effect.

Intentions and goals are further factors that have a crucial bearing on the regulation and control of thinking. There are goals that are amenable to personal awareness and form part of the person's volitional strategies. There are also internal, implicit, systemic goals that provide reference points for more automatic homeostatic cognitive processes. There may be conflict in the pursuit of different volitional goals, and conflict between volitional goals and in-built systemic goal-directed responses. I will argue that such conflict in self-regulation processes can be a source of persistence of psychopathology. An example of conflict can be seen in the metacognitive model of GAD (Wells, 1994, 1999), in which patients hold opposing positive and negative beliefs about worry, leading to vacillation in attempts to engage and avoid worry.

In summary, formulating the control of cognition—and consequently the dysfunction in control seen as perseveration in emotional disorder—requires an understanding of several elements, including (1) metacognitions, (2) intentions/goals, and (3) conflict in self-regulation. Later in this chapter, we will see how these factors contribute to GAD and PTSD.

EMOTIONAL DISORDER AND THE SELF-REGULATORY EXECUTIVE FUNCTION MODEL

The "self-regulatory executive function" (S-REF) model (Wells & Matthews, 1994, 1996; Wells, 2000) of emotional disorder explicitly includes the elements identified above. This model asserts that vulnerability to disorder and the persistence of disorder are linked to the activation of a pattern of cognition. The pattern is referred to as the "cognitive attentional syndrome" (CAS) and consists of worry/rumination, attentional strategies of threat monitoring, and coping behaviors that fail to restructure maladaptive beliefs. The CAS is a cognitive-behavioral style that is difficult to bring under control and, once activated, "locks" the individual into emotional disturbance. A marker for the CAS is often excessive and adhesive self-focused attention. The CAS is a process or cognitive style that can be viewed as independent of the content of cognition, and is directed by the individual's metacognitions. Much of the knowledge on which processing draws is metacognitive in nature and includes propositional beliefs about thinking (e.g., "Certain thoughts are bad and must be controlled"), as well as plans that guide processing. Although plans can be verbally expressed as assumptions or directives (e.g., "I must mentally plan the future in order to cope," "If I pay due attention to my body, I'll detect any serious problems"), much of the metacognitive knowledge on which processing draws is not amenable to consciousness. In order to have an impact on self-regulation, plans contain directives and goals, so that they represent a program for cognition and action. For example, an adaptive plan for handling social criticism can be represented as follows:

"If the boss criticizes my work
THEN
politely ask how I can improve it
THEN
if the boss gives reasonable feedback
THEN
focus on problem solving and changing my performance until my boss is satisfied."

However, a maladaptive plan of a depression-prone individual that gives rise to the CAS and persistent depression may be written as follows:

"If the boss criticizes my work
THEN
Focus on my weaknesses and failings, and review my memory of past failures
THEN
If this is a reasonable appraisal
THEN
Focus on analyzing what's wrong with me, until I have a feeling of understanding."

Schema theory of emotional disorder (Beck, 1976; Beck, Rush, Shaw, & Emery, 1979), with its emphasis on non-metacognitive beliefs (e.g., "I'm a failure"), does not readily account for the difference in cognitive-behavioral styles as exemplified above. In the S-REF model, attentional strategies, and worry/ruminative styles of cognition are forms of coping that are represented differently from the concept of the traditional dysfunctional schema. The propensity to engage in maladaptive patterns of thinking is guided by metacognitive knowledge. The S-REF model proposes that psychological disorder is maintained by a pattern of cognition consisting of attentional monitoring for threat, repetitive negative thinking styles of worry/rumination, and coping behaviors that fail to restructure maladaptive beliefs. The metacognitive formulation provided by the S-REF model suggests that psychological vulnerability is located predominantly at the level of volitional (strategic) processing driven by metacognitions, and linked to the activation of negative, self-perpetuating processing configurations that fail to modify dysfunctional self-beliefs. However, these processes (i.e., the CAS) have an impact on lower-level processing and can in some cases thwart more reflexive self-regulatory processes. In the remainder of this chapter, I will elucidate in detail these dimensions, and the consequences of metacognitive control of processing as they relate to the persistence and treatment of GAD and PTSD.

THE METACOGNITIVE MODEL OF GAD

GAD is characterized by chains of subjectively uncontrollable and distressing worry, with a range of psychomotor and somatic symptoms. Worrying is a repetitive, negative, and predominantly verbal conceptual activity (Borkovec, Robinson, Pruzinsky, & DePree, 1983) that has been differentiated from other types of repetitive thoughts, such as depressive rumination

(Papageorgiou & Wells, 1999) and obsessional thoughts (Clark & Claybourn, 1997; Wells & Morrison, 1994). Cognitive-behavioral therapy for GAD has relatively modest effects, with only approximately 50% of patients achieving significant clinical improvement (Fisher & Durham, 1999) at the end of this type of treatment. Perhaps the main reason for this disappointing outcome has been the absence of a cognitive model that explains the occurrence, persistence, and uncontrollable worry characteristic of the disorder. GAD appears to be a relatively "pure" manifestation of the CAS explained by the S-REF theory. Recently, the metacognitive model of GAD (Figure 9.1) grounded in this theory has received empirical support.

The metacognitive model of GAD (Wells, 1995, 1997) proposes that individuals suffering from this disorder use worrying as a predominant means of coping with anticipated dangers and threats to the self and personal world. The central components of the model are depicted in Figure 9.1. Worrying consists of a series of "What if . . . " catastrophizing questions, and conceptual planning in which the person attempts to generate a series of coping responses. This "Type 1" worrying is triggered by intruding thoughts or stresses that activate positive beliefs about the usefulness of engaging Type 1 worrying. Such worrying continues until the individual is distracted by concurrent concerns, or until some internal goal-related criterion signaling that it is safe to stop worrying is achieved. The internal criterion is often a feeling state or a sense that all currently available possibili-

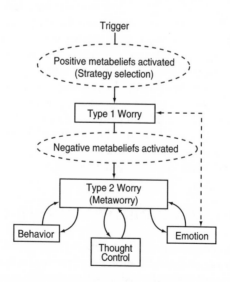

FIGURE 9.1. The metacognitive model of GAD. Adapted from Wells (1997, p. 204). Copyright 1997 by John Wiley & Sons Limited. Adapted by permission.

ties for negative outcomes have been dealt with. Positive metacognitive beliefs about the power and usefulness of worrying and negative conceptual activity support the sustained use of worrying as a predominant means of coping. Examples of positive beliefs include "Worrying helps me cope," "If I worry I'll be prepared," "Worrying keeps me in control," and "Worrying protects me from danger." The existence of positive beliefs is not in itself problematic, although the process of repeated worrying may be in some situations. However, people prone to GAD tend to be less flexible in their use of worrying, choosing the strategy as a preferred mode of preparation and coping.

For GAD to develop fully, negative appraisals of worrying have to occur. These are closely linked to the acquisition of negative metacognitive beliefs about the nature, danger, and consequences of worrying. Negative beliefs center on two themes: (1) the uncontrollability of worry; (2) and the danger of worry, which includes concerns about its emotional sequelae and its effects on mental, physical, and/or social well-being. Examples of negative beliefs are "Worrying is uncontrollable," "Worry can cause mental illness," "Worrying can lead to loss of control," and "Worrying can damage my body." Once negative beliefs are established, there is a tendency to interpret the worry process negatively when it is activated. The negative interpretation of worrying is termed "metaworry" (i.e., worry about worry) or "Type 2 worry." Once negative appraisals are activated during a worry episode, anxiety and other emotional responses are intensified. When individuals appraise worrying as imminently catastrophic, rapid intensifications of anxiety can result, culminating in panic attacks. The emotional consequences of metaworry mean that it is more difficult for these individuals to obtain an internal state signaling that it is safe to stop worrying. Moreover, anxiety symptoms may become triggers for new episodes of Type 1 worrying as the individuals attempt to analyze and cope with their subjective state.

Two additional processes contribute to problem maintenance once metaworry and negative beliefs are established. These processes are the metacognitive strategies used by an individual, which can be usefully separated into behaviors and thought control strategies. People with GAD have conflicting beliefs about worrying, believing that it is both beneficial but also potentially uncontrollable and harmful. One way to deal with this conflict is to try to avoid the need to worry in the first place. This can be accomplished by avoiding the triggers for worrying (such as medical programs, television news, magazine articles, etc.). An individual may also transfer responsibility for the control of worrying to a significant other, such as a spouse or partner. For instance, a patient avoided uncertainty concerning the welfare of her partner by asking him to provide frequent reassurances that he was safe when he was away from home. The problem with these strategies is that they remove an opportunity to discover that worrying is subject to self-control; thus negative beliefs concerning uncontrollability fail to be revised. By removing the triggers for worrying, individuals may also fail to encounter situations that challenge beliefs concerning the dangers of worrying. For instance, if reassurance effectively terminates a worry episode, an individual is unable to discover that the worry episode does not culminate in mental breakdown.

Strategies separated out for individual attention in the model are an individual's thought control strategies. These are distinguished from other behaviors in Figure 9.1 because of an important dynamic that perpetuates metaworry and negative beliefs. Because the individual holds conflicting positive and negative beliefs about worrying, there is ambivalence or vacillation in attempts to control worrying. When positive beliefs are activated, the individual does not make a concerted effort to interrupt worrying; however, when negative beliefs and metaworry are activated, the individual may attempt not to think worrying thoughts. Unfortunately, thought suppression strategies of this kind are rarely effective, and their ineffectiveness may be appraised as further evidence of loss of control over thinking. This situation deprives the person of experiences that would challenge negative beliefs about uncontrollability. However, even if worrying was successfully interrupted, problems would still remain, because successful interruption of worrying would not allow the person to discover that worrying is not dangerous.

The metacognitive model of GAD incorporates the different elements of cognitive control identified earlier, and it describes their interrelationship in contributing to the development and persistence of pathological worrying. Metacognitive beliefs are important in promoting the execution of worrying as a coping strategy, and metacognitive beliefs contribute to negative interpretation of the nature and consequences of worrying. The motivations and goals of the individual are multiple in nature. However, the most central motivation and goal is generation of coping responses and plans for dealing with anticipated future threats and challenges to the self. In GAD, many of these threats are located in the future, and so the individual is faced with the problem of knowing in the present that he or she will be able to cope in the future. Since no objective criteria for assessing coping effectively with imagined threats are available, the individual uses internal criteria as a signal that it is appropriate to stop worrying. Thus an immediate self-regulatory goal is the attainment of an internal feeling state or state of knowing that signals that the work of worrying has been effectively accomplished. Conflict in self-regulation is evident in the opposing influences of positive and negative metacognitive beliefs on thinking processes and thought control attempts. Moreover, as we will see later in the chapter, a preponderance of worry may impair lower-level processes, such as those supporting emotional processing.

EMPIRICAL SUPPORT FOR THE GAD MODEL

Research on nonpatients with high levels of GAD-like worry, and on patients with GAD, has provided support for central aspects of this model.

A colleague and I (Wells & Carter, 1999) used the Anxious Thoughts Inventory to test the relationships among Type 1 worries (social and health worries), Type 2 worry (metaworry), and pathological worry in nonpatients. Pathological worrying was measured with the Penn State Worry Questionnaire (Meyer, Miller, Metzger, & Borkovec, 1990), which assesses proneness to chronic, excessive, and general worry like that found in GAD. According to the model, Type 2 worry should predict pathological worrying independently of Type 1 worrying. Consistent with this hypothesis, Type 2 worry and trait anxiety made significant and independent contributions to pathological worrying. Social and health (Type 1) worries were nonsignificant.

In another study (Wells, in press), I developed a specific measure of metaworry—focusing on danger-related appraisals of worrying, and omitting the uncontrollability dimension to prevent confounds with GAD as defined in the *Diagnostic and Statistical Manual of Mental Disorders*, fourth edition (DSM-IV). The Meta-Worry Questionnaire consists of seven items, samples of which are as follows: "I am going crazy with worrying," "My worrying will escalate and I'll cease to function," and "My body can't take the worrying." Nonpatient participants were classified as meeting criteria for DSM-IV GAD, somatic anxiety, or no anxiety on the basis of scores on the Generalized Anxiety Disorder Questionnaire (GADQ; Roemer, Borkovec, Posa, & Borkovec, 1995). Individuals meeting criteria for GAD showed significantly higher metaworry frequency scores than participants in the groups with somatic anxiety or no anxiety. The groups with GAD also differed significantly from the nonanxious group in metaworry belief level. Even when the frequencies of Type 1 (social and health) worries were treated as covariates, the differences in metaworry remained. In a third study, we (Wells & Carter, 2001) showed that negative beliefs about worry and metaworry significantly distinguished patients with DSM-III-R GAD from patients with panic disorder or social phobia and from nonpatient controls. Moreover, discriminant-function analysis indicated that patients with GAD were best discriminated from those in the other three groups by scores on negative metacognitions.

Taken together, the above-described studies suggest that pathological worrying and the presence of GAD are associated with negative metacognitions at the appraisal and belief level. Such metacognitions appear to be more specific to pathological worry and GAD than are the frequencies of different Type 1 worries. Other questionnaire studies of nonpatients support these relationships (Cartwright-Hatton & Wells, 1997; Wells & Papageorgiou, 1998).

Although negative metacognitions are a central aspect of GAD in the metacognitive model, the model also holds that patients have positive beliefs about worrying. In two studies investigating the reasons given for worrying by students, Borkovec and Roemer (1995) showed that subjects rated motivation, preparation, and avoidance as the most characteristic reasons for their worry. Individuals meeting criteria for GAD (based on scores on the GADQ) rated using worry for distraction from more upsetting things significantly more than nonanxious subjects did. In a second study, participants with GAD gave significantly higher ratings than nonworried, anxious, or nonanxious subjects for using worry as distraction from more emotional topics. The subjects with GAD also gave significantly higher ratings for superstitious reasons for worrying and the use of worry for problem solving than nonanxious subjects did. In summary, individuals meeting criteria for GAD report positive reasons for worrying (Borkovec & Roemer, 1995), and such reasons appear to resemble positive attitudes toward or beliefs about worrying. Several correlational studies have shown that positive beliefs about worrying are associated with proneness to pathological worry (Cartwright-Hatton & Wells, 1997; Wells & Papageorgiou, 1998).

The causal role of negative metacognitions in the development of DSM-III-R-defined GAD was explored in a study by Nassif (1999). In this study, nonpatient participants were tracked over a 12- to 15-week period and were administered the GADQ and metacognition measures. Consistent with the model, negative beliefs about worrying in the uncontrollability and danger domains assessed at Time 1 positively predicted the development of GAD 12–15 weeks later when diagnostic status at Time 1 was controlled for.

The metacognitive model of GAD suggests that because of conflicting positive and negative beliefs about worry, patients are likely to vacillate between attempts to control and permit worrying. A study by Purdon (2000) has produced evidence appearing to support the suggestion that positive and negative metacognitions are linked to differential and potentially conflicting thought control responses. She examined the effects of in vivo negative appraisal of worrying in nonpatients. Negative appraisals of worry were associated with greater attempts at thought control. However, positive beliefs about worrying emerged as concurrent predictors of a reduced motivation to get rid of thoughts; thus positive and negative beliefs appear to have concurrent and conflicting effects on thought control responses and motivations. Finally, numerous studies support the idea that attempts to suppress thoughts are not particularly effective (Wegner, Schneider, Carter, & White, 1987; Purdon, 1999); it should be stressed, however, that most of these studies have not investigated the effect specifically in GAD. According to the model, not only the effectiveness of strategies, but their effects on preventing change in negative beliefs, are important. This area remains to be investigated.

The studies reviewed above suggest that pathological worrying and GAD are associated with positive and negative metacognitive beliefs. Moreover, negative metacognitions distinguish patients with GAD from patients with other anxiety disorders and from nonpatients. Preliminary indications are that negative metacognitions appear to be causally linked to the development of GAD, and that the existence of positive and negative beliefs appears to be associated with conflicting motivations and attempts to get rid of worrying thoughts. These results are consistent with the metacognitive model of the development and maintenance of GAD. Later in this chapter, I will review evidence from further studies that worrying has negative consequences for self-regulation. Individuals who use worrying as a coping strategy report elevated emotional vulnerability scores on a self-report level and appear to show an increased propensity to develop PTSD symptoms following trauma.

METACOGNITIVE THERAPY FOR GAD

The disappointing effects obtained in standard cognitive-behavioral interventions for GAD can be explained in terms of traditional treatments' not targeting the metacognitive factors (erroneous beliefs about worry and associated behaviors) that maintain excessive, out-of-control worrying. The new approach suggests that treatment should shift from focusing on modifying the content of individual Type 1 worries to modifying beliefs about and interpretations of worrying itself. The model also predicts that relapse following treatment should be positively associated with the persistence of metacognitive beliefs.

The model presented in Figure 9.1 is the basis of constructing an individual case formulation. Treatment techniques focus first on challenging negative beliefs concerning uncontrollability, and then on challenging negative beliefs concerning the dangers of worrying. Beliefs about uncontrollability are modifiable by verbal reattribution methods involving reviewing the evidence and counterevidence for absence of control. The natural modulators of worrying are discussed in this context to show how competing or distracting activities can displace the act of worrying. Such events are used as examples that worrying is subject to control and therefore is not completely uncontrollable. Patients are also questioned about how worrying typically stops. For instance, "When you start worrying, how does it come to an end? Why doesn't it continue permanently?" Such questions can be used to show how worry states are not permanent and can be modulated by other activities or events.

Behavioral experiments provide a powerful means of challenging beliefs about uncontrollability. Worry postponement experiments are used for this purpose. A patient is asked to notice a trigger for worrying, and then—rather than engaging in the Type 1 worry sequence—to choose not to worry and postpone the worrying until a set period of time later in the day. During a later allotted worry period, patients can chose to worry for a set time of 10 minutes, which can be used to provide further evidence that worrying can be controlled. After some initial skepticism, patients are typically surprised to find that they can postpone worrying, and many of them forget to use or choose not to use the worry period. This technique is presented as a specific strategy for challenging beliefs about uncontrollability, and levels of these beliefs are monitored throughout this phase of treatment. The next stage in behavioral experiments concerns using the allotted worry episode—during which time patients are instructed to try deliberately to lose control of worrying—to demonstrate that this is not possible.

Once uncontrollability beliefs have been effectively challenged beliefs about the dangers of worrying, such as the belief that it may lead to mental breakdown or bodily damage, are targeted. Questioning the evidence and counterevidence for these beliefs is useful. The reinforcement of conscious cognitive dissonance by highlighting the coexistence and conflict of positive and negative beliefs about worrying is used to weaken the metacognitive belief system. Verbal reattribution consists of questioning the mechanism by which such deleterious effects can occur, linked with providing education to correct faulty knowledge. For example, some patients believe that worrying will lead to mental breakdown or mental illness. The role of anxiety- and worry-based responses in preparing the individual to deal effectively with threat can be described as a means of decatastrophizing the consequences of worrying and anxiety. A point made here is that worry and anxiety are part of the individual's coping mechanism—part of the fight-or-flight response. It is not reasonable to assume, therefore, that they will cause paralysis or mental breakdown. This may be broadened to a wider discussion of stress effects, as many patients present with general fears about the adverse consequences of emotions and stress responses. It is useful to point to the literature suggesting that stress and strong emotion themselves are not necessarily problematic. Moreover, worry and stress are not accurately conceptualized as synonymous. Behavioral experiments provide a means of unambiguously testing predictions concerning the dangerous consequences of worrying. Here, participants are asked to worry more in situations in order to try to produce a feared mental or physiological catastrophe.

Following the successful abolition of negative beliefs, therapy focuses on positive beliefs about worrying and the tendency that patients have to use worrying as an inflexible means of dealing with threat. Positive metacognitive beliefs are challenged by reviewing the evidence and counter-evidence for them, and by using a variety of specific procedures. One procedure consists of asking patients to engage in activities normally associated with worrying while deliberately modulating the level of worry. For example, when an individual believes that worrying assists performance and coping, manipulations of the level of worrying on a day-to-day basis can be examined in the context of whether or not it improves or impairs performance or coping outcomes. If the patient is correct in believing that worrying improves coping, then abandonment of worrying for 1 or 2 days should lead to evidence of poorer coping, while increasing worrying for 1 or 2 days should lead to evidence of improved coping. To maximize the effectiveness of experiments of this type, it is beneficial to operationalize in observable and testable terms precisely what is meant by "coping" and what would be a sign of lowered or increased levels.

Finally, the therapist reviews with the patient alternative strategies for dealing with threat and negative intrusive cognitions that may trigger worrying. Since many patients have been worriers for most of their lives, it is helpful to explore alternative thinking strategies. For instance, patients may be asked to respond to a negative thought intrusion by imagining a positive ending relating to that intrusion, rather than engaging in their normal Type 1 "What if . . . " catastrophizing sequence. Similarly, patients may be asked to practice engaging in activities without protracted worrying or analysis of potential future consequences. This can be described as a strategy of "doing without thinking."

This brief section on treatment is intended only to provide an overall impression of metacognitive therapy for GAD, and the interested practitioner should consult more detailed treatment guidelines (e.g., Wells, 1997, 2000).

THE METACOGNITIVE MODEL OF PTSD

The S-REF model has been applied to conceptualizing failures in emotional processing following trauma (Wells & Matthews, 1994). Intrusions following trauma are thought to be adaptive in their normal form, since they interrupt ongoing processing activities and stimulate the selection and modification of upper-level knowledge and plans for dealing with threat. However, such intrusions can become problematic and can stall emotional processing when they are themselves appraised negatively on the basis of dysfunctional metacognitive beliefs, and when the CAS of worry/rumination, threat monitoring, and maladaptive coping is activated.

An important question in formulating emotional processing mechanisms concerns the precise goal of emotional processing. In the S-REF
model (Wells, 2000), the goal of emotional processing following stress or
trauma is the development of a mental configuration or plan that can be
called upon when similar stresses are encountered in the future. This is normally achieved through a process that has been dubbed the "reflexive adaptation process" (RAP; Wells & Sembi, in press). The RAP involves dynamic
interactions between lower-level processing activity and online processing,
often involving mental simulations of dealing with the stressor. Such simulations are capable of helping a person form a rudimentary plan for cognition and action in the future. However, the CAS interferes with this process.
Excessive self-focused attention, worry/rumination, threat monitoring, and
maladaptive thought control strategies such as avoidance interfere with the
RAP. For instance, threat-monitoring strategies are problematic because
they repeatedly present threat-related or arousal-related information to
consciousness, and they use processing resources that could otherwise be
effectively used for the development of an alternative plan for coping. Strategies such as worry and threat monitoring lock the patient into a "threat
configuration" of processing, which paradoxically maintains anxiety and
strengthens metacognitive plans for processing danger. Under these circumstances, the individual's cognitive system is unable to retune to the normal
threat-free environment. A number of factors can enhance worry and
threat monitoring: (1) aspects of the posttraumatic psychosocial environment, such as lack of social support or criticism; (2) subsequent life stresses
that contribute to worry and threat monitoring; (3) negative appraisals of
the effectiveness with which the individual dealt with the stressor; (4)
negative beliefs about symptoms and about emotional responses; and (5)
positive metacognitive beliefs about the need to focus on threat and engage
worry/rumination.

Several different categories of positive and negative metacognitive beliefs are implicated in this model. Individuals with PTSD possess positive
metacognitive beliefs (1) that it is necessary to ruminate, or analyze the
meaning, nature, and consequences of the trauma; (2) that threat monitoring and hypervigilance are effective means of coping; and (3) that worry
about future dangers is a useful preemptive coping/avoidance strategy. On
the negative belief side, metacognitions concern the abnormal or dangerous
consequences of emotional responses and intrusions. Metacognitive control
strategies that are problematic include attempts to suppress thoughts concerning the trauma or to avoid situations or reminders of the trauma.

In contrast to maladaptive processing that interferes with the RAP,
adaptive processing includes cognitive simulations that culminate in a plan
for coping, the disengagement of negative conceptual activity (worry/rumi-
nation), the acceptance of symptoms, the flexible use of attention, and the

redirection of attention away from threat and onto nonthreatening aspects of the environment.

The metacognitive model of PTSD incorporates the elements of cognitive control identified at the outset of this chapter. Metacognitive beliefs promote worry/rumination and threat monitoring as coping strategies, and they contribute to negative interpretations of stress symptoms. The motivations and goals of the individual consist of developing plans and strategies for dealing with threat. Whereas some goals are volitional and under top-down control, others are features of homeostatic lower-level processes. Achievement of these goals is signaled by conscious appraisals of current safety, and by internal feeling states (such as arousal level) generated through more reflexive processes. In the model, conflict is apparent in the tension that exists between lower-level processes (which repeatedly reintroduce threat-related material into consciousness in the form of intrusions/arousal) and upper-level processes (which attempt to exclude such material and lead to a fixation of processing on danger, exemplified by worry and threat monitoring). Thus lower-level reductions of arousal due to natural habituation, and retuning of cognition to the normal threat-free environment, are thwarted.

EMPIRICAL SUPPORT FOR THE PTSD MODEL

The metacognitive model of PTSD suggests that metacognitive coping strategies should be linked to PTSD symptoms and negative outcomes following stress. Studies of both a cross-sectional and a longitudinal nature have examined the relationship between thought control strategies and posttrauma stress symptoms. Individual differences in strategies used to control distressing thoughts can be measured with the Thought Control Questionnaire (TCQ; Wells & Davies, 1994). This instrument consists of five factorially derived domains: distraction, social control, worry, punishment, and reappraisal. The use of worry and punishment (which involves negative self-appraisal and negative behaviors) to control thought is positively associated with stress vulnerability and appears elevated in clinical disorders.

Research with the TCQ provides evidence concerning the effects of using worry as a strategy for coping with more distressing thoughts. TCQ worry is only modestly correlated ($r = .49$) with symptomatic worry, supporting its conceptualization and measurement as a coping strategy rather than just a symptom of anxiety. The endorsement of worry as a thought control strategy is positively associated with various indices of emotional disorder (Wells & Davies, 1994).

We (Reynolds & Wells, 1999) found that particular TCQ strategies distinguished recovered and nonrecovered patients with major depression and PTSD, and that change in TCQ strategies was associated with recovery. The recovered patients were more likely to use distraction and reappraisal, and less likely to use punishment and worry. Warda and Bryant (1998) assessed thought control strategies in individuals involved in road traffic accidents. Those with acute stress disorder endorsed greater use of worry and punishment than those who did not have acute stress disorder.

In a prospective study of the development of PTSD following road traffic accidents and hospitalization, we (Holeva, Tarrier, & Wells, 2001) measured thought control strategies and social support within 4 weeks of an accident and examined these factors as predictors of PTSD 4–6 months later. The presence of stress symptoms (i.e., acute stress disorder) at Time 1 was controlled for. The use of worry to control thoughts at Time 1, a change in perceived social support, and an interaction between perceived social support and the use of social thought control strategies significantly predicted subsequent PTSD. In cross-sectional analyses of symptoms, thought control strategies were predictive of acute stress disorder at Time 1 and of PTSD at Time 2. Both the distraction and social control TCQ subscales were negatively correlated with acute stress disorder and PTSD caseness, suggesting a possible benefit of these metacognitive control strategies. However, worry and punishment both emerged as positive predictors of acute stress disorder and PTSD. Taken together, these data support the prediction that worry is associated with the persistence and development of stress-related symptoms and disorder, and that particular metacognitive control strategies are associated with stress outcomes. Although some control strategies may confer a benefit for the individual as predicted by the model, perseverative or worry-based strategies appear to be detrimental. Interestingly, social control and distraction were negatively correlated with acute stress symptoms and PTSD symptoms in the cross-sectional analyses of the Holeva et al. (2001) data, suggesting that distraction and social control may be associated with short-term situational reductions in symptoms.

Other self-report and manipulation studies have provided strong support for the hypothesis that worrying or rumination may be problematic for self-regulation. These studies have explored the effects of worrying generally, rather than the effects of worrying used as a thought control strategy. In two studies, Borkovec et al. (1983) and later York, Borkovec, Vasey, and Stern (1987) demonstrated that brief periods of worry increased the frequency of subsequent negative thought intrusions. We (Butler, Wells, & Dewick, 1995) demonstrated that following exposure to a stressful film, individuals who were asked to worry for a brief period of time reported significantly more intrusive images than individuals asked to engage in imagery or settle down after the film over a subsequent 3-day period. In another study, we (Wells & Papageorgiou, 1995) introduced five different mentation strategies following exposure to a stressful film. The strategies were intended to differ in the extent to which they were problematic, and were as follows: (1) worry about the film, (2) worry about usual concerns, (3) distraction, (4) imaging the film, or (5) settling down (control condition). Those individuals who worried about the film reported significantly more intrusive images over the next 3 days than those in the control condition. The other mentation conditions showed an intermediate frequency of intrusions, which did not differ significantly from that in either the control condition or the worry-about-the-film manipulation condition. Taken together, these results suggest that worrying is associated with an increase in intrusive thoughts. We have seen how direct experimental manipulations of poststress thinking style leads to an increase in intrusive images about the stressor over a subsequent 3-day period (Butler et al., 1995; Wells & Papageorgiou, 1995). These results are consistent with the idea that worrying interferes with adaptation, and they are consistent with more naturalistic studies of predisposition to rumination. In self-report studies, individuals high in rumination report poorer adaptation following life stresses such as bereavement (Nolen-Hoeksema, Parker, & Larson, 1994) and natural disasters such as an earthquake (Nolen-Hoeksema & Morrow, 1991).

In conclusion, empirical evidence from a range of studies provides support for the idea that an aspect of the CAS—namely, worry-based processing—is associated with stress symptoms and the development of acute stress and PTSD following trauma. Furthermore, there is preliminary evidence that individual differences in specific metacognitive thought control strategies may be differentially related to stress outcomes.

METACOGNITIVE THERAPY FOR PTSD

One implication of the metacognitive approach to PTSD is that prolonged imaginal reliving of trauma may not be necessary in treatment. The goal of treatment is to "free up" the traumatized individual's natural capacity for self-regulation and adaptation following trauma—that is, to remove the conflict that exists between homeostatic lower-level processing (which is attempting to retune back to "threat-free" processing) and upper-level processes (which lead to persistence of threat-related cognitions). This consists of enabling individuals to shift to a metacognitive mode of processing in which they can discontinue worry/rumination strategies, discontinue threat monitoring, and establish a strategy of detached mindfulness in dealing with symptoms. "Detached mindfulness" (Wells & Matthews, 1994) refers to disengaging worry or ruminative responses from intruding thoughts. The presence of such thoughts is acknowledged, and cognition is then left to run its own course—without attempts to engage in conceptual analysis of events represented by intrusions, and without attempts to control thoughts or analyze the meaning of them.

The metacognitive treatment has been described in detail elsewhere (Wells, 2000; Wells & Sembi, in press), and is only briefly described here. The core treatment is divided into three phases. The first phase consists of case conceptualization and socialization. The therapist emphasizes that symptoms following stress are normal and are part of the cognitive system's adaptive mechanism for dealing with trauma and developing new knowledge. However, several factors can impede such an adaptive process. These include worry, threat monitoring, and avoidance. The therapist introduces the idea that worry and threat monitoring are driven by positive beliefs about the usefulness of these strategies, as well as by negative beliefs about symptoms. The presence of these components is identified in the individual case and presented as a specific case conceptualization.

The second phase is to help clients to see that engaging in worry/ rumination serves no purpose. An advantages–disadvantages analysis of worry/rumination is used to illustrate this, and it serves as a means of further exploring positive and negative metacognitive beliefs. Once the disadvantages of ruminative worry-based thinking are established, the concept of detached mindfulness (Wells & Matthews, 1994) is introduced. As noted above, this refers to taking a perspective on one's thought processes in which they are observed in a detached way without efforts to interpret, analyze, or control them. Patients are instructed to experience intrusive thoughts in a detached way and to disconnect any worry-based analysis or ruminative processing from the intrusion. A range of strategies have been developed to facilitate the acquisition and practice of detached mindfulness, including prescriptive "mind wandering," free-association exercises, and imagery tasks. It should be noted that these do not involve direct exposure to trauma-related memories. The emphasis on detached mindfulness is coupled with worry/rumination postponement. The therapist tells patients that whenever intrusive symptoms (thoughts, flashbacks, nightmares, etc.) occur, the patients should acknowledge to themselves that the symptoms have occurred, and tell themselves that they are not going to worry or ruminate about the trauma or symptoms now; they will just let the symptoms fade in their own time and actively think about them later. Patients are asked to allocate a half hour each evening as a designated worry/rumination or analysis time. If patients happen to remember what they have been worrying about earlier, they should engage in as much worry/rumination as they feel they need to over this 30-minute period. However, this controlled, deliberate worry time is not compulsory, and many patients choose not to use it or forget to do so.

The third phase of treatment consists of attentional modification. This is introduced when patients have mastered the use of detached mindfulness and report consistent success in using the strategy in response to intrusive symptoms. In this phase of treatment, the focus is on hypervigilance and startle reactions. Systematic manipulations of attention are important, since they shift patients out of a "threat configuration" of processing. The continuous search for threat is not synonymous with having a plan for dealing with threat or allowing cognition to "retune" to the normal (nonthreatening) environment. Here, the advantages and disadvantages of threat monitoring and hypervigilance are reviewed. The aim is to emphasize problems that exist with constantly scanning situations or the internal or external environment for signs of threat. Once the problems with threat monitoring are understood, the therapist asks the patient to consciously acknowledge the direction of attention the next time he or she feels anxious in a situation, and to stop threat monitoring. In order to apply this technique, patients are encouraged (1) to return to their normal routine of daily life; and (2) to redirect attention away from themselves and away from threat, and onto nonthreatening aspects of the external environment.

In some cases, the therapist encounters reluctance on the patients' part to give up worry or threat-monitoring strategies. In these circumstances, careful analysis of positive metacognitive beliefs about the usefulness of these strategies should be undertaken, and these beliefs should be challenged with appropriate behavioral and verbal reattribution strategies. It should be noted that the therapist is required to undertake detailed analysis during treatment to ensure that patients are abandoning a full range of worry/rumination and threat-monitoring strategies, and that they are doing so consistently.

SUMMARY AND CONCLUSIONS

In this chapter, important issues confronting attempts to advance cognitive theory toward a more comprehensive model of cognitive self-regulation have been considered. The emphasis on cognitive content in schema theory directs the conceptual spotlight away from formulating the multiplicity of cognitive elements contributing to cognitive style and cognitive regulation. However, dynamic cognitive models like the S-REF, which encompass metacognition, intentions, goals, and architecture, offer a synthesis of schema theory and information-processing theory. They provide a platform for building predictions concerning the interactions between cognitive elements that underlie persistence and change in psychological disorder. Such models are capable of specifying how cognitive change can be best accomplished. Schema theory tells us what we should do in cognitive therapy: formulate and modify the content of negative automatic thoughts and beliefs. However, it has little to say about how this can be achieved. In contrast, self-regulatory multilevel theories such as the S-REF, and the disorder-specific models derived from it, provide a range of specific new treatment strategies that not only focus on the content of general cognitions, but focus on modifying the content of metacognitions, cognitive processes, and cognitive style.

In this chapter, I have described the generic CAS of psychological disorder, and have shown how it operates in GAD and PTSD in particular. Strategies for conceptualizing and treating aspects of the CAS have been developed and provide the basis for metacognitive therapy. It is beyond the scope of this chapter to describe a full range of metacognitive treatment techniques, but new and emerging strategies for assessing and treating mechanisms underlying the CAS are described in detail elsewhere (see Wells, 2000).

The metacognitive approach is not limited to the disorders discussed in this chapter. The approach has been an impetus for explorations of metacognitive factors in a range of diverse disorders, including major depression (Papageorgiou & Wells, 2001) schizophrenia (Morrison, Wells, & Nothard, 2000), and obsessive–compulsive disorder (Wells & Papageorgiou, 1998; Emmelkamp & Aardema, 1999; Purdon & Clark, 1999). Recently, Leahy (2002) has drawn on metacognitive principles in his analysis of emotions, proposing important individual differences in knowledge about emotions and plans for coping linked to depression and anxiety. Preliminary findings also suggest that the effects of diverse cognitive vulnerabilities, such as the looming cognitive style (Riskind, 1997; see also Riskind, Chapter 4, this volume), may be influenced by metacognitive factors (Balaban, Joswick, Chrosniak, & Riskind, 2001).

The metacognitive analysis has provided a basis for conceptualizing the development and persistence of specific disorders. It is a basis for generating new treatment strategies, and for conceptualizing change processes in cognitive therapy. If progress in this new area continues, we could be on the verge of witnessing the "metacognitive age" in cognitive therapy. At such a time we will become more concerned with *what* patients think and believe in the metacognitive domain, and with *how* patients think in the cognitive or "object" domain. This approach presents exciting new possibilities in the treatment of psychological disorders.

REFERENCES

Balaban, M. S., Joswick, S. M., Chrosniak, L. D., & Riskind, J. M. (2001, July). *The effects of cognitive vulnerability to anxiety and metaworry on memory.* Poster presentation to the World Congress of Behavioral and Cognitive Therapies, Vancouver, British Columbia, Canada.
Beck, A. T. (1972). *Depression: Causes and treatment.* Philadelphia: University of Pennsylvania Press. (Original work published 1967)

Beck, A. T. (1976). *Cognitive therapy and the emotional disorders*. New York: International Universities Press.

Beck, A. T., Rush, A. J., Shaw, B., & Emery, G. (1979). *Cognitive therapy of depression*. New York: Guilford Press.

Borkovec, T. D., Robinson, E., Pruzinsky, T., & DePree, J. A. (1983). Preliminary exploration of worry: Some characteristics and processes. *Behaviour Research and Therapy, 21*, 9–16.

Borkovec, T. D., & Roemer, L. (1995). Perceived functions of worry among generalized anxiety subjects: Distraction from more emotionally distressing topics? *Journal of Behavior Therapy and Experimental Psychiatry, 26*, 25–30.

Butler, G., Wells, A., & Dewick, H. (1995). Differential effects of worry and imagery after exposure to a stressful stimulus: A pilot study. *Behavioural and Cognitive Psychotherapy, 23*, 45–56.

Cartwright-Hatton, S., & Wells, A. (1997). Beliefs about worry and intrusions: The Meta-Cognitions Questionnaire and its correlates. *Journal of Anxiety Disorders, 11*, 279–296

Clark, D. A., & Claybourn, M. (1997). Process characteristics of worry and obsessive intrusive thoughts. *Behaviour Research and Therapy, 35*, 1139–1141.

Emmelkamp, P. M. G., & Aardema, A. (1999). Metacognition, specific obsessive compulsive beliefs and obsessive compulsive behaviour. *Clinical Psychology and Psychotherapy, 6*, 139–146.

Fisher, P., & Durham, R. (1999). Recovery rates in generalized anxiety disorder following psychological therapy: An analysis of clinically significant change on the STAI-T across outcome studies since 1990. *Psychological Medicine, 29*, 1425–1434.

Flavell, J. H. (1979). Metacognition and metacognitive monitoring: A new area of cognitive-developmental inquiry. *American Psychologist, 34*, 906–911.

Holeva, V., Tarrier, N., & Wells, A. (2001). Prevalence and predictors of acute stress disorder and PTSD following road traffic accidents: Thought control strategies and social support. *Behavior Therapy, 32*, 65–84.

Leahy, R. L. (2002). A model of emotional schemas. *Cognitive and Behavioral Practice, 9*, 177–191.

Matthews, G., & Wells, A. (2000). Attention, automaticity and affective disorder. *Behavior Modifications, 24*, 69–93.

Meyer, T. J., Miller, M. L., Metzger, R. L., & Borkovec, T. D. (1990). Development and validation of the Penn State Worry Questionnaire. *Behaviour Research and Therapy, 28*, 487–495.

Morrison, A. P., Wells, A., & Nothard, S. (2000). Cognitive factors in predisposition to auditory and visual hallucinations. *British Journal of Clinical Psychology, 39*, 67–78.

Nassif, Y. (1999). *Predictors of pathological worry*. Unpublished master's thesis, University of Manchester, UK.

Nelson, T. O., & Narens, L. (1990). Metamemory: A theoretical framework and some new findings. In G. H. Bower (Ed.), *The psychology of learning and motivation* (Vol. 26, pp. 125–173). San Diego, CA: Academic Press.

Nolen-Hoeksema, S., & Morrow, J. (1991). A prospective study of depression and posttraumatic stress symptoms after a natural disaster: The 1989 Lorna Pikta earthquake. *Journal of Personality and Social Psychology, 61*, 115–121.

Nolen-Hoeksema, S., Parker, L. E., & Larson, J. (1994). Ruminative coping with depressed mood following loss. *Journal of Personality and Social Psychology, 67,* 92–104.

Papageorgiou, C., & Wells, A. (1999). Process and meta-cognitive dimensions of depressive and anxious thoughts and relationships with emotional intensity. *Clinical Psychology and Psychotherapy, 6,* 156–162.

Papageorgiou, C., & Wells, A. (2001). Metacognitive beliefs about rumination in recurrent major depression. *Cognitive and Behavioral Practice, 8,* 160–164.

Purdon, C. (1999). Thought suppression and psychopathology. *Behaviour Research and Therapy, 37,* 1029–1054.

Purdon, C. (2000, July). *Metacognition and the persistence of worry.* Paper presented at the annual conference of the British Association of Behavioural and Cognitive Psychotherapy, Institute of Education, London.

Purdon, C., & Clark, D. A. (1999). Metacognition and obsessions. *Clinical Psychology and Psychotherapy, 6,* 102–110.

Reynolds, M., & Wells, A. (1999). The Thought Control Questionnaire: Psychometric properties in a clinical sample, and relationships with PTSD and depression. *Psychological Medicine, 29,* 1089–1099.

Riskind, J. M. (1997). Looming vulnerability to threat: A cognitive paradigm for anxiety. *Behaviour Research and Therapy, 35,* 685–702.

Roemer, L., Borkovec, M., Posa, P., & Borkovec, T. D. (1995). A self diagnostic measure of generalized anxiety disorder. *Journal of Behavior Therapy and Experimental Psychiatry, 26,* 345–350.

Warda, G., & Bryant, R. A. (1998). Cognitive bias in acute stress disorder. *Behaviour Research and Therapy, 36,* 1177–1183.

Wegner, D. M., Schneider, D. J., Carter, S. R., & White, T. L. (1987). Paradoxical effects of thought suppression. *Journal of Personality and Social Psychology, 53,* 5–13.

Wells, A. (1994). Attention and the control of worry. In G. C. L. Davey & F. Tallis (Eds.), *Worrying: Perspectives on theory, assessment and treatment* (pp. 91–114). Chichester, UK: Wiley.

Wells, A. (1995). Meta-cognition and worry: A cognitive model of generalized anxiety disorder. *Behavioural and Cognitive Psychotherapy, 23,* 301–320.

Wells, A. (1997). *Cognitive therapy of anxiety disorders: A practice manual and conceptual guide.* Chichester, UK: Wiley.

Wells, A. (1999). A metacognitive model and therapy for generalized anxiety disorder. *Clinical Psychology and Psychotherapy, 6,* 86–95.

Wells, A. (2000). *Emotional disorders and metacognition: Innovative cognitive therapy.* Chichester, UK: Wiley.

Wells, A. (in press). The metacognitive model of GAD: Assessment of metaworry and relationship with DSM-IV generalized anxiety disorder. *Cognitive Therapy and Research.*

Wells, A., & Carter, K. (1999). Preliminary tests of a cognitive model of GAD. *Behaviour Research and Therapy, 37,* 585–594.

Wells, A., & Carter, K. (2001). Further tests of a cognitive model of generalized anxiety disorder: Metacognitions and worry in GAD, panic disorder, social phobia, depression, and nonpatients. *Behavior Therapy, 32,* 85–102.

Wells, A., & Davies, M. (1994). The Thought Control Questionnaire: A measure of individual differences in the control of unwanted thoughts. *Behaviour Research and Therapy, 32,* 871–878.

Wells, A., & Matthews, G. (1994). *Attention and emotion: A clinical perspective.* Hove, UK: Erlbaum.

Wells, A., & Matthews, G. (1996). Modelling cognition in emotional disorder: The S-REF model. *Behaviour Research and Therapy, 32,* 867–870.

Wells, A., & Morrison, T. (1994). Qualitative dimensions of normal worry and normal intrusive thoughts: A comparative study. *Behaviour Research and Therapy, 32,* 867–870.

Wells, A., & Papageorgiou, C. (1995). Worry and the incubation of intrusive images following stress. *Behaviour Research and Therapy, 33,* 579–583.

Wells, A., & Papageorgiou, C. (1998). Relationships between worry and obsessive–compulsive symptoms and meta-cognitive beliefs. *Behaviour Research and Therapy, 36,* 899–913.

Wells, A., & Sembi, S. (in press). Metacognitive therapy for PTSD: A core treatment manual. *Cognitive and Behavioral Practice.*

York, D., Borkovec, T. D., Vasey, M., & Stern, R. (1987). Effects of worry and somatic anxiety induction on thoughts, emotion and physiological activity. *Behaviour Research and Therapy, 25,* 523–526.

$$\boxed{Chapter\ 10}$$

Substance Abuse

Cory F. Newman

The use of cognitive therapy in the treatment of substance abuse[1] is not intended to replace existing models of treatment. Rather, cognitive therapy complements other approaches, such as those involving pharmacotherapy, 12-step facilitation (12SF), and related social learning applications. Since the early stages of its development as a therapy for substance abuse (see Beck & Emery, 1977), cognitive therapy has contributed conceptual and practical advances that may dovetail with these alternative models.

With regard to pharmacological approaches, cognitive therapy introduces improved methods for understanding patients' nonadherence to chemical treatments, such as disulfiram (Antabuse), methadone, and naltrexone. Specifically, patients may maintain maladaptive beliefs about pharmacological treatments that dissuade them from collaborating optimally with their treatment programs. For example, patients sometimes view their medications as a form of authoritarian control over their behavior, which they resent and resist. Cognitive therapists can help patients reassess and modify such interpretations. This approach to the bolstering of pharmacotherapy has been shown to produce clinically significant results with other disorders as well, most notably bipolar disorder (e.g., Lam et al., 2000).

In cognitive therapy, a collaborative set between practitioner and patient is established, so that concurrent pharmacotherapy is not merely an

---

[1]Throughout this chapter, the term "substance abuse" is used in its more general sense of "substance misuse." That is, it subsumes the formal diagnoses of both "substance abuse" and "substance dependence" as defined by the American Psychiatric Association.

exercise in taking a therapeutic chemical to replace a harmful chemical. Patients who are both receiving cognitive therapy and taking medication feel empowered, in that they are simultaneously learning self-help skills and actively addressing a full range of therapeutic concerns.

Patients who take part in 12SF are often instructed to adhere to a uniform model of recovery. Cognitive therapy helps patients to individualize their approach to recovery by teaching them the methods of assessing evidence and weighing pros and cons in decision making. This approach teaches patients to make an empirical examination of their lives, rather than believing that they must follow a single script that fits all. For example, some patients in cognitive therapy who are also participants in 12SF have expressed relief that they do not necessarily have to view the rules of their fellowship meetings in an all-or-none fashion. For example, they do not have to think of their antidepressant medications as "simply another chemical dependency," but rather as a natural part of an appropriate treatment plan for comorbid depression. Similarly, they may feel more hopeful in learning that a single relapse episode does not necessarily mean that all previous gains in treatment are lost, or that they are back to "square one." Instead, they can examine the damage that drinking or using other drugs is causing once again in their lives, and decide to implement the full range of their self-help skills and social supports in order to put the brakes on the downward slide. Great emphasis is placed on getting back into the problem-solving mode once again, rather than falling prey to feelings of catastrophization.

Although cognitive therapists are quick to encourage their substance-abusing patients to respect the power of addictive cravings, and to take stock of the illogic of rationalizing why it's okay to drink or use, they do not require their patients to adopt a position statement of powerlessness in fighting the addiction. Within a cognitive therapy framework, it is very important for patients to gain the skills that will bolster their sense of empowerment and self-efficacy. Thus patients in cognitive therapy are taught how to take responsibility for their actions, and to take systematic steps to reduce the likelihood of continued use or relapse. Being independent of the support of a group or sponsor is not seen as a setup for a fall, as long as an individual is utilizing his or her "tools."

Cognitive therapy advances general social learning models by introducing a special emphasis on patients' belief systems, especially their beliefs about substances per se, the nature of cravings, their "relationship" with substances, and the risks involved in being in various situations or states of mind (Beck, Wright, Newman, & Liese, 1993). Thus patients can work on modifying their harmful misconceptions that would otherwise allow or lure them into choosing to drink or use other drugs.

Cognitive therapy also brings its strength in treating mood, anxiety, and personality disorders into the clinical picture, such that patients with multiple diagnoses can be helped across all facets of their psychological problems simultaneously. Some of the major outcome studies on cognitive therapy for substance abuse (to be discussed below) have included populations from low socioeconomic groups, thus transporting effective clinical applications to help underserved patients. Demonstrations of empirical efficacy are especially valid for work "in the trenches."

In order to assess the unique contributions of cognitive therapy, some outcome studies (again, to be discussed later in the chapter) have tested cognitive therapy *against* such treatments as 12SF and pharmacotherapy (e.g., Anton et al., 1999, 2001; Maude-Griffin et al., 1998). However, as implied above, from either a practical or a theoretical standpoint, there is no reason why cognitive therapy cannot be used in conjunction with supplemental treatments. Although feasibility and availability issues sometimes get in the way, patients who are motivated to overcome their problems with addictions often express gratitude for being able to receive multiple sources of treatment. Thus, for example, it is hypothesized that cognitive therapy can be readily woven into a comprehensive program in which patients take methadone and also attend Narcotics Anonymous meetings. In such cases, it is most important that the treatment providers in each modality support each other's work—a goal that is sometimes difficult to achieve. Nevertheless, collaborative approaches to comprehensive psychiatric care are greatly enhanced when multiple practitioners view each other positively (see Moras & DeMartinis, 1999).

An overarching benefit that cognitive therapy brings to the treatment of substance abuse is its emphasis on long-term maintenance. Because patients who abuse alcohol and other drugs are often subject to relapse episodes, treatment needs to teach these patients a new set of attitudes and skills on which to rely for the long run. Along these lines, treatment outcome is often measured in terms of "length of abstinence" or "percentage of patients reaching [specified length of time abstinent]." Cognitive therapists help their patients achieve success in this manner by focusing on the acquisition of such skills as self-monitoring, goal setting, problem solving, assertiveness (rather than aggression or passive aggression), time management, and rational responding (instead of reflexive, impulsive acting out). These skills not only improve patients' sense of self-efficacy; they also lead to a reduction in life stressors that might otherwise increase the risk of relapse.

THE COGNITIVE APPROACH: MAIN POINTS OF INTERVENTION

Cognitive therapy is not an etiological model of substance abuse—thoughts do not cause addiction per se. The etiology of substance abuse is complex, multivariate, and not entirely understood (Woody, Urschel, & Alterman,

1992). Factors such as heredity, cellular adaptation, modeling of parents and peers, socioeconomic disadvantage, low self-esteem, illusory sense of personal control, ease of accessibility to substances, avoidance through self-medication, and others can account (either alone or interactively) for the onset of substance abuse (Newman, 1997b).

Instead, cognitive therapy makes its most meaningful contributions in terms of providing potentially fruitful points of intervention, and identifying the cognitive-behavioral variables that can trigger relapse. The following are seven of such variables, each of which represents a potentially "weak link" that could lead to drug use, and each of which suggests a potential area for therapeutic intervention.

High-Risk Stimuli

External

External high-risk stimuli include the "people, places, and things" that are commonly discussed in 12SF, but that are equally relevant in cognitive therapy. Examples may include a patient's neighbor who often comes to his or her house, suggesting that they get high together; the particular street corner where the patient used to purchase dope; and the kitchen cleaning fluid the patient used to inhale "for a buzz." Many of these external high-risk stimuli can be identified and avoided. Unfortunately, others are fairly ubiquitous (e.g., beer commercials), and some are sadly too close to home (e.g., when a patient's immediate family members abuse substances). In such instances, it may not be realistic to expect patients to avoid these external high-risk stimuli altogether. The best they may be able to do are (1) to minimize exposure; and (2) to learn a repertoire of rational self-statements that support sobriety, to go along with assertive refusal statements to prevent joining others in using substances. To borrow loosely from the "Serenity Prayer," patients have to have the awareness to avoid the high-risk stimuli they *can* avoid, the coping skills to deal with the high-risk stimuli they *cannot* avoid, and the wisdom to know the difference (Beck et al., 1993).

Internal

Perhaps even more challenging than external high-risk situations are the problematic emotions, thoughts, and sensations that comprise internal high-risk stimuli. In the vernacular of 12SF, the acronym "HALT" has been used to signify being "hungry, angry, lonely, and tired." These internal states are hypothesized to be major areas of vulnerability to relapse. Cognitive therapists would add that any subjectively troublesome emotional state would qualify in the same way. Patients who feel depressed, anxious, or guilt-ridden (among other emotions) are also at risk of using alcohol and other drugs in order to self-medicate.

Most unfortunately, internal high-risk stimuli are not limited to negative emotional states. Patients have reported having "drug dreams," in which they experience the sensations of drug use in their sleep. They may then wake up drenched in sweat, in a state of marked craving for the relevant drug. Furthermore, some patients will experience an increased desire to use substances as a result of feeling *good*, such as when they want to celebrate. As one patient rhetorically asked, "How can I have a 'happy hour' in my life without the alcohol that is always supposed to go with that?" Similarly, some patients will have gotten into the habit of trying to enhance the hedonic value of certain situations (e.g., sex) by getting high. However, a conceptualization of these cases often finds that the situation is even more problematic than that. For example, not only are these persons trying to maximize their sexual arousal via drugs; they are also escaping from their fear of the intimacy that they would experience if they tried to make love in an unaltered state of mind. This requires intervention on multiple issues.

Needless to say, patients cannot avoid their feelings entirely, nor should they. Emotions are an important part of life, and often cue persons into being more aware of key issues that need their attention. Thus, rather than encouraging patients somehow to get rid of their high-risk emotional states, it is preferable that they learn to recognize, manage, and deal with these emotions productively. Cognitive therapy is especially strong in this area, as illustrated by studies in which its application in the treatment of substance abuse was differentially effective for patients who were also depressed (Carroll, Rounsaville, Gordon, et al., 1994; Maude-Griffin et al., 1998).

Maladaptive Beliefs about Substances

Cognitive therapists assess and help patients modify their faulty beliefs about substances. Some of these problematic beliefs are about the substances themselves (e.g., "Beer doesn't really count as alcohol," or "Cocaine is only addictive if you smoke it"), and others are about how patients view themselves in relation to drugs (e.g., "I need to get high in order to face people in a social situations," or "I don't deserve to have a normal life, so I might as well use drugs, and to heck with what happens to me"). Interventions run the gamut from the simple provision of psychoeducation (e.g., "You can relapse on beer, because there is alcohol in beer") to more complex methods that address patients' core schemas of defectiveness, unlovability, social exclusion, and other schemas (Young, 1999). What all interventions in this area have in common is the examination of evidence, in an attempt to shed light on the fallacies behind patients' views about alcohol and other drugs.

Therapists can ascertain some of their patients' maladaptive beliefs about drugs via self-report measures, such as the Beliefs about Substance Use inventory and the Craving Beliefs Questionnaire (Beck et al., 1993, Appendix 1, pp. 312–314); by listening carefully to patients' comments in session; and via examination of the implicit meanings behind the patients' actions. For example, patients' responses to the written inventories may reveal that they believe strongly that cravings can escalate dangerously if left unsatisfied, and that life without substances would be boring and depressing. These beliefs then become targets for intervention. Likewise, a patient may make a spontaneous statement in session, such as "I would be all alone if I stopped using alcohol and drugs, because all my friends drink and drug." Such a lamentation would cue the therapist to discuss the full scope of the patient's personal relationships—past, present, and (potentially in the) future—with the intention of finding and creating exceptions to the patient's rule. The therapist and patient in this example would aim toward helping the patient develop a new social support system, perhaps starting with the people he or she might meet at a 12SF meeting.

In addition, therapists can infer patients' dysfunctional beliefs about substances by conceptualizing their behavior in terms of implicit, underlying assumptions. For example, "Ms. Grey" often seemed to plan her substance-using episodes hours or days in advance, reporting to her therapist after the fact that "I *knew* I was going to use this weekend," or "I was at work, but my mind was already at the bar, and nothing was going to stop me." The therapist hypothesized that the patient maintained a particular belief—namely, that once she had the inkling that she was going to drink or use other drugs, she did not believe it was possible, important, or necessary for her to use cognitive-behavioral self-help skills to avert the planned episode of substance use. She simply believed that a relapse was "inevitable," and "that was that." It did not occur to her that she could change her mind or dodge the risk. This revelation opened up a new area of potential interventions to be used when the patient began thinking of her next episode of alcohol or other drug use.

Perhaps the most challenging aspect of this area of intervention has to do with the interaction of maladaptive beliefs that are indicative of dual diagnoses. For example, it is difficult enough for a patient to change the belief that "I cannot be happy unless I get high on drugs," but it is even more so when this patient simultaneously believes that "I am a loser who will never get what I want out of life." This depressive, self-derogating belief will intensify the patient's belief that drug use is the only way to get into a good mood. Thus interventions must target not only the problematic exaltation of the effects of the drugs, but also the patient's low self-esteem and helplessness.

For example, "Wes" argued that he could not see the purpose in giving up his addictive behaviors, since he believed he had already damaged his life so much that there was nothing left to save anyway. The therapist empathized with the patient's sense of loss and shame, but invited Wes to examine what might indeed be worth saving by becoming clean and sober. First, by turning his life around for the better, Wes could preserve his legacy for his descendants. Rather than going to his grave as a substance-abusing person, he could live, and demonstrate that recovery was possible no matter what the difficulties. Second, being an avid sports fan, Wes was encouraged to examine his life thus far (metaphorically) as a very poorly played first half of football. Now, in therapy (analogous to halftime in the locker room), Wes was being coached to "get out there for the second half and play like you're capable of playing, and give the fans something to cheer about." This intervention provided the cognitive reframe necessary for Wes to believe that he had something worth trying to achieve; thus he engaged in his treatment for substance abuse more earnestly.

Automatic Thoughts

Automatic thoughts are the instantaneous ideas and images patients get about a situation in which they have the opportunity to use alcohol and/or other drugs. Often these are brief internal exclamations, such as "Party time!," "Go for it!," or "F-ck it!" Similarly, they can be represented by mental images of the act of drinking or using, or the perceptual distortions that may occur in the aftermath. Although the experience of these automatic thoughts does not necessarily lead directly to drinking or using, they are hypothesized to lead to an immediate surge in arousal. Thus cravings and substance-seeking behavior become intensified, and the risk of relapse increases significantly unless an intervention (or the sober passage of time) brings the level of arousal back to baseline once again.

Cognitive therapists teach their patients to use their heightened sympathetic nervous system activity (e.g., sweating, heavy breathing) as cues to ask themselves what they are thinking at that moment that could be causing their increased desire to drink and use. Furthermore, patients are taught how these automatic thoughts affect their decision making regarding the situations into which they put themselves, and their ultimate choice about whether to reject or accept the addictive substance. It is extremely important for patients to cease viewing their automatic thoughts as "truths," and instead to question their validity before acting on them.

Given that automatic thoughts are often fleeting, patients are taught to generate rational responses that are comparably short and to the point. Some of the sayings learned in 12SF meetings serve this purpose well, such as "One day at a time," "Easy does it," and "One [use of substances] is too many, and a thousand won't be enough." Generating more of these self-statements becomes an important task, both in therapy sessions and for homework. Some additional examples of rational responses are listed below:

1. *Automatic thought*: "Go for it! Just use it, now!"
   Rational response: "Stay with the program. 'Going for it' is the same thing as 'going, going, gone.'"
2. *Automatic thought*: "It's party time!"
   Rational response: "It's time to think this through, and time to stay true. I have to find a way to have fun without drinking or using."
3. *Automatic thought*: "Who cares if I drink?"
   Rational response: "I care, my brother cares, my mother cares, my girlfriend cares, my therapist cares, and my housemates care."

It is ideal for patients to end up compiling a large stack of flashcards with their favorite rational responses for easy reference when they need quick comebacks to their automatic thoughts.

Cravings and Urges

Cravings and urges are the physiological sensations that create an uncomfortable, unresolved sense of "drive" or "appetite" to alter one's state through the use of psychoactive chemicals. Many patients maintain the faulty belief that cravings and urges are linear, escalating phenomena, such that denying them can lead to physical or mental catastrophe (e.g., "If I don't give in to my cravings, I'll go insane"). Along the same lines, they may believe that they cannot tolerate cravings, that they are compelled to act on their urges, and that nothing can be done about this. In other words, cravings bring a great deal of psychological baggage with them, including helplessness, hopelessness, and rigid adherence to a dysfunctional (albeit familiar) response set.

Part of the psychoeducation that patients receive about this problem is mixed with an appropriate amount of empathy. Yes, cravings can cause severe physical distress, sometimes requiring medical supervision; and yes, drinking or using temporarily removes the discomfort. However, by giving in to the cravings, the patients actually increase their dependence on the chemical(s), thus leading to future cravings that are more intense and more frequent. A vicious cycle results, with ultimately devastating consequences for the patients.

Cognitive therapists educate their patients about the cyclical (not linear) nature of cravings (Newman, 1997b). They help their patients to learn the techniques of "D & D," or "delay and distraction," so as to ride out the cravings until they peak and subside. Much in the same way that patients with chronic pain are taught to divert their attention from their pain onto meaningful tasks or pleasant distractions (Turk, Meichenbaum, & Genest, 1983), patients with cravings for their substance(s) of choice are asked to produce a list of constructive things to do until the urge diminishes on its own. The goals are to build self-efficacy in withstanding the sensation of craving, and to replace addictive behavior with constructive actions. In general, cravings that run their natural course (without being satisfied by a substance) come back just a little less strongly the next time, and less strongly still the time after that (Solomon, 1980). Thus patients who become skilled at delaying and distracting soon find that the cravings themselves are not as powerful. As a caveat, however, patients must always be aware of the possibility that certain high-risk situations (both external and internal) will produce strong enough associations to cause cravings to spike once again, at least temporarily.

Permission-Giving Beliefs

When cravings are strong, many patients struggle with the conflict of whether or not to drink and/or take other drugs. On the one hand, they want to work toward sobriety. On the other hand, they want to rid themselves of the discomfort of the withdrawal. This conflict is sometimes resolved maladaptively by the implementation of "permission-giving" beliefs, also known more generally as "rationalizations" or "enabling." For example, patients will tell themselves, "Nobody will find out, so it's not going to hurt anybody, and that makes it okay this time," or "I haven't had a hit in a long time, so it's only natural for me to have a little something now." Other common examples are "I'm just going to have one [drink, snort, etc.]," "I need to test myself to see if I'm still hooked," and "I deserve a break [from my sobriety]." Patients who succeed in identifying the activation of these permission-giving beliefs as they occur tend to report that they feel a sense of relief, a reduction in anticipatory guilt, and a rush of arousal, as they have now cognitively cleared the way to enjoy their substance(s) with a sense that "it's okay this time." This reinforces their dysfunctional beliefs and makes it very difficult for the patients to choose to remain abstinent at times of internal conflict.

Given that patients will be confronted with many instances in which they will experience ambivalence about taking advantage of an opportunity to drink or use, it is imperative that they learn to spot their permission-giving beliefs, and to understand their seductive and dangerous effect on the patients' decision making. Patients will need to develop clear, unambiguous, well-rehearsed rational responses to counteract the permission-giving beliefs. Patients can generate these for homework, adopt them from 12-step slogans, or role-play with therapists so that they become skilled at responding to rapid-fire permission-giving beliefs. Some examples of rational responses include "There's no such thing as *only* one drink . . . it's a drink, and that's trouble," "I can only pass the test if I don't try to test myself in the first place," and "Keep the [sobriety] streak alive . . . don't give it up without fighting for it first."

As some of the examples above may illustrate, patients are taught to watch out for the hazards of using words such as "only," "just," and "a little bit" in their self-statements. They are instructed to repeat their automatic thoughts *without* those words, and to listen for the qualitative difference. For example, "I only want one drink," becomes "I want one drink" and "I just want to use a little bit" becomes "I want to use." This exercise drives home the stark reality of what they are proposing to do, without the minimization of the problems that is part and parcel of permission giving.

Behavioral Rituals Surrounding Drinking and Using

Persons who abuse substances over a period of time often develop patterns of behavior—in essence, rituals—surrounding the substance-using episodes. Part of constructing a thorough case conceptualization with such patients is to outline the sequence of behaviors that typically leads to the episode of using, and to take inventory of the stimulus cues that go with them. At the social level, this may involve the street corner to which they go to buy drugs, and the people with whom they initiate contact. At the individual level, the rituals may involve the particular hand-held mirror they use to cut the lines of cocaine, or the process of assembling their drug paraphernalia while sitting in a locked bathroom. Whatever the patients' most common patterns entail, it is useful to identify them, emphasizing all the steps, as well as the beliefs and automatic thoughts that get activated along the way.

Interventions in this area are intended to avoid, abort, interrupt, or otherwise counteract the progression of such rituals. One strategy is to have the patients structure their lives so as to make the acquisition and use of substances as inconvenient as possible. This involves everything from emptying their residences of alcohol, other drugs, and drug equipment, to structuring their daily activities so that they spend most of their time with sober individuals. A standard example is the patient who used to have the ritual of stopping at the local tavern on the way home from work, but now stops at a support group meeting or goes to a gym. If feasible, some patients decide to take up residence elsewhere, in order to reduce their exposure to familiar substance cues in their environment.

Some individuals are hesitant to make these changes. They will argue that they "have to" meet their friends in situations where alcohol is available, or that "it is safe" to keep old stashes of drugs in their household. When this occurs, therapists can suggest that the patients look at their statements as reflecting permission-giving beliefs, and that they question their own intent. For example, the patients can ask themselves, "Why am I giving myself permission to keep bags of marijuana and barbiturates in my closet? What makes it so important and necessary to keep these substances handy? If I am committed to sobriety, what is actually lost by getting rid of these substances? What message am I sending to others (and to myself) by insisting that the drugs should be kept on hand for easy access?" These are important questions to address openly and thoroughly.

When patients can succeed in breaking their substance-using routines, they will buy themselves time so that they can implement their self-help skills and seek appropriate social support. Any delay caused by interrupting a ritual increases the patients' chances that they will find a way to cope and remain sober in situations that might otherwise have led to a relapse in the past.

Lapses and Their Progression to Full-Blown Relapses

If patients wind up taking a drink or using another drug, the story is not over. It has only reached a new chapter. They still have the opportunity to limit the damage by deciding to stop drinking or using before the episode becomes a binge, or before it leads to successive episodes. Unfortunately, patients sometimes fall prey to the "abstinence violation effect" (Marlatt & Gordon, 1985), in which their initial lapse leads them to think in all-or-none ways that translate into binges. For example, persons who have learned in their support group meetings that a single drink of alcohol could "put them back to square one" in their recovery may reason to themselves after one drink that "I might as well go all the way, since one drink makes me a drunk." Needless to say, this type of thinking is highly problematic, since it represents a perversion of the spirit of the quest to resist getting drunk or high.

In cognitive therapy, patients are taught that the most favorable goal is absolute sobriety. However, people are human, and they sometimes have slips. When this happens, the patients should not automatically despair; nor should they activate the permission-giving belief that "I might as well go on a bender, now that I've had one slip." Instead, patients are encouraged to look at each drink, snort, injection, ingestion, and/or puff as an entirely *new decision* over which they have responsibility. Granted, this decision-making process becomes more fuzzy and distorted with each new use of a substance, but the fact remains that it is possible for patients to stop at any point in the process.

Patients in cognitive therapy learn that their therapists will not judge them or scold them if they have a lapse. Rather, patients are told to monitor and record their slips, indicating the thoughts, emotions, and situational cues that accompanied each episode. Furthermore, therapists assist their patients in utilizing techniques to limit a lapse once it has begun, and to take corrective measures in the aftermath in order to get back on track once again. Although lapses represent setbacks in therapy, patients are encouraged to view them as learning experiences, and not as reasons to abandon treatment or to feel helpless about achieving sobriety.

As a caveat, it is important to note that patients (such as the aforementioned Ms. Grey) should not be permitted to subvert the philosophy described above by *planning* to drink or use "once in a while." The patient who states (with a classic permission-giving belief) that "I only use on Saturday nights" is not following the true spirit of minimizing the scope of a lapse. A true, honest lapse is a spontaneous breakdown of coping skills in the presence of an unexpected opportunity to drink or use other drugs. By contrast, making plans to use cocaine on a weekend evening is not a lapse per se, but rather a deliberate act against the goal of sobriety and recovery. This distinction must be spelled out.

If patients learn how to do "damage control," in that they limit their lapses and reassert control over their behavior and decision making, this will reduce the likelihood of significantly setting back their therapeutic gains with each lapse. They will be less apt to feel so guilty, self-reproachful, and/or hopeless that they create a new internal high-risk stimulus that will start the cycle of abuse anew. Instead, patients will learn not to fear their mistakes, and to remain committed to the spirit and the methods of staying sober.

EMPIRICAL FINDINGS

The data on outcomes for cognitive therapy of substance abuse are promising, but still equivocal. Some studies demonstrate the decided advantages of cognitive therapy over other approaches (e.g., Maude-Griffin et al., 1998); others show that cognitive therapy works best in concert with pharmacotherapy such as naltrexone (Anton et al., 1999, 2001) and disulfiram (Carroll et al., 2000; Carroll, Nich, Ball, McCance, & Rounsaville, 1998); and some emphasize the delayed emergence of cognitive therapy's efficacy at follow-up (Baker, Boggs, & Lewin, 2001; Carroll, Rounsaville, Gordon, et al., 1994; Carroll, Rounsaville, Nich, et al., 1994). Additional studies provide evidence that cognitive therapy has therapeutic benefits, but not significantly greater ones than other active treatments (e.g., Wells, Peterson, Gainey, Hawkins, & Catalano, 1994), while a major multisite study has presented even less encouraging data (e.g., Crits-Christoph et al., 1999).

The Maude-Griffin et al. (1998) randomized controlled trial evaluated the comparative efficacy of cognitive therapy (using the Beck et al. [1993] manual) versus 12SF. This study provided a 12-week period of treatment, following which the cognitive therapy group was found more likely to achieve abstinence from crack cocaine than participants in 12SF. Significantly, the therapists in the Maude-Griffin et al. (1998) study had personally used 12SF groups to maintain their own recoveries, and thus did not present the potential confound of an allegiance effect in favor of cognitive therapy. Furthermore, the criteria for clinical improvement were stringent, in that the patients who were considered positive responders had to report at least 30 days' abstinence from cocaine and produce a cocaine-free urine sample. The sample itself represented a population often considered to be both ecologically valid and difficult to treat, since it included a large proportion of unemployed, poorly housed, minority patients. Of these patients, those who were assessed to possess "high abstract reasoning skills" were significantly more likely to achieve 4 consecutive weeks of cocaine abstinence than those with low abstract reasoning scores. In addition, the cognitive therapy condition was differentially effective for patients with a history of clinical depression. In other words, cognitive therapy was found to represent the treatment of choice for patients with both cocaine abuse and depression, but 12SF was comparably effective for those without depression.

The Maude-Griffin et al. (1998) study is significant in that it possessed many methodological strengths, including "a comparatively large sample size, manualized clinically relevant interventions . . . verification of self-reported cocaine use through urine toxicology, and a very high follow-up rate with this challenging population" (p. 836). The study also demonstrates the portability of cognitive therapy, in that the therapists had been treated and trained in 12SF prior to their education in conducting cognitive therapy.

Deas and Thomas (2001) reviewed the controlled treatment studies for adolescents with substance abuse. The authors found that the most promising results were obtained with cognitive-behavioral and family-based interventions. However, they cautioned that studies often fail to use validated outcome measures, thus clouding the interpretability of the results. As will be noted below, more research is needed in further refining existing self-report measures on variables pertinent to substance abuse.

In a randomized controlled trial, Baker et al. (2001) tested the efficacy of a very brief model of cognitive-behavioral therapy for patients with amphetamine abuse. Patients in all treatment conditions made gains, and although there were no significant differences between cognitive-behavioral treatments (either a two-session or a four-session format) and a self-help guidebook at termination, the patients who received cognitive-behavioral therapy demonstrated significantly better maintenance of abstinence at 6-month follow-up. It is expected that the main effects of treatment, as well as maintenance, would have been more robust if the intervention had been closer to a standard length.

The Crits-Christoph et al. (1999) multisite study produced data less favorable to cognitive therapy. The project evaluated four manualized treatments for cocaine addiction: (1) individual drug counseling plus group drug counseling (GDC), (2) cognitive therapy plus GDC, (3) supportive–expressive therapy plus GDC, and (4) GDC alone. Contrary to a priori hypotheses, the patients who received individual drug counseling plus GDC showed the greatest improvement on the Addiction Severity Index—Drug Use Composite (McLellan et al., 1992), as well as in the number of days of cocaine use in the past month. This finding was especially unexpected in light of the fact that these patients missed significantly more sessions than patients in the other treatments did. The authors hypothesize that individual drug counseling may have profited from its almost singular focus on achieving abstinence from cocaine. The authors also note that the therapists in the individual drug counseling condition had more clinical experience with treating substance abuse. Furthermore, the individual drug counselors included a significantly greater proportion of female and minority therapists. Regardless of whether or not these therapist differences played a role in outcome, the patients of the individual drug counselors did not show their responsivity to treatment by showing up for sessions more than in the other conditions—quite to the contrary. The scope and the rigor of the Crits-Christoph et al. (1999) study are of sufficient magnitude to make us pay close attention to these problematic findings, and to make adjustments in the content and process of the delivery of cognitive therapy for substance abuse in future trials, as described below.

FUTURE DIRECTIONS

The mixed results from randomized controlled trials indicate that although cognitive therapy offers great hope for the treatment of substance abuse, it is still a work in progress. As empirically minded practitioners, cognitive therapists have always welcomed evidence-based advancements and improvements in the treatment model; thus the cognitive therapy of substance abuse offers yet another interesting area for further development in the field.

Alliance Enhancement Strategies

One of the most important elements of doing successful cognitive therapy is facilitating a positive, collaborative therapeutic relationship. Indeed, a section of the Cognitive Therapy Rating Scale (Young & Beck, 1980), a measure of cognitive therapists' adherence and competency, is devoted entirely to issues pertinent to the therapeutic alliance. Given the difficulties in getting patients with substance abuse to attend therapy sessions regularly (Siqueland et al., 2002), it is important to explore methods to improve the therapeutic relationship with this population.

Following the completion of the Crits-Christoph et al. (1999) study (in which patients were treated during the years 1991 through 1996), a series of articles appeared in the National Institute on Drug Abuse Research Monograph Series (No. 165) that addressed the importance of improving the therapeutic relationship and patient attendance in treatment (e.g., Liese & Beck, 1997; Luborsky, Barber, Siqueland, McLellan, & Woody, 1997; Newman, 1997a). For example, it is important to acknowledge patients' ambivalence about giving up a lifestyle of getting drunk and/or high, especially if they believe that this is the only way they can find temporary relief from their life difficulties (Newman, 1997a). Along these same lines, therapists can show considerable empathy by acknowledging to patients in recovery that they may at time feel a sense of grief over giving up their use of alcohol and other drugs. In addition, therapists need to handle with great sensitivity such issues as patients' being late, missing sessions, and coming to sessions impaired. Although limits must be set in order for the therapeutic enterprise to be viable, therapists must conceptualize the patients' problematic behavior in a spirit of collaboration and acceptance. This demands the highest degree of professionalism, especially when therapists believe that their patients are being dishonest, misusing therapy, or otherwise crossing boundaries in therapy.

Liese and Beck (1997) note that patients with substance abuse tend to have serious, frequent life crises that may make it difficult for them to attend their sessions. If therapists understand this and are willing to accept patients back into treatment even after the patients have missed sessions and been out of touch, the therapeutic relationship can be salvaged, and gains can still be achieved. The Liese and Beck (1997) chapter also contains an appendix listing 50 common patient beliefs that lead to missed sessions and dropout. Therapists can utilize this list to proactively assess and address these countertherapeutic beliefs, such as "I should be strong enough to do this myself," and "I'll just get upset if I go to a psychotherapy session."

Luborsky et al. (1997) point out that material or appetitive incentives may need to be used in order to make the therapist's office more attractive to patients, and thus to retain them more effectively. Giving vouchers that can be redeemed for tangible rewards is one such method, as is the provision of food, such as sandwiches and coffee. As a clinical illustration, I once asked a patient (as a matter of routine in cognitive therapy) for feedback at the end of the session. In response to the question "What sticks in your mind the most about this session?", the patient did not recount the substantive contents of the therapeutic dialogue. Instead, he said, "I remember that you got me a soda from the machine, and that was cool."

There is evidence that the patients' views of the nature and quality of the therapeutic relationship are more predictive of outcome than their therapists' corresponding views (Barber et al., 1999). Thus it will be important to determine how substance-abusing patients view their cognitive therapists, and to find the means to address any particular problems highlighted by these views. For example, do patients have misgivings about working optimally with their therapists as a result of cultural or socioeconomic differences? Do they doubt that therapists who have not divulged that they themselves are in recovery could ever truly understand what it is like to resist the lure of substance use? Similarly, do patients believe that their therapists expect too much or too little of them? On the flip side, do cognitive therapists make faulty assumptions about their patients, and/or fail to grasp the magnitude of the challenge of sobriety that they face?

The exploration of such questions may lead to fruitful advancements in the interpersonal aspects of cognitive therapy in session. For example, it may be advantageous at the outset of treatment for therapists and patients to openly discuss their views about each other, about alcohol and other drugs, and about how they can best understand each other. Anecdotally, one of my own patients with substance abuse complained that he often reminisced about getting high, and that he believed I couldn't understand this. The patient said, "You just think that drugs are bad and that I should always want to be free of them, but sometimes I think they're *good* and I *miss* them!" I stated that I believed I understood this, but the patient was skeptical. Asked why he was so doubtful about my response, the patient said, "Only someone who has had a drug addiction can know how much you miss it when you're sober, and how hard it is to stay clean." No matter what level of "truth" exists in this comment, it represents an important belief that may interfere with the optimal formation of a therapeutic alliance. Perhaps cognitive therapists will attend to such potential patient beliefs as a more routine part of the initial interactions between therapists and patients.

In general, however, there is a limit to what the therapeutic alliance can accomplish alone. Patients will still have to learn an array of self-help skills, and they will still have to remain in treatment. The immediate, powerful gratification obtained from drugs will still prove to be a formidable opponent against the positive feelings derived from a healthy therapeutic relationship. Thus alliance enhancement strategies are not a panacea, though they may incrementally increase the overall efficacy of the treatment package, and this is valuable in itself.

Incorporation of the Stages-of-Change Model

In order to provide accurate empathy to patients, and in order to ascertain the optimal combination of validation for the status quo and action toward change, it will be important for therapists to assess each patient's "stage of change" (Prochaska, DiClemente, & Norcross, 1992). Some patients are quite committed to giving up their addictive behaviors, and thus they are at a high level of readiness for change. Others are more ambivalent and may waver in their willingness to take part in treatment. Similarly, patients who are uncertain about giving up drinking or using other drugs may present for treatment with the goal of "cutting back" on substances. Such patients may bristle at the notion that they will need to eliminate their use of psychoactive chemicals, and may decide to leave therapy. Of course, there are some patients who are remanded for treatment who otherwise would not seek treatment on their own. They may deny that they have a problem with alcohol or other drugs, and not truly engage in the therapy process at all. Therapists' understanding of each patient's stage of change will be vital in helping them to know just how much to be directive, without going too far for a particular patient to tolerate at a given time in treatment. This sort of sensitivity may allow therapists to get the maximum "mileage" out of treatment with the patients who are most motivated, while retaining less motivated patients in treatment until such time as they begin to feel more of a sense of ambition in dealing with their problem.

One of the most delicate areas that therapists must navigate is patients' denial in the face of clear evidence that they have been using (Newman, 1997a, 1997b). Confronting the denial too strongly risks rupturing the therapeutic alliance. On the other hand, *not* addressing the patients' failure to disclose or acknowledge their substance use can trivialize the process of therapy, as the most important topic is left ignored. Finding a healthy middle ground—in which the patients feel that their therapists respect them and are not shaming or competing with them, but nonetheless are challenging the veracity of their claims of sobriety—is an important yet elusive goal. Further development of both alliance enhancement strategies and stages-of-change factors will need to focus heavily and specifically on productive ways to manage and work through denial.

Further Psychometric Refinement of the Belief Scales

As noted earlier, three measures appear in the appendix of the Beck et al. (1993) volume; these are intended to assess the belief systems patients maintain about various aspects of substance abuse. Many of these beliefs are hypothesized to play an important role within a full conceptualization of the substance abuse problem. For example, in the Craving Beliefs Questionnaire, patients score 20 items on a Likert-type scale from 1 to 7 indicating degree of agreement. These items include "Once the craving starts I have no control over my behavior," and "When craving drugs it's okay to use alcohol to cope." When patients complete this questionnaire, their therapists can "eyeball" the data to determine important beliefs that need modification. If, for example, a patient scores very high on the two items quoted above, this would indicate that he or she feels helpless to deal with cravings and feels justified in using alcohol when in the throes of craving.

Such information is extremely valuable in session, where the agenda could focus on improving the patient's self-efficacy in managing cravings, and addressing his or her permission-giving beliefs surrounding alcohol.

However, a problem with this measure and its compatriot questionnaires, the Beliefs about Substance Use scale and the Relapse Prediction Scale, is that sufficient psychometric norms have not yet been established on these inventories. Refinements in the scales are necessary in order to reduce redundancy of the items, and in order to obtain the broadest range of data with the least overlap across questionnaires. Psychometric studies that aim to develop these scales further will enable cognitive therapists and researchers to improve and expand upon their current clinical use. Ultimately, these inventories can be used more effectively in outcome research as predictors of patient retention in therapy, the strength of the therapeutic alliance, the efficacy of the treatment, and maintenance. In addition, more can be learned about the proposed mechanisms of change in cognitive therapy, as disorder-specific and treatment-specific changes in beliefs can be assessed at various stages of treatment. At present, the lack of support for the psychometric robustness of these three questionnaires makes it difficult to determine how well cognitive therapy modifies the beliefs it intends to change (see Morgenstern & Longabaugh, 2000).

Combined Treatments

Similar to recent advancements in the treatment of bipolar disorder and schizophrenia (see Scott, Chapter 11, and Rector, Chapter 12, this volume), where promise has been shown in combining cognitive therapy with pharmacotherapy, refinements of substance abuse treatment will probably involve more instances of coordinated care (Onken, Blaine, & Boren, 1995). For example, the strength of medication-based treatments that diminish the patients' subjective desire for their substance(s) of choice can be paired with the strengths of cognitive-behavioral therapy in modifying faulty beliefs and maximizing skill building. Thus it may be hypothesized that patients who receive the combined treatment will be less at risk for relapse than those who receive pharmacotherapy alone and later discontinue it (Anton et al., 2001).

It is also plausible that more therapists who provide treatment as usual in the community (often involving individual drug counseling, utilizing 12SF principles) could be trained to deliver cognitive-behavioral therapy (Morgenstern, Morgan, McCrady, Keller, & Carroll, 2001). Such a development would potentially lessen the tension that at times has existed between adherents of 12SF and cognitive-behavioral approaches, and may make the benefits of cognitive-behavioral therapy more available to people in recovery who might otherwise only attend support group meetings.

There is already evidence that cognitive-behavioral principles can be incorporated successfully into a community-based program for substance-dependent and homeless veterans (Burling, Seidner, Salvio, & Marshall, 1994); this offers promise for more widespread use of cognitive-behavioral treatment practices for traditionally underserved populations.

In a similar vein, the field needs to learn more about how psychosocial treatments such as cognitive therapy may or may not need to be varied, depending on the particular chemical(s) whose abuse is being targeted. Although it is intuitive that pharmacological interventions need to be tailored to the particular neurochemical mechanisms of the addictive substance, it is less obvious how treatments such as cognitive therapy would be modified, depending on whether the patients are abusing stimulants, downers, hallucinogens, "designer drugs," alcohol, or combinations thereof. In the meantime, cognitive therapists will continue to do individualized case conceptualizations of their substance-abusing patients, so that their idiosyncratic beliefs, risks, and rituals can be addressed in the most effective manner, regardless of the substance(s) in question.

CONCLUSION

The problem of alcohol and other substance abuse poses a major health problem for society. Sufferers often experience deterioration in their life situations, and commonly meet criteria for comorbid psychiatric disorders. Cognitive therapy—an extensively researched and highly efficacious treatment across a wide range of clinical problems—has been applied to the treatment of substance abuse with promising, if equivocal, results. The treatment model elucidates many potential areas for intervention and relapse prevention, and involves teaching patients numerous self-help skills to reduce risk, boost efficacy, and change beliefs that would otherwise contribute to a substance-abusing lifestyle. Keeping patients in active treatment has posed a significant challenge; therefore, greater attention is now being paid to enhancing the therapeutic alliance and providing other incentives to increase retention and reduce attrition. Further development of the specific measures of addiction-related beliefs will also assist in our understanding of the mechanisms by which cognitive therapy can be most helpful.

REFERENCES

Anton, R. F., Moak, D. H., Latham, P. K., Waid, R., Malcolm, R. J., Dias, J. K., et al. (2001). Posttreatment results of combining naltrexone with cognitive-behavioral therapy for the treatment of alcoholism. *Journal of Clinical Psychopharmacology, 21*(1), 72–77.

Anton, R. F., Moak, D. H., Waid, R., Latham, P. K., Malcolm, R. J., & Dias, J. K. (1999). Naltrexone and cognitive behavioral therapy for the treatment of outpatient alcoholics: Results of a placebo-controlled trial. *American Journal of Psychiatry, 156*(11), 1758–1764.

Baker, A., Boggs, T. G., & Lewin, T. J. (2001). Randomized controlled trial of brief cognitive-behavioral interventions among regular users of amphetamine. *Addiction, 96*(9), 1279–1287.

Barber, J. P., Luborsky, L., Crits-Christoph, P., Thase, M. E., Weiss, R., Frank, A., et al. (1999). Therapeutic alliance as a predictor of outcome in treatment of cocaine dependence. *Psychotherapy Research, 9*(1), 54–73.

Beck, A. T., & Emery, G. (1977). *Cognitive therapy of substance abuse.* Unpublished therapy manual, University of Pennsylvania.

Beck, A. T., Wright, F. D., Newman, C. F., & Liese, B. S. (1993). *Cognitive therapy of substance abuse.* New York: Guilford Press.

Burling, T. A., Seidner, A. L., Salvio, M., & Marshall, G. D. (1994). A cognitive-behavioral therapeutic community for substance dependent and homeless veterans: Treatment outcome. *Addictive Behaviors, 19*(6), 621–629.

Carroll, K. M., Nich, C., Ball, S. A., McCance, E., Frankforter, T. L., & Rounsaville, B. J. (2000). One-year follow-up of disulfiram and psychotherapy for cocaine-alcohol users: Sustained effects of treatment. *Addiction, 95*(9), 1335–1349.

Carroll, K. M., Nich, C., Ball, S. A., McCance, E., & Rounsaville, B. J. (1998). Treatment of cocaine and alcohol dependence with psychotherapy and disulfiram. *Addiction, 93*(5), 713–727.

Carroll, K. M., Rounsaville, B. J., Gordon, L. T., Nich., C., Jatlow, P., Bisighini, R. M., et al. (1994). Psychotherapy and pharmacotherapy for ambulatory cocaine abusers. *Archives of General Psychiatry, 51,* 177–187.

Carroll, K. M., Rounsaville, B. J., Nich, C., Gordon, L. T., Wirtz, P. W., & Gawin, F. H. (1994). One-year follow-up of psychotherapy and pharmacotherapy for cocaine dependence: Delayed emergence of psychotherapy effects. *Archives of General Psychiatry, 51,* 989–997.

Crits-Christoph, P., Siqueland, L., Blaine, J., Frank, A., Luborsky, L., Onken, L. S., et al. (1999). Psychosocial treatments for cocaine dependence: National Institute on Drug Abuse Collaborative Cocaine Treatment Study. *Archives of General Psychiatry, 56,* 493–502.

Deas, D., & Thomas, S. E. (2001). An overview of controlled studies of adolescent substance abuse treatment. *American Journal on Addictions, 10*(2), 178–189.

Lam, D. H., Bright, J., Jones, S., Hayward, P., Schuck, N., Chisholm, D., et al. (2000). Cognitive therapy for bipolar disorder: A pilot study of relapse prevention. *Cognitive Therapy and Research, 24,* 503–520.

Liese, B. S., & Beck, A. T. (1997). Back to basics: Fundamental cognitive therapy skills for keeping drug-dependent individuals in treatment. In L. S. Onken, J. D. Blaine, & J. J. Boren (Eds.), *Beyond the therapeutic alliance: Keeping the drug-dependent individual in treatment* (National Institute on Drug Abuse Research Monograph No. 165, pp. 207–232). Washington, DC: U.S. Government Printing Office.

Luborsky, L., Barber, J. P., Siqueland, L., McLellan, A. T., & Woody, G. (1997). Establishing a therapeutic alliance with substance abusers. In L. S. Onken, J. D. Blaine, & J. J. Boren (Eds.), *Beyond the therapeutic alliance: Keeping the drug-depend-*

ent individual in treatment (National Institute on Drug Abuse Research Monograph No. 165, pp. 233–244). Washington, DC: U.S. Government Printing Office.

Marlatt, G. A., & Gordon, J. R. (Eds.). (1985). *Relapse prevention: Maintenance strategies in the treatment of addictive behaviors.* New York: Guilford Press.

Maude-Griffin, P. M., Hohenstein, J. M., Humfleet, G. L., Reilly, P. M., Tusel, D. J., & Hall, S. M. (1998). Superior efficacy of cognitive-behavioral therapy for urban crack cocaine abusers: Main and matching effects. *Journal of Consulting and Clinical Psychology, 66*(5), 832–837.

McLellan, A. T., Kushner, H., Metzger, D., Peters, R., Smith, I., Grissom, G., et al. (1992). The fifth edition of the Addiction Severity Index. *Journal of Substance Abuse Treatment, 9,* 199–213.

Moras, K., & DeMartinis, N. (1999). *Provider's manual: Consultation for combined treatment (CCM-P) with treatment resistant, depressed psychiatric outpatients.* Unpublished manual for National Institute of Mental Health Grant No. R21MH52737, University of Pennsylvania.

Morgenstern, J., & Longabaugh, R. (2000). Cognitive-behavioral treatment for alcohol dependence: A review of evidence for its hypothesized mechanisms of action. *Addiction, 95*(10), 1475–1490.

Morgenstern, J., Morgan, T. J., McCrady, B. S., Keller, D. S., & Carroll, K. M. (2001). Manual-guided cognitive-behavioral therapy training: A promising method for disseminating empirically supported substance abuse treatments to the practice community. *Psychology of Addictive Behaviors, 15*(2), 83–88.

Newman, C. F. (1997a). Establishing and maintaining a therapeutic alliance with substance abuse patients: A cognitive therapy approach. In L. S. Onken, J. D. Blaine, & J. J. Boren (Eds.), *Beyond the therapeutic alliance: Keeping the drug-dependent individual in treatment* (National Institute on Drug Abuse Research Monograph No. 165, pp. 181–206). Washington, DC: U.S. Government Printing Office.

Newman, C. F. (1997b). Substance abuse. In R. L. Leahy (Ed.), *Practicing cognitive therapy: A guide to interventions* (pp. 221–245). Northvale, NJ: Aronson.

Onken, L. S., Blaine, J. D., & Boren, J. J. (1995). Medications and behavioral therapies: The whole may be greater than the sum of the parts. In L. S. Onken, J. D. Blaine, & J. J. Boren (Eds.), *Beyond the therapeutic alliance: Keeping the drug-dependent individual in treatment* (National Institute on Drug Abuse Research Monograph No. 150, pp. 1–4). Washington, DC: U.S. Government Printing Office.

Prochaska, J. O., DiClemente, C. C., & Norcross, J. C. (1992). In search of how people change: Applications to addictive behaviors. *American Psychologist, 47,* 1102–1114.

Siqueland, L., Crits-Christoph, P., Gallop, R., Barber, J. P., Griffin, M. L., Thase, M. E., et al. (2002). Retention in psychosocial treatment of cocaine dependence: Predictors and impact on outcome. *American Journal on Addictions, 11*(1), 24–40.

Solomon, R. L. (1980). The opponent-process theory of acquired motivation: The costs of pleasure and the benefits of pain. *American Psychologist, 35*(8), 691–712.

Turk, D. C., Meichenbaum, D., & Genest, M. (1983). *Pain and behavioral medicine: A cognitive-behavioral perspective*. New York: Guilford Press.

Wells, E. A., Peterson, P. L., Gainey, R. R., Hawkins, J. D., & Catalano, R. F. (1994). Outpatient treatment for cocaine abuse: A controlled comparison of relapse prevention and Twelve-Step approaches. *American Journal of Drug and Alcohol Abuse, 20*(1), 1–17.

Woody, G. E., Urschel, H. C., III, & Alterman, A. (1992). The many paths to drug dependence. In M. D. Glantz & R. W. Pickens (Eds.), *Vulnerability to drug abuse* (pp. 491–507). Washington, DC: American Psychological Association.

Young, J. E. (1999). *Cognitive therapy for personality disorders: A schema-focused approach* (rev. ed.). Sarasota, FL: Professional Resource Exchange.

Young, J. E., & Beck, A. T. (1980). *The Cognitive Therapy Rating Scale*. Unpublished questionnaire, University of Pennsylvania.

Chapter 11

Cognitive Therapy of Bipolar Disorder

JAN SCOTT

Until recently, bipolar disorder (BP) was widely regarded as a biological illness that should be treated with medication (Prien & Potter, 1990; Scott, 1995a). This view is gradually changing for two reasons. First, in the past three decades, there has been a greater emphasis on stress–vulnerability models. This has led to the development of new etiological theories of severe mental disorders, which emphasize psychosocial and particularly cognitive aspects of vulnerability and risk; it has also increased the acceptance of cognitive therapy (CT) as an adjunct to medication for individuals with treatment-resistant schizophrenia and with severe and chronic depressive disorders (Scott & Wright, 1997). Second, although medication is the mainstay of treatment in BP, there is a significant efficacy–effectiveness gap (Guscott & Taylor, 1994). Mood stabilizer prophylaxis protects about 60% of individuals against relapse in research settings, but protects only 25–40% of individuals against further episodes in clinical settings (Dickson & Kendall, 1986). The introduction of newer medications has not improved clinical or social outcomes for individuals with BP. This has also increased interest in other treatment approaches.

This chapter explores why psychological treatment may be indicated, explores research into cognitive models of BP, and then gives an overview of CT in BP and the outcome studies available for it.

WHY USE PSYCHOTHERAPY?

Recent studies of clinical populations with BP identify significant types of morbidity that may impair medication response rates or may simply be medication-refractory (for reviews, see Goodwin & Jamison, 1990; Scott, 2001). Like persons with chronic medical disorders such as diabetes, hypertension, and epilepsy, 30–50% of individuals with BP do not adhere to prescribed prophylactic treatments. It is interesting to note that attitudes and beliefs about BP and its treatment explain a greater proportion of the variance in adherence behavior than medication side effects or practical problems with the treatment regimen do (Scott & Pope, 2002). From 30% to 50% of individuals with BP also meet criteria for substance misuse or personality disorders, which usually predict poorer response to medication alone. Many of these problems precede the diagnosis of and possibly the onset of BP. The median age of onset for BP is in the mid-20s, but most individuals report that they experienced symptoms or problems up to 10 years before diagnosis. Thus the early evolution of BP may impair the process of normal personality development or mean that the person engages in maladaptive behaviors or dysfunctional coping strategies from adolescence onward. Comorbid anxiety disorders (including panic disorder and posttraunatic stress disorder) and other mental health problems are common accompaniments of BP; moreover, as many as 40% of those with BP may have interepisode subsyndromal depression. Although many individuals manage to complete tertiary education and establish a career path, they may then experience loss of status or employment after repeated relapses. One year after an episode of BP, only 30% of individuals have returned to their previous level of social and vocational functioning. Interpersonal relationships may be damaged or lost as a consequence of behaviors during a manic episode, and/or the individual may struggle to overcome guilt or shame related to such acts.

The psychological and social sequelae described above identify a need for general psychological support for an individual with BP. However, for a specific psychological treatment (such as CT) to be *indicated* as an adjunct to medication in BP, it is necessary to identify a model that (1) describes how cognitive factors lead to relapse and (2) provides a clear rational for the use of CT.

COGNITIVE MODELS OF BP

Early Descriptions of BP

Beck's (1967) original description of mood disorders suggested that mania is a mirror image of depression, characterized by a positive cognitive triad regarding the self, world, and future, and by positive cognitive distortions. The self is seen as extremely lovable and powerful, with unlimited potential and attractiveness. The world is filled with wonderful possibilities, and experiences are viewed as overly positive. The future is seen as one of unlimited opportunity and promise. Hyperpositive thinking (stream of consciousness) is typified by cognitive distortions, as in depression, but in the opposite direction. Examples of manic cognitive distortions include jumping to positive conclusions, such as "I'm a winner" and "I can do anything"; underestimating risks, such as "There's no danger"; minimizing problems, such as "Nothing can go wrong"; overestimating gains, such as "I will make a fortune"; and overvaluing immediate gratification, such as "I will do this now." Thus the cognitive distortions provide biased confirmation of the positive cognitive triad. Positive experiences are selectively attended to, and Beck hypothesized that in this way the underlying beliefs and self-schemas that guide behaviors, thoughts, and feelings are maintained and strengthened. Examples of such underlying beliefs and self-schemas include "I'm special" and "Being manic helps me overcome my shyness."

Beck's original model of mania was based on the careful observation of individuals in a manic state. There are gaps in this early model; for example, there was no discussion of any similarities or differences in the specific dysfunctional beliefs held by individuals with BP as compared to unipolar disorder (i.e., major depressive disorder), and the role of personality styles (sociotropy and autonomy) was not incorporated. Also, the nature of life events that may "match" certain beliefs and uniquely precipitate mania as opposed to depression remained unexplored. However, it is important to see the model in context. It was a useful step forward from psychoanalytic models, and has recently provided an important starting point for the research that is now being undertaken. In contrast to Beck's model of depression, there have only recently been attempts to confirm or refute psychological models of mania through research. However, as is typical of Beck, he has with his associates published a manual on CT for BP (Newman, Leahy, Beck, Reilly-Harrington, & Gyulai, 2002) that formulates many of the key clinical issues and lays out an agenda for future applied and experimental research.

Brief Overview of Studies of Cognitive Style

Most studies of cognitive models in BP have used the model of unipolar disorder as a template. Apart from one early study (Silverman, Silverman, & Eardley, 1984), data on dysfunctional attitudes, personality styles, and automatic thoughts in individuals with BP demonstrate a similar pattern to those seen in individuals in the euthymic and depressive phases of unipolar disorder (Bentall, Kinderman, & Manson, in press; Scott, Stanton, Garland, & Ferrier, 2000). Hollon, Kendall, and Lumry (1986) reported that, compared to healthy control subjects, individuals with either unipolar disorder or BP who were actively depressed showed significantly higher levels of dysfunctional attitudes and negative automatic thoughts. However, there were no significant differences between the two groups in either depression or remission. Also, Hammen, Ellicott, Gitlin, and Jamison (1989) found that subjects with unipolar disorder and BP who were asymptomatic did not differ on measures of sociotropy or autonomy.

We (Scott, Stanton, et al., 2000) explored several aspects of the cognitive model simultaneously, including dysfunctional attitudes, positive and negative self-esteem, autobiographical memory, and problem-solving skills. In comparison to healthy controls, clients with BP had more fragile, unstable levels of self-esteem; higher levels of dysfunctional attitudes (particularly related to need for social approval and perfectionism); overgeneral autobiographical memory; and poorer problem-solving skills. These statistically significant differences persisted when current depression ratings were taken into account. Within the BP group, those individuals who had multiple previous mood episodes and/or earlier age of onset of BP showed the greatest level of cognitive dysfunction. We have argued that although it was not possible to determine whether these abnormalities of cognitive style were causes or consequences of relapse in BP, it was noteworthy that these differences from healthy controls persisted in clients who were fully adherent with prophylactic medication. This suggests that long-term medication alone may neither extinguish cognitive vulnerability and affective symptoms, nor fully protect clients against relapse.

A further study comparing subjects with BP and those with severe unipolar disorder supports the hypothesis of similarities in cognitive vulnerability in unipolar disorder and BP (Scott & Pope, 2003). However, labile self-esteem, with relative preservation of positive self-concept but fluctuating levels of negative self-concept, was more typical of subjects with BP. Those with severe unipolar disorder showed relatively fixed low levels of positive and negative self-esteem. Both unstable self-esteem and persistent low level of self-esteem are known to confer similar levels of risk for mood episode relapse (Kernis, Cornell, Sun, Berry, & Harlow, 1993). Furthermore, if individuals with BP have variable self-esteem, they may be particularly sensitive to life events that alter their self-evaluations.

Research on subjects experiencing mania is limited, but the available evidence highlights that subjects who are manic do show state-dependent differences from subjects in other phases of BP or unipolar disorder, as well as from healthy controls. However, they often show complex changes, with simultaneous increases in positive and negative evaluations. These findings may support the view that dysphoric mania (with increased positive and negative affect) is highly prevalent (Cassidy, Forest, Murry, & Carroll, 1998), and that some aspects of cognitive and behavioral functioning in mania do represent (partially successful) attempts to avoid a descent into depression following an initial negative dip in mood (see Lyon, Startup, & Bentall, 1999).

Life Events in BP Depression and Mania

According to Beck's cognitive theory, certain maladaptive core beliefs interact with stressors that carry a specific meaning for the individual, increasing the probability of a mood episode's occurring. In their excellent review, Johnson and Miller (1995) confirm the association between adverse life events and either an exacerbation of mood symptoms or relapse into a mood episode. However, only six studies have explored the interaction between aspects of cognitive style and life events. A study by Hammen, Ellicott, and Gitlin (1992) reported that individuals with BP who had high levels of sociotropy experienced an exacerbation of mood symptoms in response to interpersonal life events. Hammen and colleagues did not identify whether manic or depressive exacerbations were more frequent. In a similar study, Swendsen, Hammen, Heller, and Gitlin (1995) explored the relationship between life stress and personality traits known to be associated with negative cognitive style—namely, introversion and obsessionality. They demonstrated that these negative styles interacted with nonspecific stressful life events to predict relapse of BP.

Two other studies have prospectively explored symptom exacerbation in persons with subsyndromal BP or nonclinical populations. Alloy, Reilly-Harrington, Fresco, Whitehouse, and Zeichmeister (1999) reported that an internal, stable, global attributional style interacted with life stress to predict increases in affective symptoms in individuals with subsyndromal BP and unipolar disorder. In a further study, Reilly-Harrington, Alloy, Fresco, and Whitehouse (1999) screened a nonclinical sample to identify individuals with hypomanic or depressive traits. Each individual's attributional style, dysfunctional attitudes, and negative self-referent information processing were assessed at baseline interview, and then reassessed 1 month later. In individuals with hypomanic traits, negative cognitive style at initial assessment interacted significantly with a high number of negative life events to predict an increase in manic or depressive symptoms. The interaction between dysfunctional attitudes and negative life events accounted for a greater proportion of the variance in symptoms (16%) than did the interaction between attributional style and negative life events (10%).

Two recent studies explore other types of life events that may uniquely precipitate the prodromal symptoms of mania. Malkoff-Schwarz et al. (1998). demonstrated that events that disrupt an individual's social rhythms (more frequent patterns of daily interaction) pose a greater risk of circadian rhythm disruption and ultimately of a manic episode. Furthermore, such disruptions were not significantly associated with the onset of BP depression. However, the study did not explore the meaning of these events for the individual (up to 43% of events could also be classified as representing threat of loss or actual loss experiences); nor did it explore the individuals' response to their sleep disruption or early prodromal symptoms. Healy and Williams (1988) had previously commented that if individuals notice that they feel more energetic, are happier, and need less sleep than previously (changes likely to occur with circadian rhythm disruptions), it cannot be assumed that they will automatically attribute such experiences to significant ill-health. They may make causal attributions related to their own prowess, rather than thinking that they are experiencing the early symptoms of an episode of BP. Healy and Williams hypothesized that an individual who attributes the changes in functioning to dispositional as opposed to illness factors may be at greater risk of entering a vicious cycle leading to manic relapse. Those who acknowledge the symptom as an early warning sign of relapse may instigate coping strategies that reduce exposure to stimulation or actively increase relaxation, and so avert the risk of a further mood episode.

More recently, Johnson and colleagues (2000) showed that life events pertaining to goal attainment may specifically precede manic as compared to depressive relapse. This finding appears to concur with information provided by clients in clinical settings, and it also supports the hypothesis that individuals with BP may have abnormalities in the behavioral activation system (BAS; see, e.g., Depue & Zeld, 1993). This system is thought to control psychomotor activation, incentive motivation, and positive mood. The BAS may show both higher baseline level of activity and greater day-to-day variability in individuals at risk of BP. However, even healthy controls show increases in positive affect and energy after life events related to goal attainment, suggesting increased BAS activity. Individuals with BP show a greater increase in BAS activity, slower return to normal baseline levels, and consequently an increase in manic symptoms in the two months after a life event involving goal attainment. It is hypothesized that the symptoms occur in vulnerable individuals because of a failure to regulate motivation and affect after the trigger.

In summary, there are many similarities in cognitive style between unipolar disorder and BP. There is limited evidence that trait aspects of cognitive style in individuals with BP increase the likelihood of early age of first episode or influence the frequency of recurrence. There is a paucity of data on the interaction between cognitive vulnerability and specific "matching" life events in BP. However, there is a consistent trend suggesting that negative cognitive style interacts with negative life events or high levels of stress to exacerbate mood symptoms. The evidence is more robust for the prediction of depressive symptoms, but negative cognitive style and events may also interact to predict increases in manic symptoms. Events that specifically precipitate mania may relate to disrupted social rhythms or to the attainment of personal goals. These events provide an important link to biological systems—namely, circadian rhythms and the BAS. However, the attributions and coping style adopted by the individual in response to prodromal symptoms of mania will also affect whether these isolated symptoms resolve or develop into a full-blown episode.

BRIEF OVERVIEW OF CT FOR BP

An optimal course of CT begins with a cognitive formulation of the individual's unique problems related to BP, particularly emphasizing the role of core maladaptive beliefs (such as excessive perfectionism and unrealistic expectations for social approval) that underpin and dictate the content of dysfunctional automatic thoughts and drive patterns of behavior. This formulation dictates which interventions are employed with a particular individual and at what stages of therapy those interventions are used. Although each individual will define a specific set of problems, Basco and Rush (1996), Lam, Jones, Hayward, and Bright (1999), Newman et al. (2002), and I (Scott, 2001) have identified several common themes that arise in CT for patients with BP. These are summarized in Table 11.1.

At the first CT session, the individual is encouraged to tell his or her story and to identify problem areas through the use of a life chart. Current difficulties are then classified under three broad headings into intrapersonal problems (e.g., low self-esteem, cognitive processing biases), interpersonal

---

TABLE 11.1. Common Themes Arising in CT of BP

CT may be used to:
1. Facilitate adjustment to the disorder and its treatment.
2. Enhance medication adherence.
3. Improve self-esteem and self-image.
4. Reduce maladaptive or high-risk behaviors.
5. Identify and modify psychobiosocial factors that destabilize an individual's day-to-day functioning and mood state.
6. Help the individual recognize and manage psychosocial stressors and interpersonal problems.
7. Teach strategies to cope with the symptoms of depression, hypomania, and any cognitive and behavioral problems.
8. Teach early recognition of relapse symptoms, and help the individual develop effective coping techniques.
9. Identify and modify dysfunctional automatic thoughts (negative or positive) and underlying maladaptive beliefs.
10. Improve self-management through homework assignments.

problems (e.g., lack of a social network), and basic problems (e.g., symptom severity, difficulties in coping with work). These issues are explored in about 20–25 sessions of CT, which are held weekly until about Week 15 and then with gradually reducing frequency. The last two sessions are offered at about Week 32 and Week 40. These "booster sessions" are used to review the skills and techniques learned. The overall CT program comprises four stages:

1. *Socialization into the CT model, and development of an individualized formulation and treatment goals.* Therapy begins with an exploration of the patient's understanding of BP and a detailed discussion of previous BP episodes, focusing on identification of prodromal signs, events, or stressors associated with onset of previous episodes; typical cognitive and behavioral concomitants of both manic and depressive episodes; and an exploration of interpersonal functioning (e.g., family interactions). A diagram illustrating the cycle of change in BP is used to allow the individual to explore how changes in all aspects of functioning may arise (see Figure 11.1). Early sessions include development of an understanding of key issues identified in the life chart, education about BP, facilitation of adjustment to the disorder by identifying and challenging negative automatic thoughts, and development of behavioral experiments (particularly focused on ideas

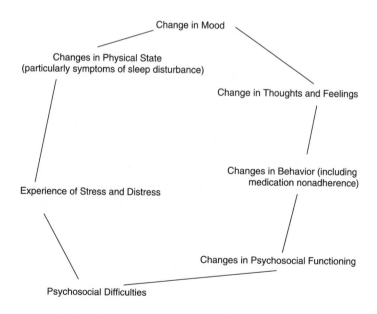

FIGURE 11.1. The cognitive-behavioral cycle of change in BP.

about stigmatization and fragile self-esteem). Other sessions include collating accurate information; enhancing understanding about the epidemiology, treatment approaches, and prognosis of BP; and beginning to develop an individualized formulation of the patient's problems, which takes into account underlying maladaptive beliefs.

2. *Cognitive and behavioral approaches to symptom management and dysfunctional automatic thoughts.* Using the information gathered previously, the therapist works during sessions to help the patient learn self-monitoring and self-regulation techniques, which enhance self-management of depressive and hypomanic symptoms, and explore skills for coping with depression and mania. These techniques and skills include, for example, establishing regular activity patterns, daily routines, and regular sleep patterns; developing coping skills, time management skills, and the use of support; and recognizing and tackling dysfunctional automatic thoughts about self, world, and future, using automatic thought diaries.

3. *Dealing with cognitive and behavioral barriers to treatment adherence, and modifying maladaptive beliefs.* Problems with adherence to medication and other aspects of treatment are tackled, for example, through exploring barriers (automatic thoughts about drugs, beliefs about BP, excessive self-reliance, or attitudes to authority and control) and using behavioral and cognitive techniques to enhance treatment adherence. The data gathered in these ways and from previous sessions are used to help the patient identify maladaptive assumptions and underlying core beliefs, and to commence work on modifying these beliefs.

4. *Antirelapse techniques and belief modification.* Further work is undertaken on recognition of early signs of relapse and coping techniques (fortnightly sessions). Examples of this work include developing self-monitoring of symptoms; identifying possible prodromal features (the "relapse signature"); developing a list of at-risk situations (e.g., exposure to situations that activate specific personal beliefs) and high-risk behaviors (e.g., increased alcohol intake), combined with a hierarchy of coping strategies for each; identifying strategies for managing medication intake and obtaining advice regarding it; and planning how to cope and self-manage problems after discharge from CT. Sessions also include typical CT approaches to the modification of maladaptive beliefs, which may otherwise increase vulnerability to relapse.

OUTCOME STUDIES OF CT OF BP

Encouraging anecdotal and single-case reports on the use of CT in clients with BP have been published over the last 20 years (Chor, Mercier, &

Halper, 1988; Scott, 1995b). These have been followed by nine reports on the use of individual and group CT in small-scale open studies or randomized controlled trials (Cochran, 1984; Palmer, Williams, & Adams, 1995; Bauer, McBride, Chase, Sachs, & Shea, 1998; Perry, Tarrier, Morriss, McCarthy, & Limb, 1999; Zaretsky, Segal, & Gemar, 1999; Lam et al., 2000; Weiss et al., 2000; Scott, Garland, & Moorhead, 2001; Scott & Tacchi, 2002). This section gives an overview of these studies, and the chapter concludes by considering the role of CT in individuals with BP.

Studies of Group Cognitive Therapy

The aim of Cochran's (1984) study was to add CT to standard clinical care, in order to enhance adherence to prophylactic lithium treatment. It compared 28 clients who were randomly assigned to six sessions of group CT plus standard clinic care or to standard clinic care alone. Following treatment, enhanced lithium adherence was reported in the intervention group, with only three patients (21%) discontinuing medication as compared with eight patients (57%) in the group receiving standard clinic care. There were also fewer hospitalizations in the group receiving CT. Unfortunately, no information was available on the nature of any mood episode relapses.

In Palmer et al.'s (1995) initial exploratory study, six clients with BP were offered CT in a group format. The focus of the program was on providing psychoeducation, describing the process of change, enhancing coping strategies, and dealing with interpersonal problems. Overall findings indicated that group therapy combined with mood-stabilizing medications was effective for some but not all of the participants. All participants improved on one or more measures of symptoms or social adjustment, but the pattern of change varied greatly across individuals.

The Life Goals program developed by Bauer et al. (1998). is a structured, manual-based intervention that seeks to improve patients' management skills, as well as their social and occupational functioning. The program utilizes a number of cognitive and behavioral techniques. Although outcome data are not yet available, a recent study of 29 clients suggested that the program was acceptable (70% of clients remained in treatment) and resulted in a significant increase in knowledge about BP.

Weiss et al. (2000) used a group format to deliver therapy to individuals with comorbid BP and substance dependence. The therapy was described as "integrated group therapy," but incorporated a number of cognitive and behavioral elements. Twenty-one individuals receiving group therapy were compared with 24 clients receiving usual treatment and regular assessments. The main outcome measures were severity of addiction and number of months abstinent. The subjects receiving group therapy showed statistically significantly greater improvement on both of these measures at a 6-month follow-up.

Studies of Individual CT

Zaretsky et al. (1999) used a matched case–control design to compare the benefits of 20 sessions of CT plus mood stabilizer medication for individuals with BP depression (n = 11) to an equivalent course of CT for individuals with unipolar depression (n = 11). Both groups achieved similar reductions in level of depressive symptoms, but Zaretsky et al. reported that only the subjects with unipolar depression showed a significant posttherapy reduction in levels of dysfunctional attitudes.

A colleague and I (Scott & Tacchi, 2002) applied the ideas proposed by Cochran (1984) to undertake a pilot study of a brief CT intervention (seven sessions of 30 minutes each) for individuals with BP who were poorly adherent to lithium treatment. We reported significant improvements in how the individuals viewed the disorder, improvements in medication adherence, and increases in serum lithium levels. These changes were all maintained at 6 months after therapy. Perry et al. (1999) undertook the largest study so far (n = 69), using cognitive and behavioral techniques to help people identify and manage early warning signs of relapse. The participants were clients at high risk of further relapse of BP who were in regular contact with mental health services. The results demonstrated that in comparison to the control group, the intervention group had significantly fewer manic relapses (27% vs. 57%), significantly fewer days in hospitals, significantly longer time to first manic relapse, higher levels of social functioning, and better work performance. However, the most fascinating finding was that the intervention did not have a significant impact on depression. The possible reasons for this and the implications of this study are discussed further below.

Lam et al. (2000) undertook a small randomized controlled study of 12–20 sessions of outpatient CT for BP. The model particularly utilizes CT techniques to cope with the prodromal symptoms of a mood episode. This has some similarities to Perry et al.'s (1999) model, but Lam and colleagues also targeted longer-term vulnerabilities and difficulties arising as a consequence of the disorder. Twenty-five subjects were randomly allocated either to individual CT as an adjunct to mood-stabilizing medication, or to usual treatment alone (mood stabilizers plus outpatient support). Independent assessments demonstrated that after gender and illness history were controlled for, the intervention group had significantly fewer mood relapses than the control group, with a significant reduction in episodes of hypomania, but nonsignificant reductions in the number of episodes of mania and of depression. The intervention group also showed significantly greater improvements in social adjustment and better coping strategies for managing prodromal symptoms.

We (Scott et al., 2001) examined the effect of 20 sessions of CT in 42 clients with BP. Subjects could enter the study during any phase of BP. Clients were initially randomly allocated to the intervention group or to a waiting-list control group (which then received CT after a 6-month delay). The randomized phase (6 months) allowed assessment of the effects of CT plus usual treatment as compared with usual treatment alone. Individuals from both groups who received CT were then monitored for a further 12 months after the end of therapy. At initial assessment, 30% of participants met criteria for a mood episode: 11 subjects met diagnostic criteria for a depressive episode, three for rapid-cycling BP, two for hypomania, and one for a mixed state. As is typical of this client population, 12 subjects also met diagnostic criteria for drug and/or alcohol problems or dependence, two met criteria for other Axis I disorders, and about 60% of the sample met criteria for a personality disorder. The results of the randomized controlled phase demonstrated that, compared with subjects receiving treatment as usual, those who received additional CT experienced statistically significant improvements in symptom levels, global functioning, and work and social adjustment. Data were available from 29 subjects who received CT and were followed up for 12 months afterward. These demonstrated a 60% reduction in relapse rates in the 18 months after commencing CT as compared with the 18 months prior to receiving CT. Hospitalization rates showed parallel reductions. We concluded that CT plus treatment as usual may offer some benefit and is a highly acceptable treatment intervention to about 70% of clients with BP. However, we also sounded a note of caution, as we found that CT for individuals with BP is often more complex than CT for unipolar disorder, requiring more flexibility and greater expertise on the part of therapists.

CONCLUSIONS

The studies reviewed in this chapter indicate that research into cognitive theory and therapy for BP is at an early stage. There is preliminary evidence that cognitive factors may influence vulnerability to BP relapse. The events associated with the onset of BP depression have many similarities to those linked with unipolar depression. Mania may arise in association with negative life events such as bereavement, but also may develop after events that disrupt an individual's day-to-day social rhythms, the sudden cessation of mood-stabilizing medication, or life events involving goal attainment. A number of researchers suggest that a common underlying link between these events is that they all can significantly disrupt circadian rhythms or induce variation in the BAS. In turn, circadian dysrhythmia or BAS dysregulation may lead to sleep disturbance, changes in motivation, and mood shifts. This model would suggest that the changes in levels of dysfunctional beliefs, attributional style, and thinking processes seen in BP episodes are secondary to biologically driven processes. However, it should be remembered that cognitive style will influence why individuals choose to stop their medication, how meaningful a loss is to them specifically, what unique causal attributions they make about any prodromal symptoms they experience, and how they react to or cope with the early warning signs of impending relapse. As such, even if there is at present no specific and unique cognitive model of BP, the use of CT and medication together may be a more fruitful approach than either treatment alone.

A review of therapy studies suggests that brief CT interventions mainly utilize a fixed set of cognitive and behavioral strategies that may facilitate change in individuals' attitudes toward and beliefs about the disorder and its treatment, or may enhance their self-management skills to allow early intervention at the first signs of prodromal symptoms. However, their role is limited to those individuals who need "fine-tuning" of their skills to allow them to cope with BP. As demonstrated by Lam's and my own groups and by Zaretsky and colleagues, there is also a role for CT in BP to utilize an individualized cognitive case conceptualization approach that provides a coherent and integrated understanding of each patient, his or her cognitive style and general coping behaviors, the patient's adjustment to BP, and the risk factors for relapse. My colleagues and I particularly target beliefs about social desirability, perfectionism, and autonomy. The evidence so far suggests that this triad may be important in subjects with BP. Lam and coworkers have targeted similar constructs—namely, dysfunctional beliefs that are characterized by an "overpositive" sense of self and an excessive desire for personal goal attainment. Given the extreme thinking styles that characterize depression and mania, it is noteworthy that Teasdale et al. (2001) demonstrated that some of the benefits of CT in more complex mood disorders might be mediated by changes in the style rather than just the content of thinking. They demonstrated that a persistently absolutistic, dichotomous thinking style predicted early relapse in chronic depression. Given that this thinking style is typical of subjects with BP, these data point to important areas of future research and developments in the process of CT in BP.

In the next 3 years, four large-scale randomized controlled trials will be published that will identify the benefits and limitations of CT for BP.

Early indications are that the intervention can reduce depressive and manic relapses and improve social adjustment. However, it may work best for those who begin treatment when they are euthymic, and who have less complex disorders or fewer (or no) comorbid disorders. We will need to review whether the large effect sizes reported in pilot studies of CT of BP are maintained when prescribed medications and clinical management are provided at an optimal level; all the treatment trials so far report deficits in the standard of treatments offered to individuals with BP. Finally, it is noteworthy that CT may be particularly beneficial in treating BP depression. It is ironic that despite few differences in cognitive style between unipolar and BP depression, individuals with BP have always been excluded from treatment studies of depression. Although modification of the CT protocol may be needed for BP depression, it is possible that CT will become a crucial alternative to antidepressant medication for this difficult-to-treat clinical condition. Large-scale trials of CT for BP depression are warranted. Such research also affords an opportunity to further explore cognitive models of depression and the similarities and differences between individuals with unipolar disorder and BP.

REFERENCES

Alloy, L., Reilly-Harrington, N., Fresco, D., Whitehouse, W., & Zeichmeister, J. (1999). Cognitive styles and life events in subsyndromal unipolar and bipolar mood disorders: Stability and prospective prediction of depressive and hypomanic mood swings. *Journal of Cognitive Psychotherapy, 13*, 21–40.

Basco, M. R., & Rush, A. J. (1995). Cognitive-behavioural therapy for bipolar disorder. New York: Guilford Press.

Bauer, M. S., McBride, L., Chase, C., Sachs, G., & Shea, N. (1998). Manual-based group psychotherapy for bipolar disorder: A feasibility study. *Journal of Clinical Psychiatry, 59*, 449–445.

Beck, A. T. (1967). *Depression: Clinical, experimental, and theoretical aspects.* New York: Harper & Row.

Bentall, R. P., Kinderman, P., & Manson, K. (in press). Self-discrepancies in bipolar disorder. *Cognitive Therapy and Research.*

Cassidy, F., Forest, K., Murry, E., & Carroll, B. J. (1998). A factor analysis of the signs and symptoms of mania. *Archives of General Psychiatry, 55*, 27–32.

Chor, P. N., Mercier, M. A., & Halper, I. S. (1988). Use of cognitive therapy for the treatment of a patient suffering from a bipolar affective disorder. *Journal of Cognitive Psychotherapy, 2*, 51–58.

Cochran, S. (1984). Preventing medical non-adherence in the outpatient treatment of bipolar affective disorder. *Journal of Consulting and Clinical Psychology, 52*, 873–878.

Depue R., & Zeld D. (1993). Biological and environmental processes in non-psychotic psychopathology: A neurobehavioral perspective. In C. G. Costello (Ed.), *Basic issues in psychopatholgy* (pp. 127–237). New York: Guilford Press.

Dickson, W., & Kendall, R. (1986). Does maintenance lithium therapy prevent recurrence of mania under ordinary clinical conditions. *Psychological Medicine, 16,* 521–530.

Goodwin, F., & Jamison, K. (1990). *Manic–depressive illness.* Oxford: Oxford University Press.

Guscott, R., & Taylor, L. (1994). Lithium prophylaxis in recurrent affective illness: Efficacy, effectiveness and efficiency. *British Journal of Psychiatry, 164,* 741–746.

Hammen, C., Ellicott, A., & Gitlin, M. (1992). Stressors and sociotropy/autonomy: A longitudinal study of their relationship to the course of bipolar disorder. *Cognitive Therapy and Research, 16,* 409–418.

Hammen, C., Ellicott, A., Gitlin, M., & Jamison, K. R. (1989). Sociotropy/autonomy and vulnerability to specific life events in patients with unipolar depression and bipolar disorders. *Journal of Abnormal Psychology, 98,* 154–160.

Healy, D., & Williams, J. (1988). Moods misattributions and mania. *Psychiatric Developments, 1,* 49–70.

Hollon, S., Kendall, P., & Lumry, A. (1986). Specificity of depressive cognitions in clinical depression. *Journal of Abnormal Psychology, 95,* 52–59.

Johnson, S., & Miller, I. (1995). Negative life events and time to recovery from episodes of bipolar disorder. *Journal of Abnormal Psychology, 106,* 449–457.

Johnson, S. L., Sandrow, D., Meyer, B., Winters, R., Miller, I., Solomon, D., & Keitner, G. (2000). Increases in manic symptoms after life events involving goal attainment. *Journal of Abnormal Psychology, 109*(4), 721–727.

Kernis, M. H., Cornell, D. P., Sun, C. R., Berry, A., & Harlow, T. (1993). There's more to self-esteem than whether it is high or low: The importance of stability of self-esteem. *Journal of Personality and Social Psychology, 61,* 80–84.

Lam, D. H., Bright, J., Jones, S., Hayward, P., Schuck, N., Chisolm, D., et al. (2000). Cognitive therapy for bipolar illness: A pilot study of relapse prevention. *Cognitive Therapy and Research, 24*(5), 503–520.

Lam, D. H., Jones, S., Hayward, P., & Bright, J. (1999). *Cognitive therapy for bipolar disorder.* New York: Wiley.

Lyon, H. M., Startup, M., & Bentall, R. P. (1999). Social cognition and the manic defense: Attributions, selective attention, and self-schema in bipolar affective disorder. *Journal of Abnormal Psychology, 108,* 273–282.

Malkoff-Schwartz, S., Frank, E., Anderson, B., Sherrill, J. T., Siegel, L., Patterson, D., et al. (1998). Stressful life events and social rhythm disruption in the onset of manic and depressive bipolar episodes: A preliminary investigation. *Archives of General Psychiatry, 55,* 702–707.

Newman, C., Leahy, R., Beck, A. T., Reilly-Harrington, N., & Gyulai, L. (2002). *Bipolar disorders: A cognitive therapy approach.* Washington, DC: American Psychological Association.

Palmer, A., Williams, H., & Adams, M. (1995). Cognitive behaviour therapy in a group format for bipolar affective disorder. *Behavioural and Cognitive Psychotherapy, 23,* 153–168.

Perry, A., Tarrier, N., Morriss, R., McCarthy, E., & Limb, K. (1999). randomized controlled trial of efficacy of teaching patients with bipolar disorder to identify early symptoms of relapse and obtain treatment. *British Medical Journal, 318*, 149–153.

Prien, R., & Potter, W. (1990). NIMH workshop report on the treatment of bipolar disorders. *Psychopharmacology Bulletin, 26*, 409–427.

Reilly-Harrington, N., Alloy, L., Fresco, D., & Whitehouse, W. (1999). Cognitive style and life events interact to predict unipolar and bipolar symptomatology. *Journal of Abnormal Psychology, 108*, 567–578.

Scott, J. (1995a). Psychotherapy for bipolar disorder: An unmet need? *British Journal of Psychiatry, 167*, 581–588.

Scott, J. (1995b). Cognitive therapy for clients with bipolar disorder: A case example. *Cognitive and Behavioural Practice, 3*, 1–23.

Scott, J. (2001). *Overcoming mood swings.* New York: New York University Press.

Scott, J., Garland, A., & Moorhead, S. (2001). A pilot study of cognitive therapy in bipolar disorder. *Psychological Medicine, 31*, 459–467.

Scott, J., & Pope, M. (2002). Nonadherence with mood stabilizers: Prevalence and predictors. *Journal of Clinical Psychiatry, 63*, 384–390.

Scott, J., & Pope, M. (2003). Cognitive style in bipolar disorders. *Psychological Medicine, 33*, 1081–1088.

Scott, J., Stanton, B., Garland, A., & Ferrier, I. (2000). Cognitive vulnerability in bipolar disorders. *Psychological Medicine, 30*, 467–472.

Scott, J., & Tacchi, M. (2002). A pilot study of concordance therapy for individuals with bipolar disorders who are non-adherent with lithium prophylaxis. *Journal of Bipolar Disorders, 4*, 386–392.

Scott, J., & Wright J. (1997). Cognitive therapy with severe and chronic mental disorders. In A. Frances & R. Hales (Eds.), *Review of psychiatry* (Vol. 16, pp. 249–267). Washington, DC: American Psychiatric Press.

Silverman, J. S., Silverman, J. A., & Eardley, D. A. (1984). Do maladaptive attitudes cause depression? *Archives of General Psychiatry, 41*, 28–30.

Swendsen, J., Hammen, C., Heller, T., & Giltin, M. (1995). Correlates of stress reactivity in patients with bipolar disorder. *American Journal of Psychiatry, 152*, 795–797.

Teasdale, J., Scott, J., Moore, R., Hayhurst, H., Pope, M., & Paykel, E. (2001). How does cognitive therapy prevent relapse in residual depression? *Journal of Consulting and Clinical Psychology, 69*, 347–357.

Weiss, R. D., Griffin, M. L., Greenfield, S. F., Najavits, L. M., Wyner, D., Soto, J. A., et al. (2000). Group therapy for patients with bipolar disorder and substance dependence: Results of a pilot study. *Journal of Clinical Psychiatry, 61*, 361–367.

Zaretsky, A. E., Segal, Z. V., & Gemar, M. (1999). Cognitive therapy for bipolar disorder: A pilot study. *Canadian Journal of Psychiatry, 44*, 491–494.

Chapter 12

Cognitive Theory and Therapy of Schizophrenia

NEIL A. RECTOR

Schizophrenia is a devastating illness characterized by severe impairments in cognition, affect, and behavior. Although pharmacotherapy is largely effective in treating acute psychosis and in preventing frequent relapses, from 25% to 50% of patients continue to experience substantial problems even while adhering to optimal medical interventions. There is a clear need to develop effective psychological interventions that target persistent delusions, hallucinations, negative symptoms, and frequently occurring comorbid conditions (such as depression and anxiety). Interestingly, case studies on the use of cognitive therapy for the treatment of delusions and hallucinations have been reported for over 50 years, although a silent revolution in the cognitive therapy of schizophrenia has occurred primarily in the past decade with the development of comprehensive cognitive therapy interventions (Beck & Rector, 2000; Chadwick, Birchwood, & Trower, 1996; Fowler, Garety, & Kuipers, 1995; Kingdon & Turkington, 1994; Rector & Beck, 2002; Tarrier, 1992) and their empirical examination (Drury, Birchwood, Cochrane, & MacMillan, 1996a, 1996b; Kuipers et al., 1997, 1998; Tarrier et al., 1998, 2000; Sensky et al., 2000; Pinto, La Pia, Mannella, Domenico, & De Simone, 1999; Rector, Seeman, & Segal, 2003). In a recent quantitative review of controlled studies, it was determined through meta-analytic procedures that cognitive therapy in tandem with pharmacological treatments leads to statistically large and clinically significant reductions in hallucinations, delusions, and negative symptoms

(Rector & Beck, 2001). As seen in Figure 12.1, patients receiving cognitive therapy plus standard treatment showed significantly greater improvement than did patients receiving supportive therapy plus standard treatment; this finding suggests that the unique cognitive approach is what accounts for the superior effects on positive and negative symptoms.

It is fitting that a book prepared to honor Professor Aaron T. Beck should include a chapter on cognitive therapy for schizophrenia, since the first description of cognitive therapy occurred in the context of treating paranoid delusions (Beck, 1952). It is also fitting, given that some of the most recent groundbreaking developments in cognitive therapy have occurred in the cognitive therapy of schizophrenia; many of these publications have been authored by Dr. Beck himself. The current review aims to provide a selective outline of the cognitive conceptualization of delusions, hallucinations, and negative symptoms, and the specific cognitive therapy approaches aimed at their reduction. In the following sections, the cognitive approaches to these groups of symptoms are considered separately, although these are typically synchronized in actual practice.

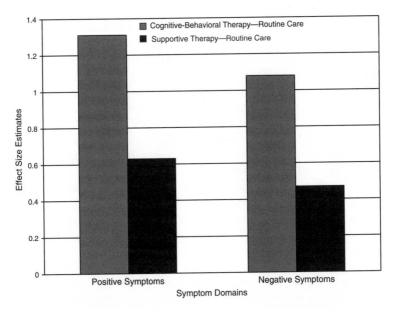

FIGURE 12.1. Effects on positive and negative symptoms following cognitive-behavioral therapy versus supportive therapy. Adapted from Rector and Beck (2001). Copyright 2001 by Lippincott Williams & Wilkins. Adapted by permission.

COGNITIVE THEORY OF DELUSIONS

According to the Diagnostic and Statistical Manual of Mental Disorders (4th ed.–text rev.) (American Psychiatric Association, 2000), a "delusion" is defined as follows: "A false belief based on incorrect inference about external reality that is firmly sustained despite what almost everyone else believes and despite what constitutes incontrovertible and obvious proof or evidence to the contrary. The belief is not one ordinarily accepted by other members of the person's culture or subculture (e.g., it is not an article of religious faith)" (p. 821). This definition continues to reflect the historical conceptualization of delusions as representing *abnormal* beliefs that are qualitatively different from *normal* beliefs. However, examination of the nature of delusions within the context of what we know about the role of specific beliefs in nonpsychotic conditions shows that delusions have many of the same dimensions as these other beliefs. Among these are the dimensions of "pervasiveness" (how much of the patient's consciousness is controlled by a belief), "conviction" (how strongly the patient endorses the belief), "significance" (how important the belief is in the patient's overarching meaning system), "intensity" (to what degree it prevents/displaces more realistic beliefs), and "inflexibility" (how impervious the belief is to contradictory evidence, logic, or reason) (Beck & Rector, 2002). These dimensions vary over time (Chadwick & Lowe, 1994) and change independently in response to cognitive therapy (Hole, Rush, & Beck, 1979).

Delusions have been said to be "empty speech acts, whose informational content refers to neither world nor self. They are not the symbolic expression of anything" (Berrios, 1991). Yet it is possible to make sense of the seeming bizarreness of the content of delusions and hallucinations when understood within the interpersonal context of a person's life. Everyday concerns about being rejected and manipulated may become amplified into paranoid delusions, whereas somatic hypervigilance and preoccupation may set the context for the development of somatic delusions. The content of delusions often reflects the patient's predelusional beliefs. Strong religious beliefs provide the foundation for delusions about Jesus, whereas a network of beliefs about the paranormal may lead to delusions about alien control. The understanding of the patient's predelusional belief system provides direct clues to the formation and content of the delusions. For instance, grandiose delusions may develop as a compensation for an underlying sense of loneliness, unworthiness, or powerlessness, whereas the proximal antecedents of a paranoid delusion may include the fear of retaliation for having done something that offended another person or group (Beck & Rector, 2002). Consistent with the hypothesis that paranoid delusions are associated with schemas reflecting interpersonal vulnerability, a recent cross-sectional study demonstrated that excessive need for others' acceptance and approval (i.e., sociotropy), as measured by the Dysfunctional Attitude Scale, significantly predicted the presence and severity of persecutory delusions (Rector, in press). Other research has shown that individuals with paranoid delusions preferentially attend to social threat-related stimuli (Bentall & Kaney, 1989; Fear, Sharp, & Healy, 1996), especially when the threat stimuli are emotionally salient (Kinderman, 1994). The person who regards him- or herself as socially unacceptable is more likely to be hypervigilant to potential rejection, and, in turn, more likely to interpret ambiguous social information as an indication of social hostility and/or rejection.

In contrast to the mechanistic framing of delusions as representing *fixed* neuropsychological deficits, the cognitive approach aims to understand the way common cognitive biases may distort perceptions of life experiences. Although delusions may arise through a number of different mechanisms, they are typically formed in response to negative interpersonal life events. For example, two patients had very similar (traumatic) experiences that resulted in very distinct delusional beliefs. The differences in the content and form of the delusional beliefs can be readily understood in relation to their differing pre-existing beliefs and their initial response to the situational trigger. In both cases, the patients reported being attacked by a small gang of boys in the playground in their early teens. For the first patient, who had a pre-existing fear of being criticized, judged, and rejected by others, the experience consolidated the belief that he was socially inadequate, broadly disliked, and consequently vulnerable to everyone's attack. The second patient grew up in a religious family and had strong religious beliefs. While being punched and kicked by the gang of boys, he saw a flash of light (as he looked at the sun), which he interpreted as the presence of a guardian angel there to protect him. Both patients presented for treatment approximately 10 years later—the first with a highly elaborate paranoid delusion that included the fear of being attacked by groups of people, and the latter with intense religious delusions incorporating a network of beliefs about guardian angels.

Once activated, delusional beliefs are maintained by a combination of factors that include cognitive distortions and biases, impairments in cognitive processing, and coping responses (including safety behaviors). Common cognitive biases, such as selective abstraction, all-or-none thinking, and catastrophizing, play a role in maintaining delusional beliefs similar to the role they have been found to play in maintaining depressogenic and anxiogenic beliefs. A number of cognitive biases seem especially prominent in the thinking of delusional patients. For instance, cross-sectional analysis of delusional thinking demonstrates several common cognitive characteristics—including an *egocentric* bias, by which patients become locked into an egocentric perspective and construe even irrelevant events as self-relevant; an *externalizing* bias, in which internal sensations or symptoms are attributed to external agents; and an *intentionalizing* bias, which leads the patients to attribute malevolent and hostile intentions to other people's behavior (Beck & Rector, 2002). In support of the importance of the externalizing bias, for instance, research has shown that when some patients with persecutory delusions attempt to make sense of relevant life experiences, they have an exaggerated tendency to blame extraneous factors (particularly other people) when things do not go well (Bentall, Kinderman, & Kaney, 1994). This exaggerated *self-serving* bias is especially prominent when the negative event is significant to a person (Kaney & Bentall, 1989; Bentall, Kaney, & Dewey, 1991), highlighting its potential protective function.

Another striking characteristic of delusional patients is their tendency to jump to conclusions (Garety, Hemsley, & Wessely, 1991; Fear & Healy, 1997; Peters, Day, & Garety, 1997). A number of experimental studies have demonstrated that patients with schizophrenia make overly rapid and overconfident judgments based on equivocal evidence (see Garety & Freeman, 1999, for a review). These patients appear prone to make impulsive judgments without seeking data to reach an informed decision; if an interpretation "feels right," they are likely to accept it at face value. Interestingly, a number of studies have also shown that when delusional patients are presented with an alternative hypothesis, they are equally impulsive in abandoning their existing hypotheses and forming new ones on the basis of little evidence. This impairment is most pronounced under high cognitive load and in the midst of "hot" situations when the patient is experiencing personal threat.

Finally, the various strategies that patients employ to cope with the fear, embarrassment, anger, and sadness generated by the delusional beliefs often serve to prevent corrective feedback. Just as patients with anxiety avoid situations that trigger fear, patients with delusions avoid "hot" situations that are likely to provoke their fears. Those with persecutory fears often avoid situations where they expect to be demeaned or attacked, whereas patients with religious delusions may escape from situations that are perceived to be sacrilegious (e.g., they may exit a conversation that makes reference to sexual themes). Patients with delusions also engage in subtle avoidance strategies that are similar to the detailed safety behaviors common in the various anxiety disorders. For instance, a patient refused to take off a headband because it was perceived to be holding his mind together. Another patient, with delusions of thought withdrawal, engaged in a neutralizing strategy by blurting out "I love music and movies" as a way of preventing passers-by from stealing away his love of music and movies. In a more dramatic example, a couple that shared a delusional belief about persecution from the Federal Bureau of Investigation (FBI) took turns staying up throughout the night to prevent a surprise attack. The absence of actual persecution from the FBI during "day shifts" or "night shifts," in turn, was seen to be a result of their watertight monitoring system.

The interacting roles of these different factors in the production and maintenance of a paranoid delusion, for example, can be seen in Figure 12.2 and enumerated in a case example. James presented with a 5-year history of paranoid schizophrenia. He grew up in a family where honesty, openness, and responsibility were core values. He believed that he had lived

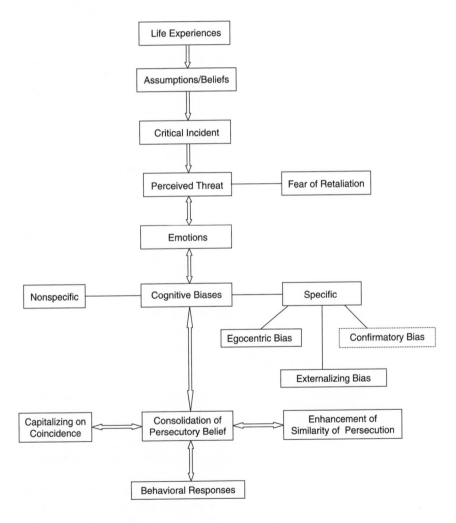

FIGURE 12.2. Development of persecutory delusions. Based on Beck and Rector (2002).

true to these values until his late teens, when, faced with mounting stress at college, he had plagiarized an essay. The essay was not only evaluated positively, but it was subsequently recommended for a writing award. James went on to complete his bachelor's degree and then a graduate degree at a teacher's college, but this incident had a transforming effect: he had come to see himself as a "dishonest fraud living a lie." As with others with persecutory delusions, the sequence started with a fear of retaliation: Officials at the school where James worked announced that they were going to take serious action against student plagiarism. James's automatic thought in response to the announcement was "I've done that too." He next thought, "What if they knew I had done that?" Over the next several days, he slept little and was preoccupied with "being a fraud just like the cheating students." The seeds of an elaborated conspiracy theory took form: Colleagues met to discuss joint action against "suspected" students, and the discussion evolved into their "disgust" with academic dishonesty. James thought, "I should be taught a lesson too," and began to experience a combination of heightened fear and guilt. Coincidentally, a book was missing in the school, and the principal asked James whether he had seen it. James first thought, "Do they think that I stole the book?" and then later, "They think I stole the book." The previous thought "I should be taught a lesson" made a similar transition to "I am being taught a lesson." These experiences crystallized the belief that "I bent the rules; now others are going to teach me the consequences." Subsequently, even remote events were seen as self-relevant. For instance, James read a headline in the newspaper—"European Swimmer Caught Cheating"—and he saw the message as pertaining to him in light of his distant European ancestry and his love of aquatics (i.e., egocentric bias). He further noted that conversations with colleagues in the lunchroom seemed to focus on the plagiarism issue only when he was present, and he thought, "They're sending me a message—aren't they?" He minimized disconfirming evidence (i.e., other topics were also discussed, conversations about plagiarism also took place in his absence). The biased perception of ongoing coincidental events served to consolidate the persecutory belief. The principal sent him new guidelines on plagiarism, and he (mis)interpreted this as confirmation that the principal knew of his past. There was enhancement of similarity in the persecutors: James's fear that his past was known extended from the principal, to his colleagues, to his students' parents. In response, he began to avoid the lunchroom, colleagues, and eventually classes, as he awaited being removed from the school and public shaming.

Conceptualizing delusions in terms of predelusional beliefs, activation of cognitive distortions and biases, and behavioral responses provides a road map for their clinical assessment and treatment with cognitive and behavioral strategies.

COGNITIVE THERAPY OF DELUSIONS

The therapeutic approach to delusions involves a number of cognitive and behavioral strategies aimed at undermining the rigid conviction, pervasiveness, and intensity of the delusions in an effort to reduce the distress and interference that they create in the person's life. Therapy begins with a focus on engagement and assessment. The initial sessions are relatively unstructured and focused on empathic listening and gentle questioning to communicate acceptance and support. A strong therapeutic alliance has been shown to have an impact on the process and outcome of cognitive therapy for schizophrenia (Rector, Seeman, & Segal, 2002). Next, the therapist completes a thorough structured assessment and a problem list, before attempting to shift the patient to a questioning mode. During the cognitive assessment, the therapist attempts to identify proximal events critical to the formation of the delusions (i.e., critical incidents—"How were things going in your life when you started having this idea?"), as well as current events that are likely to trigger the delusions. Specific triggers for delusions can be both external (e.g., a passing car) and internal (e.g., a headache). The specific emotional (e.g., fear) and behavioral consequences (e.g., avoidance, safety behaviors) created by the activation of the delusion are also assessed. In the assessment phase, the patient's predelusional beliefs are also ascertained by inquiring into the person's view of self, others, and the world, as well as any specific fantasies or daydreams the person had prior to the development of the delusion. The therapist aims to identify the range and severity of cognitive distortions in response to day-to-day life experiences and the extent to which these experiences have been misconstrued as providing supporting evidence for the delusional beliefs.

The next phase of therapy is aimed at socializing the patient to the cognitive model. Through guided discovery, the therapist begins to help the patient identify cognitive biases and distortions. Once the therapist has a cognitive conceptualization of the patient's delusional beliefs, an understanding of the past and most recent events that are interpreted as supporting the belief, gentle questioning of the evidence for the delusional beliefs is undertaken. The approach is collaborative and Socratic, and *never* challenging.

Initially, the therapist deals with interpretations and explanations that are peripheral to more central and highly charged beliefs. Take, for example, a patient with an elaborate paranoid delusional system that includes government officials, family members, and (more peripherally) the local phone company because of an earlier disagreement over an unpaid bill. Although there is a range of purported evidence to support the patient's beliefs, the therapist determines that her fear of persecution by the phone company is less charged than her fears of persecution by family members and government officials. So the therapist begins by discussing beliefs about the phone company. The patient describes the following events in the past week that are seen to support persecution by the phone company: The phone rang, and then stopped before she could pick it up; she could hear faint interference on the line during several phone calls; there was a telephone cable truck in front of the house 2 days earlier; and, finally, someone "pretended" to call with the wrong number. The therapist assesses the range of automatic thoughts (delusional inferences) in response to each of these events, along with a belief conviction rating. The patient is least convinced of the importance of the truck incident. The therapist asks a series of questions: "What was it about the truck's presence that led you to believe that it was there for you?," "Did anything else happen that day that led you to doubt this, by chance?," "Has anything else happened in the past couple of days that led you to doubt this?", and "Are there any other possible explanations why the truck may have been on your street that day?" Through this questioning of inferences, the patient considers a range of alternative evidence: "Well, the truck driver did go in and out of the neighbor's house . . . he was carrying equipment . . . he seemed pretty busy," "The neighbors did just move in . . . they might need a new line," and "He didn't take notice of me when I came outside . . . I guess if he was following me, he'd try to hide." The therapist helps to elicit an alternative/balanced explanation as the patient states, "Maybe he was just installing new cable." With repeated practice in generating alternative explanations for the range of evidence—first in session, and then increasingly as part of assigned homework—the patient begins to see his or her interpretations and inferences as hypotheses to be tested rather than as statements of fact.

Other cognitive approaches routinely employed to instill a questioning perspective include the survey method (e.g., "Can you ask your three good friends whether they ever get static [wrong numbers, hangups, etc.] on their phone line?") and pie charts (e.g., "Let's summarize all the different possible reasons why the phone would ring and then stop ringing before you could pick it up"). Through the downward-arrow technique, the therapist also aims to uncover the underlying core beliefs (e.g., "I'm worthless" and "I'm vulnerable") and assumptions (e.g., "If I'm not watchful 100% of the time, then I'm likely to be taken advantage of") that give rise to the misinterpretations of others' intentions and behaviors.

In addition, the cognitive therapist aims to change delusional thinking (and, later, negative core beliefs) by setting up behavioral experiments to directly test the accuracy of different interpretations. With the patient described above, an experiment included having him record the level of interference during calls that he made outside his home (e.g., at friends' houses, at the hospital) and inside the home over a 2-week period. The finding that there is considerable variation in the quality of the line both outside and in-

side his home provided disconfirming evidence that interference only occurred on his line and was the result of phone tapping. Finally, behavioral
experiments and other belief modification strategies (e.g., positive event
logs, core belief records) are introduced to target and reduce dysfunctional
beliefs and assumptions.

COGNITIVE THEORY OF HALLUCINATIONS

Similar to the mechanisms described above for the development and maintenance of delusions, the mechanisms involved in the formation and persistence of hallucinations require consideration of how the various
subcomponents connect to the broader cognitive organization of the person—schemas pertaining to the self, others, and the world (Beck & Rector,
2003). The important subsystems and their interplay in the production and
persistence of hallucinations are outlined in Figure 12.3.

Hallucinations are generally defined as perceptual experiences in the
absence of external stimulation and may involve any of the sensory modalities, although they are most common in the auditory sphere. Although auditory hallucinations are the most frequently reported symptoms in schizophrenia (World Health Organization, 1973), they are also present in a wide
variety of disorders, including psychotic depression, bipolar disorder, and
posttraumatic stress disorder. Auditory hallucinations are also commonly
reported during periods of bereavement, as a consequence of sleep deprivation, and in such adverse situations as solitary confinement and hostage
taking. Community-based studies indicate that from 5% to 25% of the
general population report hearing voices at some time in their lives (Slade
& Bentall, 1988; Tien, 1992), whereas surveys of college students show
even higher rates (Posey & Losch, 1983; Barrett, 1992). A comparison of
nonpatients who hear voices and psychiatric patients indicates great similarity in the physical characteristics of the voices, suggesting that
hallucinations may lie on a continuum with normal experience.

Just as in other forms of psychopathology, when certain idiosyncratic
schemas become activated, they play a role in information processing and
drive the cognitions that are typical of the disorder (such as self-denigration
in depression or perceived danger in anxiety). The voice content reported
by patients with hallucinations consist of a wide variety of comments, criticisms, commands, ruminations, and worries that are similar to the automatic thoughts observed in other psychiatric conditions. A differentiating
feature of the hallucinated cognitions is that the self is perceived as the object rather than the initiator or the subject. For instance, the automatic
thought "I'm worthless" following perceived failure becomes converted
into an externalized voice in the second person: "You're worthless." A

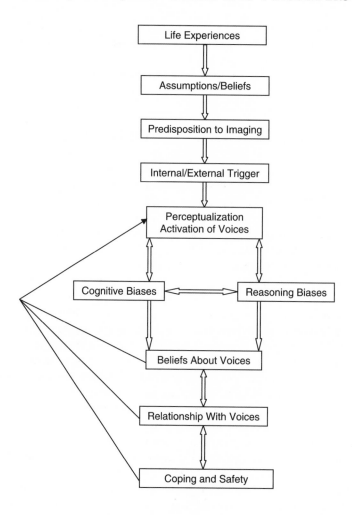

FIGURE 12.3. Cognitive model of auditory hallucinations. Based on Beck and Rector (2003).

question then emerges: Why do some thoughts become perceptualized as voices?

A number of studies demonstrate that patients who hear voices have an unusual propensity for imagery in the auditory modality. For instance, Bentall and Slade (1985) tested patients with and without hallucinations in a signal detection paradigm in which the task was to listen to white noise and determine whether or not a voice was present (when a voice was present 50% of the time). The patients with hallucinations showed the expected bias of assuming that a voice was present when, in fact, it had not been presented. In an extension of this work, Young, Bentall, Slade, and Dewey (1987) found that when the suggestion "Close your eyes and listen to the recording 'Jingle Bells'" (when, in fact, it was never played) was given to hallucinating and nonhallucinating patients, the ones who hallucinated were more likely than the ones who did not to report hearing the music.

A number of other studies highlight the tendency for hallucinating patients to misattribute internal cognitive events to an external source (Johns et al., 2001; Brebion, Smith, & Gorman, 1996; Franck et al., 2000). This externalizing bias is similar to the externalizing bias observed in paranoid delusions (Bentall, 1990; Young et al., 1987; Beck & Rector, 2002). For instance, Morrison and Haddock (1997) showed that patients with hallucinations, in comparison to delusional patients without hallucinations and to normal controls, were more likely to attribute their own thoughts in a word association task to the investigator. Use of functional magnetic resonance imaging (Shergill, Cameron, & Brammer, 2001) has demonstrated that the pattern of activation during auditory hallucinations is remarkably similar to that observed when healthy volunteers imagine another person talking to them. This finding provides further support to the hypothesis that auditory hallucinations are an expression of "internal speech" that becomes misattributed to an external source.

Yet a further question arises: How can internally generated phenomena be experienced as identical to externally derived phenomena? The inconsistency in the experience of hallucinations suggests a corresponding *threshold* for perceptualization. This threshold may vary considerably, depending on endogenous and external factors (e.g., fatigue, stress, and isolation, as well as emotional factors—anxiety, sadness, etc.). The likelihood of a thought's "crossing the sound barrier" (Beck & Rector, 2003) to become a voice is dependent on the emotional salience of the thought—the extent to which it represents a "hot" cognition. Hoffman (2002) has reported that Broca's and Wernicke's areas are excessively coupled in patients who hear voices, so that the production of language occurring in Broca's area is "dumping" language representations into Wernicke's area as a speech perception area, thereby creating hallucinated percepts of spoken speech.

Given that reality-testing functions tend to be compromised in the hallucinating patient, the ability to consider alternative explanations, suspend judgment until more sufficient information is collected, and create distance from the delusional beliefs and voices is underactive. The dearth of these functions may be instrumental in both the generation of voices and their maintenance. Other factors involved in the persistence of hallucinations include the formation of beliefs about the voices, the nature of the relationship with the voices, and the behavioral responses to the voices. Chadwick and Birchwood (1994, 1995) suggest that the disturbance associated with hearing voices is in part dependent on the idiosyncratic beliefs the person has about the voices' identity. For instance, the extent to which the agent of the voices is perceived as powerful, controlling, and all-knowing has been found to be more predictive of the emotional and behavioral consequences of the voices than the frequency, duration, and form of the voices. Furthermore, patients who hear voices tend to appraise their voices in the same way as obsessional patients appraise intrusive thoughts: as signs of danger and future harm (Baker & Morrison, 1998; Morrison & Baker, 2000). This appraisal process contributes to the emotional and behavioral reactions to the voices, and the subsequent maintenance of voice activity—just as similar appraisals have been shown to maintain the distress associated with intrusive thoughts in obsessional patients.

Early core beliefs and assumptions about the self influence both the content and the appraisal of voices. An underlying belief regarding oneself as worthless, for example, may lead to automatic thoughts of being a "failure" and demeaning hallucinations following a failure at school or work. Many patients who hear critical, demeaning, and insulting comments report having similar automatic thoughts pertaining to "worthlessness." For example, the content of the automatic thoughts of one patient who saw herself as incompetent ("I can't do anything right") paralleled that of her critical voice ("You can't do anything right"). Finally, patients may build up relationships with their voices just as they would with other people: positive, ambivalent, or negative (see Benjamin, 1989).

Patients who hear voices report staying away from public places, watching television, and keeping busy with household chores as a way of minimizing the voices (Romme & Escher, 1989). Unfortunately, the effort spent on avoiding or neutralizing the voices leads to a curtailment in the scope of activities, creating isolation and a paradoxical increase in voice activity. Of significance is the finding that engagement in these coping behaviors prevents the patients from disconfirming negative appraisals about the consequences of hearing the voices (e.g., "If I hadn't followed the command, God would have killed me"). Furthermore, the safety strategies deprive patients of the opportunity to determine whether their beliefs about the source of the voices are true. By foreclosing the process of reality testing, the coping behaviors may make the experience of hearing voices worse.

These findings have provided the impetus for developing a cognitive therapeutic intervention that helps patients (1) identify, test, and correct cognitive distortions in the content of voices, with the assumption that this content is similar to the patient's own (negative) thinking (which has been externally attributed); and (2) identify, question, and construct alternative beliefs about the nature, purpose, and meaning of the voices.

COGNITIVE THERAPY OF VOICES

Prior to implementing cognitive and behavioral strategies to help the patient construct an alternative view of his or her voices, a thorough assessment is undertaken with careful questioning of the frequency, duration, intensity, and variability of the voices. What situations or circumstances are likely to trigger the voices? Are there circumstances where the patient does not experience voices or where they are attenuated? Stressful situations are most likely to trigger voices. For instance, patients report hearing voices more frequently in the context of interpersonal difficulties, daily hassles, and negative life events (e.g., financial strain, housing crises). Internal cues, particularly emotional upset, can also trigger voices. As part of the early assessment phase, patients can monitor the relationship among situational triggers, mood states, and the activation of voices, using a modified thought record.

The cognitive therapist attempts to get verbatim accounts of what the voices say. Typically, patients will report hearing critical one-word utterances (e.g., "Bastard," "Goof") or similar two-word utterances (e.g., "You're worthless," "You're ugly"). Voices may offer a running commentary on a patient's activities or deliver commands instructing the patient to perform certain activities ranging from the mundane (e.g., "Take out the garbage") to more threatening edicts. Patients are taught to record the specific voice content between sessions, using the modified thought record.

The therapist also aims to elicit all of the beliefs a patient has about his or her voices. What agents (God, the devil, dead relatives, etc.) are purportedly talking to the patient? Beliefs about the origins of voices can range from the bizarre to the ordinary, and can vary from known, unknown, and deceased persons to supernatural entities and even machinery. A significant number of patients interpret their voices positively and experience positive emotions when they occur. For instance, receiving direct communication from God, Jesus, or a Knight of the Round Table sets the person apart from others and is accompanied by feelings of excitement and power. The therapist asks how the patient would feel if the voices were not present, as a way of unmasking the underlying feelings of loneliness and inadequacy from which these voices may be providing compensatory protection. The therapist tries to identify the life circumstances both distal and proximal to the initial onset of the voices, and to determine how the specific voice content (and the secondary delusional beliefs about the voices) reflect the person's prehallucinatory fears, interests, and fantasies.

Finally, the therapist assesses the patient's reactions to the voices. The patient's behavioral responses can include shouting back at the voices and/ or escaping specific situations in order to extinguish the voices. As described, patients first respond to their voices with surprise and puzzlement, but over time they tend to establish a personal relationship with the voices. For instance, if the voices are seen to be benevolent, they are frequently followed by positive emotions and the patients engage with them, whereas if they are seen as malevolent, patients are likely to experience a range of negative emotions and to cope by resisting the voices (Birchwood & Chadwick, 1997). All coping responses and safety behaviors are identified.

Following the assessment phase and the establishment of a strong therapeutic alliance, the therapist begins to employ gentle questioning to elicit alternative perspectives on both the voice content and the beliefs held about the voices. It is better with some patients to start by focusing on the beliefs about the voices, whereas with other patients it may be better to target the voice content first. The approach to undermining a patient's beliefs about voices is similar to the cognitive approach in treating delusions. The therapist begins by gently questioning the evidence that the patient takes as support for his or her interpretation. For instance, a patient believed that the neighbors were conspiring to have him removed from his apartment complex, and that he heard them speaking to him on a daily basis (Rector & Beck, 2002). As the neighbors arrived home from work and ascended the stairs of the building, the creaking of the stairs would activate the voices. When asked in session how he knew it was his neighbors' voices, he responded, "They sound just like my neighbors, and they speak to me every time they pass my door." To generate alternative explanations for the evidence "every time they pass my door," the therapist could ask these questions:

1. "Are there any possible alternative explanations?"
2. "Has it ever been the case that you heard the creaking stairs and not the voices?"
3. "Has it ever happened that you heard the creaking stairs and then the voices—and then you checked and found that it wasn't your neighbors passing your door?"
4. "If this did by chance happen, would it change your view?"

The therapist could also ask, "Do you ever expect to hear the voices when people come up the stairs?" and provide education (and normalizing) about the role of expectations and hearing voices. It is important that inconsistencies in the network of beliefs be addressed in a gentle and collaborative way, and not as a direct challenge. Behavioral experiments can also be incorporated to test whether the voice heard as someone passed the door actually corresponded to the person's passing by the door at that moment.

In addition to working with the evidence, patients are asked directly (as in the first question above) whether they have ever considered other explanations for their voices. Through collaboration, the therapist and patient attempt to generate as many alternative explanations as possible. The therapist also highlights any inconsistencies in the beliefs. Often the consequences of the voices are taken as proof of the interpretation of the voices (i.e., circular reasoning bias). For instance, one patient heard the voices of two men he had fought with in a bar. He believed that the voices were a form of punishment for fighting. The activation of the voices led to feelings of frustration and anger that, in turn, were taken as evidence of being punished. Alternative explanations for these feelings (e.g., not being able to control the voices) helped to reduce what would otherwise be taken as confirmatory evidence.

As suggested, beliefs pertaining to the omnipotence, omniscience, and uncontrollability of the voices are especially important and can be alleviated by a number of strategies. The Uncontrollability beliefs can be addressed by demonstrating to patients that they can initiate, diminish, or terminate the voices (Chadwick et al., 1996). Based on knowledge from the assessment phase, a patient can be presented with the cues that activate the voices (e.g., discussing an important past relationship) and then directed to engage in an activity that is known to terminate the voices (e.g., speaking with the therapist). This experiment can chip away at the belief that the voices are uncontrollable. The omnipotence and omniscience beliefs can be tackled by setting up experiments to demonstrate that the patient can ignore commands without consequence.

Alternative perspectives to the voice content are generated through exploring the evidence for what the voices actually say. For instance, a patient heard several voices telling her that she was "worthless." The patient was first asked, "What evidence do you have that supports the truth of this statement made by the voices?" With repeated practice, she was able to identify the cognitive distortions in the voices' comments (e.g., all-or-none thinking, catastrophizing, labeling) and to generate an alternative perspective when they occurred. Having patients keep separate thought records—one for their automatic thoughts and another for recording what the voices say—can convincingly demonstrate the overlap.

COGNITIVE THEORY AND THERAPY OF NEGATIVE SYMPTOMS

Just as delusions and hallucinations are not specific to schizophrenia and can be seen on a continuum with normality, aspects of the negative syndrome—such as apathy, anergia, avolition, affective flattening, and anhedonia—are not specific to schizophrenia (Rector, Beck, & Stolar, 2004). They have been found to be more prevalent in depressed inpatients than in hospitalized patients with schizophrenia (Siris et al., 1988). The distinction between negative symptoms and depression in schizophrenia is complicated, because they share many features.

In describing personal vulnerability to psychopathology, Beck (1983) characterized the highly autonomous person as having poor susceptibility to external feedback; low openness to corrective influences; a dislike of externally imposed directives, demands, and pressures; and a dislike of asking for help. All these aspects are commonly noted in those with prominent negative symptoms. Furthermore, excessive autonomy in nonpsychotic individuals has been found to be associated with symptoms that focus on the theme of defeat, including hopelessness, self-blame, anhedonia, feeling like a failure, and withdrawal of emotional interest in others (Robins, Bagby, Rector, Lynch, & Kennedy, 1997). In a recent cross-sectional study examining the relations between autonomous and sociotropic vulnerabilities and selective symptoms in patients diagnosed with chronic schizophrenia, it was found that patients scoring higher on autonomy-related concerns reported a greater breadth and severity of negative symptoms, even when the presence of concurrent depression levels was taken into account (Rector, in press). Patients who maintain unrealistic standards for their performance may be at particular risk of becoming avoidant and withdrawn if they perceive that they are persistently falling short of their own and others' expectations. Avoidance and withdrawal, in turn, may further contribute to perceived failure and hopelessness, creating a steady downward spiral of disengagement. For instance, a patient with a 15-year history of prominent negative symptoms without positive symptoms would respond to opportunities for enjoyment (e.g., watching television, playing a game, attending a day group) with such automatic thoughts as these: "No point in trying if I can't get better at it," "What's the point? I'll still have schizophrenia," and "It doesn't feel as good as it used to, so why bother?"

It is true that many patients with prominent negative symptoms experience other people (i.e., family, friends, and health care professionals) as demanding more from them in terms of activity and engagement then they are capable of giving. This may be especially pernicious for some patients who, prior to becoming ill, also held (excessively) dysfunctional performance beliefs, so that they now see themselves as failing to live up to both their own and others' expectations. Repeated unmet demands may further impact on perceived self-efficacy and fuel the cycle of hopelessness. The first step for the therapist is to reduce this pressure.

Negative symptoms can also be simple consequences of other problems, including depressed mood, distressing positive symptoms, anxiety conditions (including, but not limited to, panic disorder with or without agoraphobia, social phobia, posttraumatic stress disorder, and obsessive–compulsive disorder), and/or medication side effects (APA, 2000). Conceptualizing negative symptoms in terms of interacting cognitive, emotional, and behavioral factors, rather than irremediable *deficits*, provides a platform for the cognitive assessment and treatment of these symptoms with similar strategies to those that have proven effective in harnessing depressed patients' motivation and social and emotional reengagement (Beck, Rush, Shaw, & Emery, 1979). Prior to implementing change, cognitive therapists aim to complete a thorough functional analysis of patients' behavior. How are the patients spending their time? What do they take pleasure in? What helps create feelings of mastery? What would they like to do more of but currently find difficult to do? What do they not like to do? What do people in their lives want them to do more often?

The cognitive approach to treating negative symptoms follows from the cognitive and behavioral strategies previously described in the treatment of depression (Beck et al., 1979). These include behavioral self-monitoring, activity scheduling, mastery and pleasure ratings, graded task assignments, and assertiveness training methods. Cognitive strategies also include eliciting a patient's reasons for inactivity and testing these beliefs directly with behavioral experiments; direct attempts to stimulate interests (either new interests or a reactivation of previously held interests); and identifying, testing, and changing low expectancies for pleasure and efficacy in task pursuits.

SUMMARY AND CONCLUSIONS

This chapter has been a selective review of developments in the cognitive theory and therapy of schizophrenia. Attention to the phenomenology of delusions, hallucinations, and aspects of emotional disengagement reveals the importance of personal and interpersonal schemas and information-processing biases in their production and maintenance. Patients' beliefs about themselves, others, and the world shape the idiosyncratic form and content of the delusions and hallucinations. They also influence action tendencies that may help to account for the persistence of negative symptoms. The conceptualization of the symptoms of schizophrenia in cognitive as opposed to neurobiological terms provides a framework for therapeutic interventions, and there is increasing evidence for the efficacy of cognitive therapy as an important adjunct to standard treatments. A. T. Beck first described the cognitive therapy of psychotic symptoms, and half a century later he continues to pioneer developments in the field.

ACKNOWLEDGMENTS

The author would like to thank Dr. Eilenna Denisoff for her helpful comments on a draft of this chapter, and Magdalena Turlejski and Kate Szacun-Schimizu for their editorial assistance. Finally, the author would like to thank Aaron T. Beck for his encouragement, mentorship, and friendship.

REFERENCES

American Psychiatric Association (APA). (2000). *Diagnostic and statistical manual of mental disorders* (4th ed., text rev.). Washington, DC: Author.

Baker, C., & Morrison, A. (1998). Metacognition, intrusive thoughts and auditory hallucinations. *Psychological Medicine, 28,* 1199–1208.

Barrett, T. R. (1992). Verbal hallucinations in normals: I. People who hear "voices." *Applied Cognitive Psychology, 6*(5), 379–387.

Beck, A. T. (1952). Successful outpatient psychotherapy of a chronic schizophrenic with a delusion based on borrowed guilt. *Psychiatry, 15,* 305–312.

Beck, A. T. (1983). Cognitive therapy of depression: New perspectives. In P. J. Clayton & J. E. Barrett (Eds.), *Treatment of depression: Old controversies and new approaches* (pp. 265–290). New York: Raven Press.

Beck, A. T., & Rector, N. A. (2000). Cognitive therapy of schizophrenia: A new therapy for the new millennium. *American Journal of Psychotherapy, 54,* 291–300.

Beck, A. T., & Rector, N. A. (2002). Delusions: A cognitive perspective. *Journal of Cognitive Psychotherapy: An International Quarterly, 16,* 455–468.

Beck, A. T., & Rector, N. A. (2003). A cognitive model of hallucinations. *Cognitive Therapy and Research, 27,* 19–52.

Beck, A. T., Rush, A. J., Shaw, B. F., & Emery, G. (1979). *Cognitive therapy of depression.* New York: Guilford Press.

Benjamin, L. S. (1989). Is chronicity a function of the relationship between the person and the auditory hallucination? *Schizophrenia Bulletin, 15*(2), 291–310.

Bentall, R. P. (1990). The illusion of reality: A review and integration of psychological research on hallucinations. *Psychological Bulletin, 107*(1), 82–95.

Bentall, R. P., & Kaney, S. (1989). Content specific information processing and persecutory delusions: An investigation using the emotional Stroop test. *British Journal of Medical Psychology, 62*(4), 355–364.

Bentall, R. P., Kaney, S., & Dewey, M. E. (1991). Paranoia and social reasoning: An attribution theory analysis. *British Journal of Clinical Psychology, 30,* 13–23.

Bentall, R. P., Kinderman, P., & Kaney, S. (1994). Self, attributional processes and abnormal beliefs: Towards a model of persecutory delusions. *Behaviour Research and Therapy, 32,* 331–341.

Bentall, R. P., & Slade, P. D. (1985). Reality testing and auditory hallucinations: A signal-detection analysis. *British Journal of Clinical Psychology, 24,* 159–169.

Berrios, G. (1991). Delusions as 'wrong beliefs': A conceptual history. *British Journal of Psychiatry, 159*(Suppl.), 6–13.

Birchwood, M., & Chadwick, P. D. J. (1997). The omnipotence of voices: Testing the validity of a cognitive model. *Psychological Medicine, 27,* 1345–1353.

Brebion, G., Smith, M. J., & Gorman, J. M. (1996). Reality monitoring failure in schizophrenia: The role of selective attention. *Schizophrenia Research, 22*(2), 173–180.

Chadwick, P. D. J., & Birchwood, M. J. (1994). Challenging the omnipotence of voices: A cognitive approach to auditory hallucinations. *British Journal of Psychiatry, 164,* 190–201.

Chadwick, P. D. J., & Birchwood, M. (1995). The omnipotence of voices: II. The Beliefs About Voices Questionnaire (BAVQ). *British Journal of Psychiatry, 166*(6), 773–776.

Chadwick, P. D. J., Birchwood, M., & Trower, P. (1996). *Cognitive therapy for delusions, voices, and paranoia.* New York: Wiley.

Chadwick, P. D. J., & Lowe, C. F. (1994). A cognitive approach to measuring and modifying delusions. *Behaviour Research and Therapy, 32,* 355–367.

Drury, V., Birchwood, M., Cochrane, R., & MacMillan, F. (1996a). Cognitive therapy and recovery from acute psychosis: A controlled trial. I. Impact on psychotic symptoms. *British Journal of Psychiatry, 169,* 593–601.

Drury, V., Birchwood, M., Cochrane, R., & MacMillan, F. (1996b). Cognitive therapy and recovery from acute psychosis: A controlled trial. II. Impact on recovery time. *British Journal of Psychiatry, 169,* 602–607.

Fear, C. F., & Healy, D. (1997). Probabilistic reasoning in obsessive–compulsive and delusional disorders. *Psychological Medicine, 27,* 199–208.

Fear, C., Sharp, H., & Healy, D. (1996). Cognitive processes in delusional disorders. *British Journal of Psychiatry, 168,* 1–8.

Fowler, D., Garety, P., & Kuipers, E. (1995). *Cognitive behavior therapy for psychosis: Theory and practice.* New York: Wiley.

Franck, N., Rouby, P., Daprati, E., Dalery, J., Marie-Cardine, M., & Georgieff, N. (2000). Confusion between silent and overt reading in schizophrenia. *Schizophrenia Research, 41,* 357–368.

Garety, P. A., & Freeman, D. (1999). Cognitive approaches to delusions: A critical review of theories and evidence. *British Journal of Clinical Psychology, 38,* 113–154.

Garety, P. A., Hemsley, D. R., & Wessely, S. (1991). Reasoning in deluded schizophrenic and paranoid patients: Biases in performance on a probabilistic inference task. *Journal of Nervous and Mental Disease, 179,* 194–202.

Hoffman, R. E. (2002). Slow transcranial magnetic stimulation, long-term depotentiation, and brain hyperexcitability disorders. *American Journal of Psychiatry, 159*(7), 1093–1102.

Hole, R. W., Rush, A. J., & Beck, A. T. (1979). A cognitive investigation of schizophrenic delusions. *Psychiatry, 42,* 312–319.

Johns, L. C., Rossell, S., Frith, C., Ahmad, F., Hemsley, D., Kuipers, E., et al. (2001). Verbal self-monitoring and auditory hallucinations in people with schizophrenia. *Psychological Medicine, 31,* 705–715.

Kaney, S., & Bentall, R. P. (1989). Persecutory delusions and attributional style. *British Journal of Medical Psychology, 62,* 191–198.

Kinderman, P. (1994). Attentional bias, persecutory delusions and the self-concept. *British Journal of Medical Psychology, 67,* 33–39.

Kingdon, D., & Turkington, D. (1994). *Cognitive-behavioral therapy of schizophrenia.* New York: Guilford Press.

Kuipers, E., Fowler, D., Garety, P., Chisholm, D., Freeman, D., Dunn, G., et al. (1998). London–East Anglia randomized controlled trial of cognitive-behaviour therapy for psychosis: III. Follow-up and economic evaluation at 18 months. *British Journal of Psychiatry, 173,* 61–68.

Kuipers, E., Garety, P., Fowler, D., Dunn, G., Beggington, P., Freeman, D., et al. (1997). London–East Anglia randomized controlled trial of cognitive-behaviour therapy for psychosis: I. Effects of the treatment phase. *British Journal of Psychiatry, 171,* 319–327.

Morrison, A. P. (Ed.). (2002). *A casebook of cognitive therapy for psychosis.* Hove, UK: Brunner-Routledge.

Morrison, A. P., & Baker, C. A. (2000). Intrusive thoughts and auditory hallucinations: a comparative study of intrusions in psychosis. *Behaviour Research and Therapy, 38*(11), 1097–1107.

Morrison, A. P., & Haddock, G. (1997). Cognitive factors in source monitoring and auditory hallucinations. *Psychological Medicine, 27,* 669–679.

Peters, E., Day, S., & Garety, P. (1997). From preconscious to conscious processing: Where does the abnormality lie in delusions? *Schizophrenia Research, 24,* 120.

Pinto, A., La Pia, S., Mannella, R., Domenico, G., & De Simone, L. (1999). Cognitive-behavioral therapy and clozapine for clients with treatment-refractory schizophrenia. *Psychiatric Services, 50,* 901–904.

Posey, T., & Losch, M. (1983). Auditory hallucinations of hearing voices in 375 normal subjects. *Imagination, Cognition and Personality, 2,* 99–113.

Rector, N. A. (in press). Dysfunctional attitudes and symptom expression in schizophrenia: Predictors of paranoid delusions and negative symptoms. *Journal of Cognitive Psychotherapy: An International Quarterly.*

Rector, N. A., & Beck, A. T. (2001). Cognitive behavioral therapy for schizophrenia: An empirical review. *Journal of Nervous and Mental Disease,189*(5), 278–287.

Rector, N. A., & Beck, A. T. (2002). Cognitive therapy for schizophrenia: From conceptualization to intervention. *Canadian Journal of Psychiatry, 47*(1), 39–48.

Rector, N. A., Beck, A. T., & Stolar, N. (2004). *The negative symptoms of schizophrenia: A cognitive perspective.* Manuscript under review.

Rector, N. A., Seeman, M. V., & Segal, Z. V. (2002, November). *The role of the therapeutic alliance in cognitive therapy for schizophrenia.* Paper presented at the annual meeting of the Association for the Advancement of Behavior Therapy, Reno, NV.

Rector, N. A., Seeman, M. V., & Segal, Z. V. (2003). Cognitive therapy of schizophrenia: A preliminary randomized controlled trial. *Schizophrenia Research, 63,* 1–11.

Robins, C. J., Bagby, R. M., Rector, N. A., Lynch, T. R., & Kennedy, S. H. (1997). Sociotropy, autonomy, and patterns of symptoms in patients with major depression: A comparison of dimensional and categorical approaches. *Cognitive Therapy and Research, 21*(3), 285–300.

Romme, M., & Escher, D. (1989). Hearing voices. *Schizophrenia Bulletin, 15,* 209–216.

Sensky, T., Turkington, D., Kingdon, D., Scott, J. L., Scott, J., Siddle, R., et al. (2000). A randomized controlled trial of cognitive-behavioral therapy for persistent symptoms in schizophrenia resistant to medication. *Archives of General Psychiatry, 57*(2), 165–172.

Shergill, S. S., Cameron, L. A., & Brammer, M. J.(2001). Modality specific neural correlates of auditory and somatic hallucinations. *Journal of Neurology, Neurosurgergy and Psychiatry, 71*(5), 688–690.

Siris, S. G., Adan, F., Cohen, M., Mandeli, J., Aronson, A., & Kasey E. (1988). Post-psychotic depression and negative symptoms: An investigation of syndromal overlap. *American Journal of Psychiatry, 145,* 1532–1537.

Slade, P., & Bentall, R. (1988). *Sensory deception: A scientific analysis of hallucination.* Baltimore: Johns Hopkins University Press.

Tarrier, N. (1992). Psychological treatment of positive schizophrenic symptoms. In D. Kavanagh (Ed.), *Schizophrenia: An overview and practical handbook* (pp. 356–373). London: Chapman & Hall.

Tarrier, N., Wittkowski, A., Kinney, C., McCarthy, E., Morris, J., & Humphreys, L. (2000). Durability of the effects of cognitive-behavioural therapy in the treatment of chronic schizophrenia. *British Journal of Psychiatry, 174,* 500–504.

Tarrier, N., Yusupoff, L., Kinney, C., McCarthy, E., Gledhill, A., Haddock, G., et al. (1998). randomized controlled trial of intensive cognitive behaviour therapy for patients with chronic schizophrenia. *British Medical Journal, 317,* 303–307.

Tien, A. Y. (1992). Distribution of hallucinations in the population. *Social Psychiatry and Psychiatric Epidemiology, 26,* 287–292.

World Health Organization. (1973). *International pilot study of schizophrenia.* Geneva: Author.

Young, H. F., Bentall, R. P., Slade, P. D., & Dewey, M. E. (1987). The role of brief instructions and suggestibility in the elicitation of hallucinations in normal and psychiatric subjects. *Journal of Nervous and Mental Disease, 175,* 41–48.

Part IV

PERSONALITY DISORDERS

Chapter 13

Cognitive Therapy of Borderline Personality Disorder

JANET KLOSKO

JEFFREY YOUNG

In developing cognitive therapy, Aaron Beck made a major contribution to the understanding and treatment of psychiatric disorders. Cognitive therapy was revolutionary, in that it shifted the focus of therapy to the patient's life outside sessions (rather than the transference), to the present (rather than the patient's early childhood), and to the contents of consciousness (rather than the unconscious).

Beck originally created cognitive therapy to work with depression. However, it was always his plan that the cognitive model would be adapted to other disorders. Practitioners of cognitive therapy have constructed effective psychological treatments for many Axis I disorders, including mood, anxiety, sexual, eating, somatoform, and substance use disorders. These treatments have traditionally been short-term, and have focused on reducing symptoms, building skills, and solving problems in the patient's current life. Treatment outcome studies usually report success rates over 60% (Barlow, 2001).

Often, however, patients with underlying personality disorders fail to respond fully to cognitive therapy (Beck, Freeman, & Associates, 1990; Beck, Freeman, Davis, & Associates, 2004). Some patients present for treatment of Axis I symptoms, and either fail to progress in treatment or relapse. Other patients come for cognitive therapy of Axis I symptoms; then later their characterological problems become a focus of treatment once their Axis I problems are resolved. Still other patients come for cognitive therapy, but they lack specific symptoms to serve as targets of therapy. Their problems are vague or diffuse and lack clear precipitants. Because they do not have significant Axis I symptoms, or they have so many of them, cognitive therapy is difficult to apply to them.

One of the challenges facing us today is developing effective treatments for patients with these chronic, difficult-to-treat disorders. Jeffrey Young, a protégé of Beck, applied Beck's model to personality disorders. Young expanded Beck's original model in several ways to work with personality disorders, prior to developing his adaptation for borderline personality disorder (BPD). Conceptually, he incorporated the concept of core needs, expanded the emphasis on early schemas, and introduced the idea of coping styles to cognitive therapy. In terms of treatment, Young placed more stress on understanding the patient's early history and life patterns, developed several inventories, introduced Gestalt-type techniques, and placed a heightened importance on the therapy relationship. Eventually, Young named his expansion of cognitive therapy for characterological problems "schema therapy," to accentuate the importance of early life themes and patterns. As Young and his colleagues gained more experience with patients who had BPD, they recognized that the original schema model needed to be modified. These patients had almost all of the schemas, and they had frequent, dramatic mood shifts. To address these problems, Young introduced an additional construct, the "schema mode." Young also felt that the therapeutic relationship needed to be reformulated for patients with BPD, and thus introduced the concept of "limited reparenting."

ASSUMPTIONS OF TRADITIONAL COGNITIVE THERAPY VIOLATED BY PATIENTS WITH CHARACTEROLOGICAL PROBLEMS

Cognitive therapy makes several assumptions about patients that often prove untrue of those with characterological problems. One assumption is that patients will comply with the treatment protocol. Patients are motivated to reduce symptoms and build skills; therefore, with some prodding and positive reinforcement, they will undertake the necessary treatment procedures. However, for many patients with characterological problems, their motivation and approach to therapy are complicated, and they are often unwilling or unable to comply with cognitive procedures.

Another assumption in cognitive therapy is that with brief training, patients can access their cognitions and emotions and can report them to their therapists. However, patients with characterological problems are often unable to do so. They seem out of touch with their cognitions or emotions. Many of these patients engage in cognitive and affective avoidance. They thus avoid many of the behaviors and situations that are essential to their progress.

Cognitive therapy also assumes that patients can change their problematic cognitions and behaviors through such practices as empirical analysis, logical discourse, experimentation, gradual steps, and repetition. However, for patients with characterological problems, this is often not the case. In our experience, their distorted thoughts and self-defeating behaviors are extremely resistant to modification solely through cognitive techniques. Even after months of therapy, there is often no sustained improvement.

Because these patients usually lack psychological flexibility, they are much less responsive to cognitive techniques, and frequently do not make meaningful changes in a short period of time. Rather, they are psychologically rigid. According to the *Diagnostic and Statistical Manual of Mental Disorders*, fourth edition (DSM-IV), rigidity is a hallmark of personality disorders (American Psychiatric Association, 1994, p. 633). When challenged, these patients rigidly, reflexively, and sometimes aggressively cling to what they already believe to be true about themselves and the world.

Cognitive therapy also assumes that patients can engage in a collaborative relationship with their therapists within a few sessions. Difficulties in the therapeutic relationship are typically viewed as obstacles to be overcome in order to attain a patient's compliance with treatment procedures. The therapist–patient relationship is not generally regarded as an "active ingredient" of the treatment. However, patients with characterological disorders often have difficulty forming a therapeutic alliance. Lifelong disturbances in relationships with significant others are another hallmark of personality disorders (Millon, 1981). These patients thus often find it difficult to form secure therapeutic relationships.

Finally, in cognitive therapy, the patient is presumed to have problems that are readily discernible as targets of treatment. In the case of patients with characterological problems, this presumption is often not met. These patients commonly have presenting problems that are vague, chronic, and pervasive. They are fundamentally dissatisfied in love, work, or play. These very broad, hard-to-define life themes usually do not make easy-to-address targets for standard cognitive treatment.

LATER EXPANSIONS OF BECK'S COGNITIVE THERAPY

Thus far, we have discussed Beck's *original* cognitive therapy. Now we will discuss later expansions of the cognitive model by Beck and his colleagues.

Beck's "Reformulated" Model

In the revised model of cognitive therapy for personality disorders proposed by Beck and his associates, personality is defined as "specific patterns of social, motivational and cognitive–affective processes" Alford & Beck, 1997). Personality includes behaviors, thought processes, emotional responses, and motivational needs. Personality is determined by the "idiosyncratic structures," or schemas, that constitute the basic elements of personality. Alford and Beck (1997) propose that the schema concept may "provide a common language to facilitate the integration of certain psychotherapeutic approaches." According to Beck's model, a "core belief" represents the meaning, or cognitive content, of a schema.

Modes

Beck has also elaborated his concept of a "mode." A mode is an integrated network of cognitive, affective, motivational, and behavioral components. A mode can consist of many cognitive schemas. These modes mobilize individuals in intense psychological reactions, and are oriented toward achieving particular aims. Like schemas, modes are primarily automatic and also require activation. Individuals with a cognitive vulnerability who are exposed to relevant stressors may develop symptoms related to the mode.

According to Beck's view, modes consist of schemas, which contain memories, problem-solving strategies, images, and language. Modes activate "programmed strategies for carrying out basic categories of survival skills, such as defense from predators" (Alford & Beck, 1997). The activation of a specific mode is derived from an individual's genetic makeup and cultural/social beliefs.

Beck further explains that when a schema is triggered, a corresponding mode is not necessarily activated. In other words, even when a schema is triggered, mode activation may not take place; in this case, although the cognitive component of the schema has been triggered, we would not see any corresponding affective, motivational, or behavioral components.

In treatment, a patient learns to utilize the conscious control system to deactivate modes. When trigger events are reinterpreted in a manner inconsistent with the mode, the mode can be deactivated. Furthermore, modes can be modified.

Borderline Personality Disorder

Beck applies his cognitive model to BPD (Beck et al., 1990, 2004). His model is consistent with a stress–diathesis model. Patients with BPD experience ordinary life events as threatening because of their sensitivity. They react with negative affect, then cope by engaging in self-defeating behaviors. These patients' vulnerability is based upon extreme thinking, primarily due to dichotomous representations of themselves and others. Specific beliefs include "The world is malevolent and dangerous," "I am powerless," and "I am unacceptable." Patients with BPD behave in ways that support these beliefs. Treatment centers on correcting such a patient's "black-or-white," dichotomous thinking. The therapist demonstrates that the patient engages in dichotomous thinking, and that it is in the patient's best interest to modify such thinking. Patients carry out behavioral experiments to test the validity of their beliefs. Patients also receive assertiveness training.

Beck acknowledges that it is necessary for therapists to invest considerable effort in establishing a trusting and collaborative relationship with patients who have BPD. Therapists help patients identify their positive traits, and they provide positive feedback when patients show effective coping. Beck advises therapists to attend to their automatic thoughts when treating these patients, since therapists are likely to experience strong emotional reactions. If therapists allow patients to have a part in developing agendas and homework assignments, there is less likelihood of power struggles. When patients are not compliant, the therapists can explore the pros and cons of choosing to comply.

LINEHAN'S DIALECTICAL BEHAVIOR THERAPY

Linehan sets out an approach to the treatment of patients with BPD in her book *Cognitive-Behavioral Treatment of Borderline Personality Disorder* (1993). She views BPD as reflecting a pattern of behavioral, emotional, and cognitive instability and dysregulation. Her treatment, called "dialectical behavior therapy" (DBT), integrates concepts from Buddhism with a broad range of cognitive and behavioral strategies for addressing the problems of patients with BPD. The core treatment procedures are mindfulness meditation, problem solving, exposure techniques, skills training, contingency management, and cognitive modification.

Linehan and her colleagues have provided empirical support for the effectiveness of her approach (Linehan, Armstrong, Suarez, Allmon, & Heard, 1991). They compared DBT to "treatment as usual" in a group of patients with severe BPD, and found that the group receiving DBT had a significantly lower dropout rate and produced significantly less self-injurious behavior than the control group.

Linehan defines the overriding characteristic of DBT as an emphasis on "dialectics"—the reconciliation of opposites in a continual process of synthesis. The most fundamental dialectic is accepting patients just as they are, while simultaneously encouraging them to change. Treatment requires "moment-to-moment changes in the use of supportive acceptance versus confrontation and change strategies. This emphasis on acceptance as a balance to change flows directly from the integration of a perspective drawn from Eastern (Zen) practice with Western psychological practice" (Linehan, 1993, p. 19). Linehan contends that our Western culture's investment in individual autonomy promotes an invalidating bias against many female patients with BPD (and women constitute the great majority of this patient population).[1] She asserts that this investment runs against the grain of the feminine propensity toward connection and interdependence.

In DBT, the therapist actively teaches the patient emotion regulation, interpersonal effectiveness, distress tolerance, and mindfulness techniques. Linehan (1993) writes:

> In a nutshell, DBT is very simple. The therapist creates a context of validating rather than blaming the patient, and within that context the therapist blocks or extinguishes bad behaviors, drags good behaviors out of the patient, and figures out a way to make the good behaviors so reinforcing that the patient continues the good ones and stops the bad ones. (p. 97)

Schema therapy has much in common with DBT's integrative, active, and practical approach to patients with BPD. Linehan's concept of "dialectics" bears a similarity to schema therapy's concept of "empathic confrontation"; in both, the therapist strives for the optimal balance between support and acceptance on the one hand, and reality testing and confrontation of the other. Schema therapy also shares Linehan's empathic response to the intense affect and behavior of patients with BPD. Unlike clinicians who see these patients' self-destructive and impulsive behaviors as rooted in aggression or as efforts to manipulate their therapists, both DBT and schema therapy view these behaviors as attempts to cope with extreme emotional pain.

However, while Linehan stresses the need for therapists to validate patients with BPD, hers is not a reparenting model. Schema therapy focuses more directly on fulfilling the patients' unmet emotional needs. Linehan (1993) states that therapists should not "take care of patients," because the therapists' attempts to soothe and comfort patients will work against their learning to soothe and comfort themselves. As we will discuss later in this chapter, we find the opposite to be true. We find that "taking care of pa-

---

[1]Given the preponderance of women among patients with BPD, we ourselves use feminine pronouns in the remainder of this chapter to refer to such a patient.

tients," in the sense of partially meeting their needs for soothing and comforting, leads to stable improvements in most patients with BPD. Limited reparenting provides patients with leverage in the fight against their schemas, and, over time, enhances their capacities to soothe and comfort themselves. Therapists provide a model that patients gradually internalize as their own "Healthy Adult" mode.

Another difference between DBT and schema therapy in the treatment of BPD is the latter's greater focus on uncovering and expressing affect. In schema therapy, a therapist first focuses on forming an attachment to a patient's youngest and most vulnerable mode—the "Abandoned Child." The therapist encourages the patient to stay in the Abandoned Child mode, and to express her feelings fully—about present and past events, about family members, about the therapist. The therapist focuses on providing understanding and validation, and only introduces cognitive and behavioral elements later, once the patient experiences the therapeutic relationship as stable. In schema therapy of a patient with BPD, most cognitive and behavioral strategies are aimed at building the patient's "Healthy Adult" mode, modeled after the therapist. The "Healthy Adult" reparents the "Abandoned Child," defeats the "Punitive Parent," and replaces the "Detached Protector" with more adaptive coping strategies.

DBT uses contingency management to address suicidal and other acting-out behaviors. Schema therapy accomplishes this goal with increased reparenting, limit setting, mode work, and empathic confrontation. Schema therapists set limits more as circumstances call for them, as a parent would, rather than more formally in the form of contracts at the beginning of treatment. We also believe that schema therapy's conceptual model more clearly delineates the psychological structure of a patient with BPD—in terms of the four primary modes (the first four modes to be described below)—giving the therapist greater ease and depth in understanding the rapid and seemingly chaotic shifts in the patient's affective states.

YOUNG'S SCHEMA THERAPY FOR BPD

As we have noted, one problem we had applying the schema model to patients with BPD was that they seemed to have so many schemas. For example, when we give such patients the Young Schema Questionnaire (Young & Brown, 1990, 2001), it is not unusual for them to score high on almost all of the schemas. We needed a different unit of analysis, one that would group schemas together and make them more manageable to treat. Patients with BPD were also problematic for the original schema model because they continually shift from one extreme affective state to another: One moment they are angry, then the next they are sad, detached, terrified, or filled with self-hatred. Schemas, which are essentially traits, did not explain this rapid flipping from state to state. We developed the concept of modes to capture the shifting affective states of our patients with BPD. We define a "mode" as *those schemas or coping responses—adaptive or maladaptive— that are currently active for an individual.*

Patients with BPD switch continually from mode to mode in response to life events. Whereas healthier patients usually have fewer modes, spend longer periods of time in each one, and have less extreme modes, patients with BPD have more modes, switch modes from moment to moment, and have more extreme modes. Moreover, when a patient with BPD switches into a mode, the other modes seem to vanish. Unlike healthier patients, who can experience two or more modes simultaneously so that one modulates the other, the modes are dissociated from one another in patients with BPD.

Modes in the Patient with BPD

We have identified five main modes that characterize the patient with BPD:

1. Abandoned Child
2. Angry and Impulsive Child
3. Punitive Parent
4. Detached Protector
5. Healthy Adult

We now briefly describe each one.

The Abandoned Child mode is the suffering inner child. It is the part of the patient that feels the pain and terror associated with most of the schemas, including Abandonment, Abuse, Deprivation, Defectiveness, and Subjugation. In this mode, patients appear fragile and childlike. They seem sorrowful, frantic, frightened, unloved, and lost. They are obsessed with finding a parent figure who will take care of them, and engage in desperate efforts to prevent caretakers from abandoning them. They idealize nurturers and have fantasies of being rescued by them.

The Angry and Impulsive Child mode is predominant when the patient is enraged, or behaves impulsively, because her basic emotional needs are not being met. When patients are in the Angry and Impulsive Child mode, they vent their anger in inappropriate ways. They may appear intensely rageful, demanding, devaluing, controlling, abusive, or reckless; they may also make suicidal threats.

The Punitive Parent Mode is the internalized rage or hatred of one or both parents (usually). Its function is to punish the patient for doing something "wrong," such as expressing needs or feelings. Signs and symptoms include self-loathing, self-criticism, self-denial, self-mutilation, suicidal fantasies, and self-destructive behavior. Patients in this mode become their own punitive, rejecting parents, and become angry at themselves for having normal needs that their parents did not allow them to express. They punish themselves—for example, by cutting or starving themselves—and speak about themselves in mean, harsh tones, saying such things as that they are "evil," "bad," or "dirty."

In the Detached Protector mode, the patient shuts off all emotions, disconnects from others, and behaves submissively. Signs and symptoms include depersonalization, emptiness, boredom, substance abuse, bingeing, self-mutilation, psychosomatic complaints, "blankness," and robot-like compliance. Patients switch into the Detached Protector mode when their feelings are stirred up in order to cut off the feelings. Patients with BPD in this mode often appear normal; they are "good patients." In fact, many therapists mistakenly reinforce this mode. The problem is that when patients are in this mode, they are cut off from their own needs and feelings. They are basing their identity on gaining their therapists' approval, but they are not really connecting to the therapist. Sometimes a therapist spends a whole treatment with a patient who has BPD, not realizing that the patient is in the Detached Protector mode nearly the entire time. The patient never makes significant progress.

One dysfunctional mode can activate another. For example, a patient may express a need in the Abandoned Child mode, and then flip into the Punitive Parent mode to punish herself for expressing the need, and then flip into the Detached Protector to escape the pain of the punishment. Patients with BPD often get trapped in these vicious cycles, with one mode triggering another in a self-perpetuating loop.

The Healthy Adult mode is extremely weak and undeveloped in most patients with BPD, especially at the beginning of treatment. In a sense, this is the primary problem: These patients have no soothing parental mode to calm and care for them. This contributes significantly to their inability to tolerate separation. A therapist models the Healthy Adult for a patient, until the patient eventually internalizes the therapist's attitudes, emotions, reactions, and behaviors as her own Healthy Adult mode.

DSM-IV Diagnostic Criteria for BPD and Schema Modes

What follows is a paraphrase of the DSM-IV diagnostic criteria for BPD, matched to the relevant schema modes.

DSM-IV diagnostic criteria	Relevant schema modes
1. Desperate attempts to avoid abandonment (real or imagined).	Abandoned Child mode.
2. A history of erratic and intense relationships with others, marked by shifts between idealizing and devaluating extremes.	Any of the first four modes. (It is the rapid flipping from mode to mode that creates the instability and intensity. For example, the Abandoned Child idealizes nurturers, while the Angry and Impulsive Child devalues and reproaches them.)
3. Disturbed identity—a notably and chronically unstable image or sense of self.	a. Detached Protector mode. (Because these patients must please others and are not allowed to be themselves, they cannot develop a secure identity.) b. Constantly switching from one nonintegrated mode to another, each with its own view of the self, also leads to an unstable self-image.
4. Impulsive behavior (e.g., spending money, promiscuous sex, substance abuse, binge eating, reckless driving).	a. Angry and Impulsive Child mode (to express anger or get needs met). b. Detached Protector mode (to self-soothe or break through numbness).
5. Recurring suicidal threats, gestures, or behavior, or self-mutilating behavior.	Any of the first four modes (each for different reasons—see below).
6. Affective instability caused by notable mood reactivity (e.g., severe episodes of irritability, dysphoria, or anxiety).	a. Hypothesized intense, labile biological temperament. b. Rapid flipping of modes, each with its own distinctive affect.
7. Continuing feelings of emptiness.	Detached Protector mode (the cutting off of emotions and disconnection from others leads to feelings of emptiness).
8. Out-of-place, intense anger or problems with controlling anger.	Angry and Impulsive Child mode.

9. Occasional stress-related paranoid ideas or intense dissociative
symptoms

Any of the first four modes (when affect becomes unbearable or overwhelming).

When a patient with BPD is suicidal or parasuicidal, it is important for
the therapist to recognize which mode is experiencing the urge. Is the urge
coming from the Punitive Parent mode, and designed to punish the patient?
Or is the urge coming from the Abandoned Child mode, as a wish to end
the pain of unbearable loneliness? Is it coming from the Detached Protector
mode, in an effort to distract from emotional pain through physical pain,
or to pierce the numbness and feel something? Or is it coming from the Angry or Impulsive Child mode, in a desire to get revenge or hurt another person? The patient has a different reason for wanting to attempt suicide in
each of the first four modes, and the therapist addresses the suicidal urge in
accord with the particular mode that is generating it.

TREATMENT OF PATIENTS WITH BPD

In our view, the most constructive way to view patients with BPD is as vulnerable children. They may look like adults, but psychologically they are
abandoned children searching for their parents. The behave inappropriately because they are desperate. They are doing what all young children do
when they have no one who takes care of them and makes sure they are
safe. Most patients with BPD were lonely and mistreated as children. There
was no one who comforted or protected them. Often they had no one to
turn to except the very people who were hurting them. Lacking a Healthy
Adult they could internalize, as adults they lack the internal resources to
sustain themselves when they are alone.

Patients with BPD almost always need more than their therapists can
provide. This does not mean that the therapists should attempt to give
these patients everything they need. On the contrary, therapists have rights,
too. Therapists have the right to maintain private lives, to be treated re-
spectfully, and to set limits when patients infringe on these rights. A patient
with BPD has the needs of a very young child. The patient needs a parent.
Since the therapist can only provide the patient with "limited reparenting,"
it is inevitable that there will be a gulf between what the patient wants and
the therapist can give. No one is to blame for this: It is not that the patient
with BPD wants too much, and it is not that the schema therapist gives too
little. It is simply that therapy is not an ideal way to reparent. Thus there is
certain to be conflict in the therapist–patient relationship. Patients with
BPD are apt to view professional boundaries as cold, uncaring, unfair,
selfish, or even cruel.

Psychologically, the patient grows up in therapy. The patient begins as an infant or very young child and—under the influence of the therapist's reparenting—gradually matures into a healthy adult. This is why effective treatment of BPD cannot be brief. To treat this disorder fully requires relatively long-term treatment (at least 2 years and often longer).

Treatment Goals

Stated in terms of modes, the overall goal of treatment is to help the patient *incorporate the Healthy Adult mode, modeled after the therapist,* in order to do the following:

1. Empathize with and protect the Abandoned Child.
2. Help the Abandoned Child to give and receive love.
3. Fight against, and expunge, the Punitive Parent.
4. Set limits on the behavior of the Angry and Impulsive Child, and help the patient in this mode to express emotions and needs appropriately.
5. Reassure, and gradually replace, the Detached Protector with the Healthy Adult.

Tracking modes is the heart of the treatment: The therapist tracks the patient's modes from moment to moment in the session, selectively using the strategies that fit each one of the modes. The patient gradually identifies with and internalizes the therapist's reparenting as her own Healthy Adult mode.

The treatment has three main stages: (1) the Bonding and Emotional Regulation stage, (2) the Schema Mode Change stage, and (3) the Autonomy stage.

Stage I: Bonding and Emotional Regulation

Facilitating the Reparenting Bond

The therapist begins to reparent the patient's Abandoned Child, providing safety and emotional holding (Winnicott, 1965). The goal is for the therapist to create an environment that is a partial antidote to the one the patient knew as a child—one that is safe, nurturing, protective, forgiving, and encouraging of self-expression. The therapist asks about current and past problems. We have identified four predisposing factors in the early family environments of patients with BPD: (1) abuse and lack of safety, (2) abandonment and emotional deprivation, (3) subjugation of needs and feelings, and (4) punitiveness or rejection. The therapist assesses whether these factors were present in the patient's childhood history.

The therapist encourages the patient to stay in the Abandoned Child mode during this stage. Keeping the patient in the Abandoned Child mode helps the therapist develop feelings of sympathy and warmth for the patient. The patient's vulnerability encourages the therapist to bond with the patient and feel empathy for her. Later, when the other modes start emerging and the patient becomes angry or punitive, the therapist will have the caring and patience to endure it. Keeping the patient in the Abandoned Child mode also helps the patient bond with the therapist. This bond keeps the patient from leaving therapy prematurely, and it gives the therapist leverage to confront the patient's other, more problematic modes.

The patient will spontaneously hold back needs and feelings, thinking that the therapist just wants her to be "nice" and polite. However, this is not what the therapist wants. The therapist wants the patient to be herself—to say what she feels and ask for what she needs—and the therapist tries to convince the patient of this fact. This is a message the patient with BPD probably never got from a parent. In this way, the schema therapist tries to break the cycle of subjugation and detachment in which the patient is caught.

When the therapist encourages the patient to express emotions and needs, these emotions and needs generally come from the Abandoned Child mode. Keeping the patient in the Abandoned Child mode and nurturing the patient are stabilizing to the patient's life. The patient flips less often from mode to mode. If the patient is able to express her emotions and needs in the Abandoned Child mode, then she will not have to flip into the Angry and Impulsive Child mode to express them. She will not have to flip into the Detached Protector mode to shut off her feelings. And she will not have to flip into the Punitive Parent mode, because, in accepting her, the therapist replaces the Punitive Parent with a parent figure who allows self-expression. Thus, as the therapist reparents the patient, gradually her dysfunctional modes drop away.

Negotiating Limits

Limit setting is an important part of the early phase of treatment. We have established these basic guidelines:

1. *Limits are based upon the patient's safety and the therapist's personal rights.* The patient's safety is the first consideration. The therapist has to set some limits that provide safety, whether the therapist resents it or not. However, if the patient *is* safe, and she is asking the therapist to do something the therapist will resent doing, the rule of thumb is that the therapist should not agree to do it.

2. *Therapists should not start doing anything they cannot continue doing for patients, unless they expressly state that it is for a specified time period.* For example, a therapist should not read long e-mails from a patient each day for several weeks, and then abruptly announce that reading e-mails will have to stop. However, if the patient is going through a crisis, the therapist may agree to check in with the patient each day until the crisis passes. It is important that therapists determine their limits ahead of time and then adhere to them.

3. *The therapist sets limits in a personal way.* Rather then using impersonal explanations of limits (e.g., "It is my policy to forbid suicidal behavior"), the therapist communicates in a personal manner (e.g., "For the sake of my peace of mind, I have to know that you're safe"). The therapist uses self-disclosure of intentions and feelings whenever possible, and avoids sounding punitive or rigid. Patients with BPD are usually empathic and can understand their therapists' point of view.

4. *The therapist introduces a rule the first time the patient violates it.* Unless patients are extremely low-functioning, therapists do not recite their limits ahead of time to patients, nor do they set up an explicit contract. Such a list or contract sounds too clinical. Rather, a therapist states a limit the first time a patient oversteps it, and does not impose any consequences until the next time the patient oversteps it. The therapist explains the rationale for imposing the limit, and shows empathy for how difficult it may be for the patient to follow it.

5. *The therapist sets natural consequences for violating limits.* The therapist sets consequences for limit violations that follow naturally from what the patient did, whenever possible. For example, if the patient calls the therapist more often than agreed upon, then the therapist sets a period when the patient cannot call.

We tend to enforce limits more strictly as therapy progresses and the patient forms a strong attachment to the therapist. Generally, the stronger the attachment to the therapist, the greater the patient's motivation to adhere to the limits the therapist has set.

Limiting Outside Therapist–Patient Contact. We believe that therapists working with patients who have BPD must be prepared to give the patients extra time outside sessions. But how much? Therapists should give patients as much outside contact as they can without becoming angry. That is where they must draw the line. In addition to setting a limit and modeling appropriate assertion, a therapist is conveying to a patient a lesson about the nature of anger. This helps the patient understand her own pattern (i.e., her own unexpressed anger builds until she flips into the Angry and Impulsive Child mode), and shows her how to overcome the pattern.

Limiting Suicidal Crises. The therapist is the primary resource for the patient with BPD who is in crisis. Most crises occur because the patient is feeling worthless, bad, unloved, abused, or abandoned. The therapist's capacity to acknowledge these feelings and respond to them compassionately is what enables the patient to resolve the crisis. Ultimately, it is the patient's conviction that the therapist truly cares about her and respects her, in contrast with the Punitive Parent, that stops the self-destructive behavior. As long as the patient is confused about whether the therapist truly cares, she will keep acting out self-destructive behaviors.

Therapists ask patients with BPD to agree that they will not make a suicide attempt without contacting the therapists first. Their agreement is a condition of therapy. The therapists bring up the limit the first time patients say that they are suicidal or have been suicidal in the past. Patients with BPD tend to see this requirement as caring and agree to it readily. In addition, patients agree to follow the hierarchy of rules that the therapists set for dealing with suicidal crises.

Limiting Impulsive Self-Destructive Behaviors. Patients with BPD can become so inundated with unbearable affect that impulsive behaviors such as cutting themselves or abusing drugs seem the only viable forms of release. Teaching patients coping skills (such as those we describe below) can help them learn to tolerate distress, but sometimes they become too overwhelmed to benefit from their coping skills. Once patients connect to their therapists as stable, nurturing figures, and once they are able to express anger toward their therapists and others, then the impulsive self-destructive behaviors tend to reduce significantly.

Self-destructive behavior can derive from any of the first four schema modes. Many of these behaviors occur because a patient is angry at someone and cannot express it directly. The patient's anger builds, eventually coming out in the form of impulsive behavior. In addition to the Angry and Impulsive Child mode, the patient may be in the Abandoned Child mode, and attempting to use the behavior as a distraction from emotional pain; or in the Punitive Parent mode, and using the behavior as a punishment; or in the Detached Protector mode, and trying to break through the numbness to feel that she exists. The therapist sets limits in accord with the mode that is generating the behavior.

When patients with BPD refuse to comply with the limits of therapy, their noncompliance is usually not part of the Abandoned Child mode. The exception is contacting the therapist too frequently because the patient feels separation anxiety. The Abandoned Child is dependent upon the therapist, and therefore is likely to be compliant. The noncompliance usually comes from another mode—the Detached Protector, the Punitive Parent, or the Angry and Impulsive Child. In order to overcome the patient's noncompliance, the therapist works with these modes until the patient abides by the limits. For example, the therapist might ask the patient to conduct a dialogue between the noncompliant mode (such as the Detached Protector) and the Healthy Adult.

Cognitive-Behavioral Techniques for Affect Regulation

As early as possible in therapy, the therapist teaches the patient cognitive-behavioral techniques to contain and regulate affect. The more severe the patient's symptoms are (especially suicidal and parasuicidal behaviors), the sooner the therapist introduces these techniques. However, we have found that the majority of patients with BPD cannot accept and benefit from cognitive-behavioral techniques until they trust the stability of the reparenting bond. If the therapist introduces these techniques too early, they tend not to be effective. Early in treatment, the patient's primary focus is on making sure the therapist–patient bond is still there, and she lacks the free attention to focus on cognitive-behavioral techniques. Many patients reject them as too cold or mechanical. As patients increasingly trust the stability of the therapy relationship, they become more capable of utilizing these techniques.

When the patient seems amenable to cognitive-behavioral techniques, we usually begin with ones designed to enhance the patient's self-control of moods and self-soothing. These may include safe-place imagery, self-hypnosis, relaxation, self-monitoring of automatic thoughts, flashcards—whatever appeals most to the patient. The therapist also educates the patient about schemas, and begins to challenge the patient's schemas using cognitive techniques. The patient reads *Reinventing Your Life* (Young & Klosko, 1993) as part of this educational process. Through these coping techniques, the therapist seeks to reduce schema-driven overreactions and to build the patient's self-esteem. Some sample cognitive-behavioral techniques for affect regulation are described below.

Mindfulness Meditation. Mindfulness meditation is a particular type of relaxation technique that helps patients calm themselves and regulate their emotions (Linehan, 1993). Rather than shutting down or becoming overwhelmed by emotions, the patient observes the emotions but does not act on them. Feeling upset is the cue that alerts the patient to do the meditation exercise. Patients are instructed to stay focused on mindfulness meditation until they are calm and can think through the situation rationally. This way, when they act, it will be thoughtfully rather than impulsively.

Pleasurable Activities for Self-Nurturing. The therapist encourages the patient to nurture her Abandoned Child by engaging in pleasurable activities.

These vary from patient to patient, depending upon what a person finds pleasurable. Some examples include taking a bath, buying oneself a small gift, getting a massage, or cuddling with a lover. These activities counter the patient's feelings of deprivation and worthlessness.

Flashcards. Flashcards are the single most helpful coping strategy for many of our patients with BPD. These are small sheets of paper or cards that patients carry around with them and read whenever they feel upset. A therapist composes the flashcards with a patient's help. The therapist usually composes different cards for different trigger situations—such as when the patient gets angry, a friend disappoints her, her boss is angry with her, or her partner needs some space apart from her.

Here is a sample flashcard, written for a patient with BPD to read when her therapist is away on vacation, using a template we provide (Young, Wattenmaker, & Wattenmaker, 1996) as a guide:

> Right now I feel scared and angry because my therapist is away. I feel like cutting myself. However, I know that these feelings are my Abandoned Child mode, which I developed from having alcoholic parents who left me alone a lot. When I'm in this mode, I exaggerate the degree to which people will never return and don't really care about me.
>
> Even though I believe my therapist will not come back or will not want to see me again, the reality is that he will come back and will want to see me again. The evidence in my life supporting this healthy view includes the fact that every time he has gone away before, he has always come back and has always still cared about me.
>
> Therefore, even though I feel like hurting myself, instead I will do something enjoyable (take a walk, call a friend, listen to music, play a game). I will also listen to my relaxation tape.

In addition to writing down the flashcard, the therapist can dictate it onto a tape that the patient plays at home. It can be helpful for the patient to hear the therapist's voice. However, it is also important to put the flashcard into the more portable written form. That way, the patient can carry the flashcard around with her, and read it whenever she feels the need.

The Schema Diary. The Schema Diary (Young, 1993) is a more advanced technique because, unlike a flashcard, it requires patients to generate their own coping responses when they are upset. The cue for filling out the Schema Diary is that a patient feels upset and is unsure how to handle it. In some ways, it is similar to the Daily Record of Dysfunctional Thoughts in cognitive therapy (Young, Weinberger, & Beck, 2001). Filling out the form helps the patient think through a problem and generate a healthy response. The patient generally relies more on the Schema Diary later in therapy.

Assertiveness Training. It is important to provide patients who have BPD with assertiveness training throughout the therapy, so that they learn more acceptable ways to express their emotions and get their needs met. They especially need to improve their skills in expressing anger, since most tend to swing from extreme passivity to extreme aggression. Patients learn anger management in conjunction with assertiveness training: Anger management teaches patients self-control over their angry outbursts; assertiveness training teaches them appropriate ways to express anger. The therapist and patient role-play various situations in the patient's life which call upon assertiveness skills. Once the patient develops a healthy response, the therapist and patient rehearse it until the patient feels confident enough to carry it out in real life.

Before turning the patient's attention to assertiveness techniques, the therapist gives the patient the opportunity to vent all her emotions about the upsetting situation and linked situations from childhood. Patients with BPD need to vent before they can apply behavioral strategies. Until they vent, they do not have the ability to focus on appropriate assertiveness.

Stage II: Schema Mode Change

To reiterate, the therapist's general approach to treatment is to track the patient's modes from moment to moment, and utilize the strategies appropriate for the current mode. The goals are to build the patient's Healthy Adult mode (modeled on the therapist), to care for the Abandoned Child, to reassure and replace the Detached Protector, to overthrow and expunge the Punitive Parent, and to teach the Angry and Impulsive Child appropriate ways to express emotions and needs.

Educating the Patient about Modes

The therapist explains the modes to the patient. If therapists present the modes in a personal way, most patients with BPD relate to them quickly and well. However, some patients reject the idea of modes. When this happens, a therapist does not insist. Rather, the therapist drops the labels and uses some other expressions, such as "the sad side of you," "the angry side of you," "the self-critical side of you," and "the numb side of you." It is important that the therapist label these different parts of the self in some way, but it does not have to be with our labels.

The therapist also asks the patient to read relevant chapters in *Reinventing Your Life* (Young & Klosko, 1993). Although the book does not mention modes directly, it describes the experience of the schemas and the three coping styles of surrender, escape, and counterattack. It is important for therapists to assign one chapter at a time and pace the chapters, because when patients with BPD read *Reinventing Your Life,* they tend to see themselves everywhere and become overwhelmed.

The Abandoned Child Mode: Treatment

The Abandoned Child is the child part of the patient who was abused, abandoned, deprived, subjugated, and harshly punished. The therapist attempts to furnish the opposite: a relationship that is safe, secure, nurturing, encouraging of genuine self-expression, and forgiving.

The Therapist–Patient Relationship. The therapeutic relationship is central to the treatment of the Abandoned Child mode. Through limited reparenting, the therapist seeks to provide a partial antidote to the patient's toxic childhood. The therapist reparents the patient within the appropriate boundaries of the therapeutic relationship; this is what we mean by "limited reparenting." Within these boundaries, the therapist tries to satisfy many of the patient's unmet childhood needs.

Experiential Work. The therapist helps the patient work through images of upsetting events from childhood, entering the images and reparenting the child. Later in therapy, when the therapeutic bond is secure and the patient is strong enough not to decompensate, the therapist guides the patient through traumatic images of abuse or neglect. The therapist enters the images and does whatever a good parent would have done: removes the child from the scene, confronts the perpetrator, stands between the perpetrator and the child, or empowers the child to handle the situation. Gradually, the patient takes over the role of the Healthy Adult.

Cognitive Work. The therapist educates the patient about normal human needs, beginning with the developmental needs of children. Many patients with BPD have never learned what normal needs are, since their parents taught them that even normal needs were "bad." These patients do not know that all children need safety, love, autonomy, praise, and acceptance. The early chapters of *Reinventing Your Life* are helpful in this phase of treatment.

Cognitive techniques, especially flashcards, can help patients with BPD feel connected to their therapists in upsetting situations.

Behavioral Work. The therapist helps the patient practice assertiveness techniques. The goals are for the patient to learn to manage affect in productive ways, and to develop intimate relationships with appropriate significant others where she is able to be vulnerable without overwhelming the other person.

Dangers in Working with the Abandoned Child Mode. The first danger is that the patient may leave the session in the Abandoned Child mode and become depressed or upset. Patients with BPD cover a broad spectrum of functionality; what one patient can handle, another cannot. The therapist is careful not to overwhelm a patient in this mode, only gradually approaching more emotionally charged issues.

The therapist may inadvertently act in a way that causes the patient to shut off the Abandoned Child mode. If the therapist responds to the patient by trying to problem-solve or otherwise ignoring the patient's childlike side, the patient may think that the therapist wants her to be objective and rational, and flip into the Detached Protector mode. All their lives, most of these patients have been given the message that their Abandoned Child mode is not welcome in interpersonal interactions.

The therapist may become irritated with the patient's "childish" behavior and poor problem solving when she is in this mode. Any display of anger on the therapist's part will immediately shut off the Abandoned Child. The patient will flip into the Punitive Parent mode, to punish herself for making the therapist angry.

The Detached Protector Mode: Treatment

The Detached Protector mode serves to cut off the patient's emotions and needs in order to protect the patient. This mode is an empty shell of the patient, which acts to please automatically and mechanically.

The Therapist–Patient Relationship. The therapist reassures the Detached Protector that it is safe to let the patient be vulnerable with the therapist. The therapist consistently protects the patient, so the Detached Protector does not have to do it. The therapist helps the patient contain overwhelming affect by soothing the patient, so it is safe for the Detached Protector to let the patient experience her feelings. The therapist allows the patient to express all her feelings (within appropriate limits), including anger at the therapist, without punishment.

Experiential Work. The therapist must bypass the Detached Protector in order to get to the other modes, because no real progress can occur as long as the patient remains in the Detached Protector mode. As the Healthy Adult, the therapist challenges and negotiates with the Detached Protector. The therapist conducts imagery dialogues in which the Detached Protector becomes a character. The therapist's goal is to convince the Detached Protector to step aside and allow the therapist to interact with the Abandoned Child and other child modes. Once the therapist has bypassed the Detached Protector, the therapist can begin other imagery work.

Cognitive Work. Education about the Detached Protector mode is useful. The therapist highlights the advantages of experiencing emotions and connecting to other people. To live in the Detached Protector mode is to live as one who is emotionally dead. True emotional fulfillment is only available to those who are willing to feel and to want. Beyond educating the patient in this way, there is something inherently paradoxical about doing cognitive work with the Detached Protector. By emphasizing rationality and objectivity, the process of doing cognitive work itself reinforces the mode. For this reason, we do not recommend focusing on the cognitive work with the Detached Protector. Once the patient recognizes intellectually that there are important advantages to supplanting the Detached Protector with better forms of coping, the therapist moves on to the experiential work.

Behavioral Work. Distancing from people is an important aspect of this mode. The Detached Protector is extremely reluctant to open up to people emotionally. It is important for the therapist to be consistently confrontational in fighting the Detached Protector. In the behavioral work, the patient attempts to open up—gradually and incrementally—despite this reluctance. The patient practices shifting out of the Detached Protector mode and into the Abandoned Child and Healthy Adult modes with appropriate significant others. The patient can rehearse in imagery or role plays during sessions, and then carry out homework assignments.

Dangers in Treating the Detached Protector Mode. The first danger is that the therapist may mistake the Detached Protector for the Healthy Adult. The therapist believes that the patient is doing well, but the patient is merely shut down and compliant. The key distinguishing factor is whether the patient is experiencing any emotions. The patient can experience emotion in the other modes, but not in the Detached Protector.

A second danger is that the therapist may get drawn in by the Detached Protector, and get lost in problem solving without addressing the underlying mode. Many therapists fall into the trap of trying to solve the problems of their patients with BPD. Often a patient does not want solutions: She wants the therapist to empathize with the mode underlying the Detached Protector—with the hidden Abandoned Child and Angry Child modes.

A third danger is that the Detached Protector may cut off the patient's anger at the therapist, so that the therapist fails to recognize it. If the therapist does not break through the Detached Protector and help the patient express her anger, then the patient's anger will build up, and eventually the patient will act out or leave.

The Punitive Parent Mode: Treatment

The Punitive Parent is the patient's identification with and internalization of the parent (and others) who devalued and rejected the patient in childhood. By making the self-punitive part of the patient into a mode, the therapist helps the patient undo the identification and internalization processes that created it. The self-punitive part becomes ego-dystonic and external. The therapist then allies with the patient against the Punitive Parent. The goal of treatment is to defeat and cast out the Punitive Parent. The therapist battles the Punitive Parent, and the patient gradually learns to battle the Punitive Parent on her own.

The Therapist–Patient Relationship. By modeling the opposite of punitiveness—an attitude of acceptance and forgiveness toward the patient—the therapist proves the Punitive Parent false. Rather than criticizing and blaming the patient, the therapist forgives the patient when she does something "wrong." The patient is allowed to make mistakes.

Experiential Work. The therapist helps the patient fight the Punitive Parent mode in imagery. The therapist begins by helping the patient identify which parent (or other person) the mode actually represents. From then on, the therapist calls the mode by name (e.g., "your Punitive Father"). Labeling the mode in this way helps the patient externalize the voice of the Punitive Parent: It is the parent's voice, and not the patient's own voice. The patient becomes more able to distance herself from the punitive voice and fight back. Identifying the punitive voice with the parent solves the problem of how to fight the Punitive Parent without seeming to fight the patient. Once the voice is labeled as belonging to the parent, it is no longer a debate between the therapist and the patient; it is now a debate between the therapist and the parent. In this debate, the therapist verbalizes what the Angry Child has been feeling all along. The therapist finally says what the patient feels underneath, but has been unable to express because the Punitive Parent is so tyrannical.

Most patients with BPD need their therapists to step in and fight the Punitive Parent. Early in the treatment, they are too afraid of the Punitive Parent to fight back in imagery. At this point, a patient is essentially an observer of the battle between the Punitive Parent and the therapist.

Cognitive Work. The therapist educates the patient about normal human needs and feelings. Most patients with BPD believe that it is "bad" to express their needs and feelings, and that they deserve punishment when they do. The therapist teaches the patient that punishment is not an effective strategy for self-improvement, and does not support the idea of punishment as a value. When the patient makes a mistake, the therapist replaces punishment with a more constructive response involving forgiveness, understanding, and growth. The goal is for the patient to look honestly at what she did wrong, experience appropriate remorse, make restitution to anyone who might have been negatively affected, explore more productive ways of behaving in the future, and (most importantly), forgive herself. In this way, the patient can take responsibility for her mistakes without punishing herself.

The therapist works to reattribute the parent's condemnation of the patient to the parent's own issues. Over time, therapists convince patients with BPD that their parents' mistreatment of them occurred not because they were bad children, but because their parents had problems of their own, or the family system was dysfunctional. Patients with BPD cannot overcome their feelings of worthlessness until they can make this reattribution. They were good children and did not deserve mistreatment; in fact, no child deserves mistreatment. Even though their parents mistreated them, they were worthy of love and respect.

A patient struggling to make this reattribution faces a dilemma. In order to blame the parent and get angry at the parent, the patient risks losing the parent, either psychologically or in reality. This dilemma highlights once again the importance of the reparenting relationship. As the therapist becomes the (limited) substitute parent, the patient is no longer so dependent upon the real parent.

Repetition is a vital aspect of the cognitive work. Patients need to hear the arguments against the Punitive Parent over and over again. The Punitive Parent mode has developed over a long time through countless repetitions. Each time patients fight the Punitive Parent mode with self-love, they weaken the Punitive Parent mode a little bit more. Repetition slowly wears down the Punitive Parent.

Finally, it is important that the therapist and patient acknowledge the parent's good qualities. Often the parent gave the patient some love or acknowledgment, which is viewed as all the more precious by the patient because it was so rare. However, the therapist insists that the parent's positive attributes do not justify or excuse the parent's harmful behavior.

Behavioral Work. Patients with BPD expect other people to treat them the same way their parents treated them. Their implicit hypothesis is that everyone is the Punitive Parent. The therapist sets up experiments to test this hypothesis. The purpose is to demonstrate to the patient that expressing needs and emotions appropriately will usually not lead to rejection or retaliation by healthy people. For example, a patient may have the assignment of asking her close friend to listen to her when she is distressed about work. The therapist and patient role-play the interaction until the patient feels comfortable enough to attempt it, and then the patient carries it out as a homework assignment. If the therapist and patient have chosen the significant other wisely, then the patient will be rewarded for her efforts with a positive response.

Dangers in Treating the Punitive Parent Mode. The Punitive Parent may fight back by punishing the patient after the session. It is important for the therapist to keep monitoring the patient for this possibility and to take steps to prevent its occurrence. The therapist instructs the patient not to punish herself, and provides alternative activities for when the patient experiences urges to do so, such as reading flashcards or practicing mindfulness meditation.

The therapist may underestimate how frightened the patient is of the Punitive Parent, and fail to provide enough protection during the experiential exercises. Often a real-life punitive parent was also an abusive parent. The patient usually needs a great deal of protection. Similarly, the therapist may not take an active enough role in fighting the Punitive Parent. The therapist may be too passive or too calmly rational. The therapist has to fight the Punitive Parent aggressively. Dealing with the Punitive Parent is like dealing with a person who has neither good will nor empathy. One does not reason with such a person; one does not make appeals to empathy. These approaches do not work. The method that works most often is fighting back.

It is as a transitional measure that the therapist steps in and fights the Punitive Parent. The therapist gradually withdraws from this function, allowing the patient to assume an increasing level of responsibility for fighting the Punitive Parent.

The Angry and Impulsive Child Mode: Treatment

The Angry and Impulsive Child mode expresses rage about the mistreatment and unmet emotional needs that originally formed the patient's schemas. Although it is usually justified in regard to childhood, in adult life this mode of expression is self-defeating. The patient's anger overwhelms and alienates other people, and thus makes it even more unlikely that the patient's emotional needs will be met. The therapist sets limits on rageful behavior, validates the patient's underlying needs, and teaches her more effective ways of communicating.

The Therapist–Patient Relationship. Anger at their therapists is common among patients with BPD, and for many therapists it is the most frustrating aspect of treatment. A therapist often feels exhausted trying to meet a patient's needs. Thus, when the patient becomes angry at the therapist, the therapist naturally feels unappreciated. When therapists feel anger toward patients with BPD, their first priority is to attend to their own schemas. What schemas, if any, are being triggered in a therapist by a patient's behavior? How can the therapist respond to these schemas so as to maintain a therapeutic stance toward the patient? We will discuss the issue of the therapist's own schemas later in the chapter.

The therapist sets limits if the patient's anger is abusive. There is a line a patient can cross from simply venting anger, which is healthy, to being abusive toward the therapist. The patient crosses this line when she calls the therapist demeaning names, attacks the therapist personally, swears at the therapist, yells loud enough to disturb others, tries to physically dominate the therapist, or threatens the therapist or the therapist's possessions. The therapist gives the patient two messages: The first is that the therapist wants to hear the patient's anger; the second is that the patient has to express the anger within appropriate limits.

When the patient is in the Angry and Impulsive Child mode and not behaving abusively, then the therapist responds by following these four steps.

1. *Ventilating.* First, the therapist allows the patient to express the anger fully. This will help the patient calm down enough to be receptive to the next steps. The therapist allows the patient broad latitude in venting anger, even if the intensity seems unwarranted or exaggerated.

2. *Empathizing.* Next, the therapist empathizes with the patient's underlying schemas. Underneath the patient's anger is usually a sense of abandonment, deprivation, or abuse. The Angry and Impulsive Child is a response to the unmet needs of the Abandoned Child. The goal of empathizing is to shift the patient from the Angry and Impulsive Child into the Abandoned Child mode, so the therapist can reparent the Abandoned Child and remedy the source of the anger.

3. *Reality testing.* Next, the therapist helps the patient engage in reality testing related to the anger and its intensity. The therapist is neither defensive nor punitive, and acknowledges any realistic components of the patient's accusation.

4. *Rehearsal of appropriate assertiveness.* After the therapist and patient have gone through the first three steps, they practice appropriate assertion.

Experiential Work. In the experiential work, patients vent anger toward the significant others in their childhood, adolescence, or adult life who mistreated them. Venting anger helps patients release strangulated affect and place the current situation in perspective.

Cognitive Work. Education about the value of anger is an important part of the treatment. Patients with BPD tend to think of anger as "bad." Thera-

pists teach them that feeling angry and expressing it appropriately are normal and healthy. It is not that the patients' anger is "bad"; rather, their way
of expressing anger is problematic. They need to learn to express anger
more constructively. Rather than flipping from passivity to aggression, they
can find a middle ground utilizing assertiveness skills.

Therapists teach patients reality-testing techniques so that they can
formulate more accurate expectations of other people. Patients come to recognize their "black-and-white thinking," and to stop themselves from over-
reacting impulsively to emotional slights. Patients use flashcards to help
maintain self-control. When patients feel angry, they take a time out and
read a flashcard *before* responding behaviorally, and think through how
they want to express their anger. For example, one patient who frequently
paged her boyfriend became furious whenever he failed to call her back immediately. Using the template we have created (Young et al., 1996), the
therapist and patient composed the following flashcard:

> Right now I'm angry because I just paged Alan and he isn't calling me back.
> I'm upset because I need him and he's not there for me. If he could do this to
> me, I believe that he doesn't care about me any more. I feel scared that he's
> going to break up with me. I want to keep paging him over and over again
> until he answers me. I want to tell him off.
>
> However, this is my Abandonment schema making me think Alan's
> going to leave me. The evidence that the schema is wrong is that I've
> thought Alan was going to leave me a million times before, and I've al-
> ways been wrong. Instead of paging him over and over or telling him off,
> I'm going to give him the benefit of the doubt and trust that he's got a
> good reason for not calling me back right away, and that he's going to
> call me back when he can. When he finally reaches me, I am going to an-
> swer him in a calm and loving way.

Asking a patient to generate alternative explanations for the behavior
of others can also be helpful. For example, the patient described above
might have generated a list of alternative explanations for her boyfriend's
not calling her back immediately, including such items as "He's busy at
work," or "He's in a situation where there's no privacy to call me."

Behavioral Work. Using anger management and assertiveness techniques,
patients practice healthier ways to express anger in their current lives. They
utilize imagery or role plays with their therapists to work out constructive
ways to behave. They conduct negotiations between the Angry and Impulsive Child and the Healthy Adult to find compromises. Usually the compro-
mise is that the patient can express anger or assert her needs, but she must
do it in an appropriate manner.

Dangers in Treating the Angry and Impulsive Child Mode. When patients are in the Angry and Impulsive Child mode, there is a high risk that therapists will behave countertherapeutically. A therapist may counterattack—that is, retaliate by attacking the patient. This will trigger the patient's Punitive Parent mode, and the patient will join with the therapist in the attack. Alternatively, therapists may withdraw psychologically, retreating into their own Detached Protector mode. This will give a patient the message that her therapist cannot contain the patient's anger, and is likely to trigger the patient's Abandonment schema. Therapists need to work on their own schemas so that they are prepared to respond therapeutically when their schemas are triggered by the Angry and Impulsive Child.

A second danger is that a therapist may allow a patient to become emotionally abusive. Such behavior on the part of the therapist reinforces the patient's Angry and Impulsive Child in unhealthy ways. The therapist gives the patient permission to carry her anger to abusive extremes and fails to set appropriate limits.

Another risk is that the patient may flip into the Punitive Parent mode after the session to punish herself for getting angry at the therapist. Once the patient has gotten angry with the therapist, it is important for the patient to hear that she is not bad for having gotten angry, that the therapist does not want her to punish herself afterward, and that the therapist wants to help her if this is what she starts to do.

A final danger is that the patient may discontinue therapy because she is angry at the therapist. However, we have found that in most cases, if the therapist allows the patient to vent anger fully within appropriate limits and expresses empathy, the patient does not leave therapy.

Stage III: Autonomy

As they move into the third stage, the therapist and patient focus intensively on the patient's intimate relationships outside of therapy. The therapist fosters generalization from the therapy relationship to appropriate significant others outside of therapy. The therapist helps patients to select stable partners and friends, and to develop genuine intimacy with them. When the patient resists engaging in this process, the therapist responds with empathic confrontation: The therapist expresses understanding of how difficult it is for the patient to risk intimacy, but acknowledges that only through such measured risks will the patient experience meaningful intimate relationships with others. The therapist also conducts mode work with the avoidant part of the patient. That is, the therapist makes the "resistant" part a character in the patient's imagery and then carries on dialogues with that mode.

The therapist empathically confronts self-defeating social behaviors, such as clinging, withdrawal, and excessive anger. The patient learns to behave more constructively. She learns to express affect in appropriate, modulated ways, and to ask appropriately to get needs met.

The therapist helps the patient individuate by discovering her "natural inclinations." As the patient stabilizes and spends less time in the Detached Protector, Angry and Impulsive Child, and Punitive Parent modes, she gradually becomes more able to focus on self-realization. She learns to act on the basis of her genuine needs and emotions, rather than in order to please others. The therapist helps her identify her life goals and the sources of fulfillment in her life. The patient learns to follow her natural inclinations in such areas as career choice, appearance, subculture, and leisure activities.

The final step is for the therapist to encourage gradual independence from therapy by slowly reducing the frequency of sessions. On a case-by-case basis, therapist and patient address termination issues. The therapist allows the patient to set the pace for termination. The therapist permits as much independence as the patient can handle, but is there as a secure base when the patient needs refueling.

Therapist Pitfalls

Because her modes are continually shifting, a patient with BPD does not have a stable internal image of the therapist. The patient's image of the therapist shifts along with her modes. In the Abandoned Child mode, the therapist is an idealized nurturer who might suddenly disappear. In the Angry and Impulsive Child mode, the therapist is a devalued depriver. In the Punitive Parent mode, the therapist is a hostile critic. In the Detached Protector mode, the therapist is a distant, remote figure. These shifts can be highly disconcerting for the therapist. Therapists are prone to a variety of intense "countertransference" reactions, including guilt feelings, rescue fantasies, angry desires to retaliate, boundary transgressions, and profound feelings of helplessness. We now briefly discuss some pitfalls therapists face when treating patients with BPD, tied to the therapists' own schemas and coping styles.

Therapists who have Subjugation schemas, and who surrender or avoid as coping styles, face the danger of becoming too passive with patients who have BPD. They may avoid confrontation and fail to set appropriate limits. The consequences can be negative for both a therapist and a patient: The therapist becomes increasingly angry over time, and the patient feels increasingly anxious about the lack of limits and may engage in impulsive or self-destructive behavior. Therapists who have Subjugation schemas must make conscious and determined efforts to confront patients with BPD when it is indicated, and to enforce appropriate limits.

A danger for therapists with Self-Sacrifice schemas (and almost all therapists have this schema, in our experience) is that they permit too much outside contact with patients and then become resentful. Underlying most therapists' Self-Sacrifice is a sense of Emotional Deprivation: Many therapists give to patients what they wish they had been given themselves as children. Such a therapist gives too much; resentment builds; and eventually the therapist withdraws or punishes the patient. The best way for therapists with this schema to manage the situation is to know their own limits ahead of time and to adhere to them faithfully.

Therapists with Defectiveness, Unrelenting Standards, or Failure schemas risk feeling inadequate when patients with BPD fail to progress, relapse, or criticize them. It is important for these therapists to remember that the course of treatment with this population is characterized by discouraging periods, relapses, and conflicts—even under the best of circumstances, with the best of therapists. Having a cotherapist and supervision can help a therapist maintain a clear vision of what is realistic to achieve.

Schema overcompensation by therapists is a serious pitfall that can destroy therapy. If a therapist tends to counterattack, then the therapist may angrily blame or punish the patient. Therapists who tend to be schema overcompensators are at high risk for damaging patients with BPD rather than helping them, and should be closely supervised when they treat them.

Therapists who are schema avoiders may inadvertently discourage their patients with BPD from expressing intense needs and emotions. When the patients express strong affect, these therapists feel uncomfortable and withdraw or otherwise express dismay. The patients often detect these reactions and misinterpret them as rejections or criticisms. Therapists sometimes encourage termination prematurely to avoid the intense affect of these patients. In order to be effective therapists for patients with BPD, schema avoiders must learn to tolerate their own, and their patients', emotions.

Therapists who have the Emotional Inhibition schema often come across to patients with BPD as aloof, rigid, or impersonal. Therapists who are extremely emotionally inhibited may cause harm to such patients, and probably should not work with them. A patient with BPD needs to be reparented. An outwardly cold therapist is probably not going to be able to give her the nurturing she needs. If the therapist chooses to try to heal the schema, there is the possibility of overcoming the emotional inhibition through therapy.

CONCLUSION

Therapy with a patient who has BPD is a long-term process. For a patient to achieve individuation and intimacy with others often requires many years of treatment, but patients generally show improvement all along the way. We feel a sense of optimism and hope about helping such patients. Although treatment is often slow and difficult, the rewards are great. We have found that most with BPD patients make significant progress. In our opinion, the essential curative elements of schema therapy for these patients are the "limited reparenting" therapists provide, mode work, and progressing through therapy in the stages we have described.

Beck's cognitive therapy was the inspiration and starting point for his own, Linehan's, and Young's approaches to treatment of patients with BPD. There is a need for outcome research comparing these three approaches to BPD. In the future, more integration of these three models may lead to an even more effective conceptual and treatment model for BPD.

REFERENCES

Alford, B. A., & Beck, A. T. (1997). *The integrative power of cognitive therapy.* New York: Guilford Press.

American Psychiatric Association. (1994). *Diagnostic and statistical manual of mental disorders* (4th ed.). Washington, DC: Author.

Barlow, D. H. (Ed.). (2001). *Clinical handbook of psychological disorders* (3rd ed.). New York: Guilford Press.

Beck, A. T., Freeman, A., & Associates. (1990). *Cognitive therapy of personality disorders.* New York: Guilford Press.

Beck, A. T., Freeman, A., Davis, D. D., & Associates. (2004). *Cognitive therapy of personality disorders* (2nd ed.). New York: Guilford Press.

Linehan, M. M. (1993). *Cognitive-behavioral treatment of borderline personality disorder.* New York: Guilford.

Linehan, M. M., Armstrong, H. E., Suarez, A., Allmon, D., & Heard, H. L. (1991). Cognitive-behavioral treatment of chronically parasuicidal borderline patients. *Archives of General Psychiatry, 48,* 1060–1064.

Millon, T. (1981). *Disorders of personality.* New York: Wiley.

Winnicott, D. W. (1965). *The maturational processes and the facilitating environment: Studies in the theory of emotional development.* London: Hogarth Press.

Young, J. E. (1993). *The schema diary.* New York: Cognitive Therapy Center of New York.

Young, J. E., & Brown, G. (1990). *Young Schema Questionnaire.* New York: Cognitive Therapy Center of New York.

Young, J. E., & Brown, G. (2001). *Young Schema Questionnaire: Special Edition.* New York: Schema Therapy Institute.

Young, J. E., & Klosko, J. S. (1993). *Reinventing your life.* New York: Dutton.

Young, J. E., Wattenmaker, D., & Wattenmaker, R. (1996). *Schema therapy flashcard.* New York: Cognitive Therapy Center of New York.

Young, J. E., Weinberger, A. D., & Beck, A. T. (2001). Cognitive therapy for depression. In D. Barlow (Ed.), *Clinical handbook of psychological disorders* (3rd ed., pp.264–308). New York: Guilford Press.

Chapter 14

Cognitive Therapy of Personality Disorders

Twenty Years of Progress

JAMES PRETZER
JUDITH S. BECK

Twenty years ago, personality disorders were barely mentioned by behavior therapists or cognitive-behavioral therapists. The term "personality disorder" seemed to imply that the individual with such a disorder has a broken personality, and that this is the root of his or her problems. This idea was not compatible with behavioral and cognitive-behavioral conceptualizations, and many behaviorists were inclined to think of "personality disorders" as a psychoanalytic construct that either did not exist or was of little relevance.

However, significant changes in the conceptualization and treatment of personality disorders have occurred since then. First, a personality disorder has been more clearly and more behaviorally defined as "an enduring pattern of inner experience and behavior that . . . is pervasive and inflexible . . . and leads to distress or impairment" (American Psychiatric Association, 2000, p. 685). Thus it is no longer necessary to understand personality disorders as resulting from a broken personality. Second, it has been found that about 50% of clients in many outpatient settings meet diagnostic criteria for at least one personality disorder diagnosis (Turkat & Maisto, 1985). Third, some outcome studies found that cognitive therapy or cognitive-behavioral therapy (CBT) was much less effective with clients diagnosed with personality disorders than with clients in general. These findings were sobering to cognitive-behavioral therapists. Some suggested that cognitive therapy or CBT could not be used with personality disorders (Rush & Shaw, 1983). Others started to develop cognitive therapy or CBT approaches tailored to clients diagnosed with personality disorders (see, e.g., Fleming, 1983; Pretzer, 1983; Simon, 1983; Young, 1983).

THE EVOLUTION OF COGNITIVE CONCEPTUALIZATIONS OF PERSONALITY DISORDER

Therapists often find that some of their clients do not respond well to standard treatment. They may idealize their therapists, display outright hostility, overwhelm the therapists with recurrent crises, demand special treatment, or make extraordinary efforts to please. A high proportion of these individuals are found to have one or more Axis II disorders, in addition to the Axis I problems for which they originally sought treatment.

How are therapists to understand personality disorders in cognitive or cognitive-behavioral terms? The first attempts were fairly straightforward. Theorists suggested that personality disorders are complex and difficult to treat simply because individuals with these disorders have many concurrent problems (Stephens & Parks, 1981). Perhaps all a clinician needs to do is to match treatments to symptoms. For example, Table 14.1 lists the symptoms of dependent personality disorder and some interventions that could be used if one simply matched treatments to symptoms. This approach had the virtue of being simple and straightforward, and it did not require any changes in theory or therapy. Unfortunately, symptomatic treatment for in-

TABLE 14.1. Intervention Approach Suggested by Thinking of Personality Disorders as Collections of Symptoms

Symptom	Intervention
Difficulty making decisions	Improving decision-making skills
Avoidance of responsibility	Desensitization to responsibility
Difficulty disagreeing with others	Assertion training
Difficulty initiating projects	Desensitization, improving skills
Excessive reassurance seeking	"Weaning"
Discomfort with being alone	Desensitization
Urgent seeking of new relationships	Desensitization to being alone
Fear of self-reliance	Desensitization, improving skills

dividuals with Axis II disorders is often not very effective (see, e.g., Giles, Young, & Young, 1985).

The second stage of the evolution of cognitive or cognitive-behavioral approaches to personality disorders came with the realization not only that individuals with these disorders have many problems, but also that most of these problems occur in an interpersonal context. Thinking of personality disorders as disorders of social behavior provided an organizing principle that permitted a more strategic approach to intervention (see Turkat & Maisto, 1985). Rather than approaching the many problems encountered by an individual with dependent personality disorder haphazardly, one can think strategically: "What is disrupting the individual's interpersonal interactions, and what can we do about it?" Table 14.2 illustrates the intervention approach that follows from this view of personality disorders.

Up to this point, cognitive-behavioral investigators had approached personality disorders from a largely behavioral perspective. However, behavioral perspectives had some difficulty accounting for persistent, cross-situational consistencies in behavior, since most of their theoretical concepts were situation-specific. More cognitively oriented approaches (such as the one described by Beck, Rush, Shaw, & Emery, 1979) had a major advantage in explaining cross-situational consistencies in behavior, since they emphasized the central role of the individual's core beliefs and assumptions. Some cognitive concepts, such as automatic thoughts, were viewed as situation-specific; others, such as core beliefs or schemas,[1] were not.

The individual's core beliefs and assumptions, along with automatic thoughts and images, were hypothesized to be the cognitive contents of mental structures termed "schemas," which shape information processing and thereby have an important influence on emotion and behavior. In theory, once a schema is acquired, it persists. The schema is inactive when it is not relevant to the immediate situation, and it automatically becomes active when a relevant situation is encountered. Since a dysfunctional schema will have a major impact in any relevant situation, this was believed to help explain the pervasive, persistent problems that occur in a wide range of sit-

---

[1] In works on cognitive therapy, the terms "schema," "core belief," "underlying assumption," "dysfunctional belief," and so on have sometimes been used interchangeably, and at other times, distinctions have been drawn among these closely related terms. In contemporary usage, "schemas" are cognitive structures that serve as a basis for screening, categorizing, and interpreting experiences. "Core beliefs" are unconditional beliefs, such as "I'm no good," "Others can't be trusted," and "Effort does not pay off." These often operate outside of an individual's awareness and often are not clearly verbalized. "Underlying assumptions" or "dysfunctional beliefs" are conditional beliefs that shape one's response to experiences and situations—for example, "If someone gets close to me, they will discover the 'real me' and reject me." These may operate outside of the individual's awareness and may not be clearly verbalized, or the individual may be aware of these beliefs.

TABLE 14.2. Intervention Approach Suggested by Thinking of Personality Disorders as Disorders of Interpersonal Behavior

Conceptualization	Intervention
Lack of confidence in own capabilities produces excessive reliance on others, underuse of own skills, and fear of abandonment.	First increase sense of self-efficacy and improve skills; then gradually increase reliance on own skills and decrease reliance on others.
Fear of abandonment inhibits assertion and produces excessive compliance.	As confidence in own capabilities increases, increase assertion; use assertion training if necessary.

uations for individuals with personality disorders. This view had clear implications for treatment (see Table 14.3). If the symptoms of personality disorders are the results of dysfunctional schemas, then treatment should focus specifically on modifying the dysfunctional cognitions contained in the schemas.

The concept of personality disorders as products of dysfunctional schemas had considerable appeal. However, this view did little to explain why personality disorders are much more difficult to treat than Axis I disorders. After all, clients with Axis I problems often have dysfunctional schemas that play a role in their problems, and cognitive therapy routinely includes time spent identifying and modifying them (J. S. Beck, 1995). What accounts for the difference in treatment difficulty?

Young (1990; Young & Lindemann, 1992) hypothesized that, rather than having ordinary maladaptive schemas, individuals with personality disorders have what he termed "early maladaptive schemas" (EMSs), which differ in important ways from the maladaptive schemas of clients with Axis I disorders. He hypothesized that clients with Axis II disorders actively avoid activation of EMSs and use "schema coping mechanisms" (SCMs), which make it difficult for therapists to modify EMSs. See Young, Klosko, and Weishaar (2003) for a discussion of EMSs, SCMs, and a variety of intervention approaches designed to address these new concepts.

Although this modification of cognitive therapy was a plausible approach to understanding and treating personality disorders, it had the dis-

TABLE 14.3. Intervention Approach Suggested by Thinking of Personality Disorders as Products of Dysfunctional Schemas

Conceptualization	Intervention
Symptoms are due to dysfunctional schemas.	Treatment should focus on identifying and modifying dysfunctional schemas.

advantage of adding considerable complexity. Another approach to the conceptualization and treatment of personality disorders combined the idea that personality disorders are disorders of interpersonal behavior with the idea that personality disorders result from dysfunctional schemas (see Safran & McMain, 1992). This provided a basis for understanding and treating personality disorders without adding to the complexity of cognitive therapy.

In this view, as in the schema-focused approaches, dysfunctional schemas are seen as having a broad impact on cognition, emotion, and behavior. However, it also suggests that others' responses to the individual's interpersonal behavior can result in experiences that either reinforce or challenge dysfunctional beliefs and assumptions. If an individual's interpersonal behavior consistently elicits responses from others that reinforce dysfunctional beliefs and assumptions, this can result in self-perpetuating cognitive–interpersonal cycles that are quite resistant to change. Pretzer and Beck (1996) theorized that when this type of self-perpetuating cycle produces pervasive problems, this results in the cross-situational consistencies in behavior that are labeled "personality disorders."

The view of personality disorders as the product of self-perpetuating cognitive–interpersonal cycles has important implications for intervention (see Table 14.4). If dysfunctional schemas play a central role in personality disorders, one goal of intervention will be to modify the dysfunctional beliefs at some point. However, if self-perpetuating cycles continually reinforce dysfunctional beliefs, the therapist may need to moderate the self-perpetuating cycles and try to shift the individual to more adaptive interpersonal behavior before addressing the dysfunctional beliefs, or the therapist may need to address the dysfunctional beliefs and the dysfunctional interpersonal behavior simultaneously.

TABLE 14.4. Intervention Approach Suggested by Thinking of Personality Disorders as Products of Cognitive–Interpersonal Cycles

Conceptualization	Intervention
Dysfunctional schemas bias cognition, emotion, and behavior in a way that reinforces dysfunctional beliefs.	Base interventions on an individualized understanding of the cognitive–interpersonal cycles.
The client's interpersonal behavior elicits responses from others that reinforce dysfunctional beliefs.	Initially work to moderate the intensity of the self-perpetuating cycles; then work to change interpersonal behavior. Work to modify the dysfunctional beliefs after the self-perpetuating cycles have been attenuated.

MODIFYING "STANDARD" COGNITIVE THERAPY
FOR PERSONALITY DISORDERS

A number of authors have questioned whether cognitive therapy is a suitable approach for treating individuals with personality disorders (Rothstein & Vallis, 1991; Young, 1990). Vallis, Howes, and Standage (2000) examined this question empirically by analyzing the relationship between a composite measure of personality dysfunction and scores on a measure designed to assess the extent to which respondents are suitable for short-term cognitive therapy. They found that high scores on the measure of personality dysfunction were associated with low scores on the measure of suitability for short-term cognitive therapy. Although this finding might seem to support the idea that cognitive therapy is not suitable for individuals with personality disorders, it is important to note that the results were strongest for a subscale that assesses suitability for short-term therapy in general. Vallis et al. (2000) concluded that the basic cognitive therapy approach needs to be modified to take the characteristics of individuals with personality disorders into account, not that cognitive therapy is unsuitable as a treatment for individuals with personality disorders.

A number of authors have proposed ways of modifying cognitive therapy for use with individuals diagnosed with personality disorders (see, e.g., Beck, Freeman, & Associates, 1990; Beck, Freeman, Davis, & Associates, 2004; J. S. Beck, 1998; Freeman, Pretzer, Fleming, & Simon, 1990; Pretzer & Beck, 1996). Cognitive therapy for personality disorders has much in common with cognitive therapy for depression (Beck et al., 1979). Both emphasize the development of a cognitive conceptualization, a collaborative therapeutic relationship, a relatively structured therapy session, a problem-solving approach, active evaluation of clients' cognitions, psychoeducation, and actively helping clients to learn new skills and apply them in problem situations (J. S. Beck, 1997). However, clients with personality disorders typically have ingrained interaction patterns and dysfunctional cognitions that complicate many aspects of therapy (see Table 14.5). Therapists must make some adjustments in order to apply the principles of cognitive therapy effectively with such clients (J. S. Beck, 1997), as described below.

• *Principle 1: Cognitive therapy is based on a cognitive formulation.* Therapists working with clients with either Axis I or Axis II diagnoses focus on specific situations in which the clients' problems are manifested and make a cross-sectional analysis of the clients' thoughts, feelings, and actions in problem situations. This information provides a basis for developing an understanding of the ways in which the clients' cognitions, emotions, and behavior interact and contribute to the clients' problems. This cognitive conceptualization (see Figure 14.1 later in this chapter for an example) provides a basis for planning treatment to be as effective and efficient as possible. The process of data collection with clients who have personality disorders can be problematic. These individuals often hold beliefs that interfere with free and candid disclosure of their thoughts, feelings, and actions (see Table 14.5). The conceptualization that eventually emerges as a therapist and a client develop an understanding of the client's problems is often much more complex than is the case with most Axis I problems.

• *Principle 2: Cognitive therapy emphasizes a strong therapeutic alliance.* Cognitive therapy is based on a collaborative relationship in which therapist and client work together toward goals the client values. They jointly decide which issues to address and how to go about doing so. The therapist talks explicitly with the client about the goals of therapy, and works with the client to help him or her obtain symptomatic relief and acquire useful skills. With clients who have straightforward Axis I disorders, a strong collaborative relationship is usually easy to establish. However, for clients with Axis II problems, the therapeutic relationship itself often becomes a focus of therapy. These clients' dysfunctional beliefs about themselves, about their therapists, and about relationships often become activated during sessions.

During therapy sessions, it is important for a therapist to be alert for verbal and nonverbal cues of a shift in a client's mood, and then to assess the client's thoughts and feelings on the spot. Although the complexity of establishing and maintaining a strong therapeutic alliance complicates therapy with clients who have personality disorders, the time spent doing so is necessary as a foundation for effective intervention; it provides insight into dysfunctional beliefs and interpersonal strategies that affect these clients' other relationships in much the same way as they affect therapy.

• *Principle 3: Goal setting and problem solving are integral parts of cognitive therapy.* From the beginning of cognitive therapy, the therapist helps the client identify overall goals for therapy and interim steps toward those goals. Clients with Axis I disorders usually do not have much trouble doing so, but many clients with Axis II disorders have difficulty specifying goals and working to achieve them. They may express vague or unrealistic goals; they may specify goals in terms of what they want someone else to do, rather than identifying changes they want to make; or their goals may change from week to week. Also, whereas many clients with Axis I disorders have reasonably good problem-solving skills, clients with personality disorders often do not know how to solve problems effectively, or they may engage in dysfunctional problem-solving strategies. With a client who has an Axis II disorder, the therapist may need to spend extra time identifying consistent, achievable goals and helping the client learn effective problem-solving strategies.

• *Principle 4: Cognitive therapy emphasizes structured sessions.* Therapy proceeds most efficiently when the therapist actively structures the session so that the time is used productively (see Table 14.6). However, many clients with Axis II disorders hold beliefs that make it hard for them to tolerate a structured approach to therapy (see Table 14.5). Therapists should not unilaterally impose a structured approach on clients who resist it. In each case, a therapist must judge whether efforts to identify and address these beliefs when they first emerge are likely to be productive, or whether to vary the structure of the session initially and wait until the therapeutic alliance is stronger before addressing these cognitions. Some clients with Axis II disorders, particularly those who are quite isolated, may benefit from being able to talk without interruption for the initial portion of the session. It may be useful to allow time for this at the beginning of the session and then implement the more standard structure for the remainder of the session.

• *Principle 5: Cognitive therapy emphasizes cognitive restructuring.* An important part of therapy involves identifying, evaluating, and responding to the client's dysfunctional thoughts and beliefs. The therapist helps the client learn that it is not the situation per se that shapes one's reactions, but one's *interpretations* of the situation. Clients with Axis II disorders may find this concept hard to grasp, may avoid facing upsetting thoughts and feelings, or may feel invalidated by their therapists' attempts to help them look at their experiences from a different point of view. This complicates the process of cognitive restructuring.

• *Principle 6: Cognitive therapy addresses clients' developmental histories and uses specialized techniques to alter core beliefs as needed.* Most clients who have Axis I problems are able to modify their dysfunctional thoughts and core beliefs without examination of childhood events, and doing so may take time away from solving here-and-now problems. Therefore, cognitive therapy with such clients often involves spending very little time on childhood experiences. Clients with personality disorders, in contrast, often have extremely rigid beliefs stemming from childhood experiences. It often can be quite useful for a therapist to help such a client understand how his or her beliefs developed naturally from early experiences and were reinforced by other experiences over time. The same techniques are used in modifying dysfunctional beliefs with all types of clients (see J. S. Beck, 1995), but clients with Axis II disorders may need additional help in developing more positive, reality-based beliefs to replace their dysfunctional beliefs.

• *Principle 7: Cognitive therapy incorporates relapse prevention techniques.* Cognitive therapists are concerned not only with helping clients overcome their problems, but also with teaching them how to deal with problems on their own. In therapy, the clients learn how to solve problems,

TABLE 14.5. Cognitions That Can Complicate the Treatment of Clients with Personality Disorders

Stage of treatment	Examples of problematic cognitions
Conducting initial evaluation and developing a conceptualization	"If I reveal myself, I'll be rejected." "If people know about me, they'll be able to hurt me."
Developing and maintaining a therapeutic alliance	"If I trust others, I'll be hurt." "I have to rely on others to solve my problems."
Structuring the therapy session	"People must know every detail, or they won't give me the 'right' help." "If others interrupt me, it means they don't care." "If I let others direct me, it means they are controlling me."
Setting goals	"If I try to [work toward a goal], I'll fail." "If I can't accomplish something totally, it isn't worth working toward at all." "If I accomplish my goals, things will get worse."
Problem solving	"My problems can't be solved." "Others should solve my problems for me." "It is unfair that I have to deal with these problems."
Eliciting and responding to automatic thoughts	"If I think about upsetting things, I won't be able to tolerate the feelings." "If someone questions the validity of my thoughts, he or she is invalidating me."
Skills training	"If I'm assertive with others, they'll get angry and reject me." "If I try my new skills, I'll fail." "If I become more competent, I'll be abandoned."
Homework	"If I do what others tell me to, it shows that I am weak." "If I accomplish this step, others will just expect more and more of me." "If I don't feel motivated, I can't do it."
Modifying dysfunctional beliefs	"If my belief isn't true, I don't know who I am." "If I admit that my belief isn't true, it shows that I am weak."
Termination and relapse prevention	"If my therapist wants me to terminate, it means he or she doesn't care about me." "If I end therapy, I'll fall apart." "If I try to solve problems on my own, I'll fail."

TABLE 14.6. Structure of a Typical Cognitive Therapy Session

Element	Description
Mood check	Therapist briefly assesses client's mood.
Agenda setting	Therapist finds out what problems the client wants to address, and proposes any additional issues he or she wants to address as well.
Bridge from previous session	Therapist finds out about major events since previous session, assesses client's overall level of functioning, reviews what the client learned from the previous session, and reviews the client's homework.
The body of the session	Therapist and client address the items on the agenda in order of priority—collecting detailed information, utilizing a problem-solving approach, and teaching new skills.
Developing homework	Therapist and client jointly identify ways for the client to apply what he or she has learned to everyday life.
Closing	Therapist summarizes the main points covered in the session (or has the client do so) and asks for feedback about the session.

restructure their thinking, and change their behavior in order to overcome problems as they arise. This learning improves the likelihood that gains achieved through therapy will persist after the conclusion of treatment.

Relapse prevention also typically involves responding to clients' fears about ending therapy; introducing the idea that active steps are needed to maintain the gains made in therapy; anticipating high-risk situations that the clients may encounter, and planning how to cope with them; and identifying early warning signs that a problem is returning, and developing strategies for forestalling relapse. Although these things are important for all clients, they are crucially important for clients with Axis II disorders. Often negative core beliefs are modified but not completely eliminated. There is a risk that future events could reactivate dysfunctional beliefs and maladaptive behaviors. It is important for these clients to recognize this and for them to be prepared to deal effectively with this if it occurs.

Some clients with Axis II disorders express a desire to terminate therapy prematurely—perhaps because the therapeutic relationship has broken down; because their Axis I symptoms have remitted, and they do not want to engage in the hard work of modifying their core beliefs and compensatory strategies; or because they are testing how their therapists will respond. Other clients with Axis II disorders cling to therapy, even though they have achieved significant improvement and seem equipped to face life without ongoing therapy. When the number of sessions is not constrained by forces beyond a client's control (e.g., insurance), it is important for the termination of therapy to be a decision that therapist and client reach collaboratively. It is important for the therapist to take an active role in assessing the extent to which the client's goals for therapy have been accomplished, and the degree to which the client has mastered the skills needed to maintain his or her gains. In any case, it can be important for the therapist to help the client explore the pros and cons of terminating therapy versus continuing in therapy, and to address any unrealistic hopes or fears. When a client seems ready to terminate therapy but is reluctant to do so, it may be useful to schedule appointments at longer intervals, so that the client has a greater opportunity to discover whether he or she can deal with problems as they arise.

APPLYING A COGNITIVE–INTERPERSONAL PERSPECTIVE TO UNDERSTANDING AND TREATING PERSONALITY DISORDERS

An example of how this approach can be applied to understanding one particular personality disorder (in this case, borderline personality disorder) is shown graphically in Figure 14.1. Three beliefs that are central in borderline personality disorder are seen on the left side of this figure: "The world is dangerous and malevolent," "I am weak and vulnerable," and "My feelings are unacceptable and dangerous." These beliefs have important effects on cognition and behavior.

Individuals who see the world as a dangerous place, and themselves as vulnerable, have specific fears in many different situations. They often become hypervigilant for signs of danger and overlook or discount signs of safety. This bias in information processing generally occurs outside of the individuals' awareness (until therapy), and strengthens their conviction that the world is a dangerous place.

One strategy for remaining safe in a dangerous world is to be continually vigilant, on guard, and ready to defend oneself. Individuals who are hypervigilant for signs of danger and who rely on this interpersonal strategy may well develop paranoid personality disorder. However, individuals with borderline personality disorder have a second core belief: They typically see themselves as weak and vulnerable—as not being competent to handle the dangers which they see around them. This belief blocks them from relying on their own capabilities.

Individuals who see themselves as weak, vulnerable, and incompetent have a low sense of self-efficacy and are likely to avoid situations that they fear. This avoidance, in turn, reinforces the belief that they cannot cope with the feared situation. When individuals see themselves as being weak and vulnerable in a dangerous world, one solution is to find someone capa-

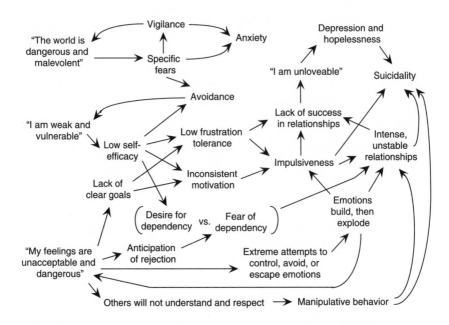

FIGURE 14.1. A cognitive–interpersonal conceptualization of borderline personality disorder.

ble to rely on. Individuals who consistently rely on others and subjugate themselves to assure that others will not withdraw their help may develop dependent personality disorder.

But individuals with borderline personality disorder hold a third belief, "My feelings are unacceptable and dangerous," which blocks this solution. Because they see themselves as inadequate and weak, the idea of finding someone strong and capable to take care of them is appealing. However, because they see themselves as inherently unacceptable, relying on a protector seems unacceptably risky. They anticipate that they will be rejected and abandoned once their protector really gets to know them. As a result, they have strongly conflicting feelings about depending on someone else.

In addition, since individuals with borderline personality disorder see their emotions as dangerous and unacceptable to others, they often engage in extreme attempts to avoid, control, or escape from strong emotions. They suppress, avoid, or deny emotions, but then suddenly manifest them at full intensity. This results in recurrent problems in relationships, which reinforce the belief that these emotions are unacceptable and dangerous, and which encourage further attempts to avoid, control, or escape emotions.

Because clients with borderline personality disorder have a proclivity toward intense emotional reactions, have conflicting feelings about depending on others, and have a low frustration tolerance, their relationships tend to be intense and unstable. They anticipate that others will not understand and respect their feelings if they speak up directly. Therefore, they are likely to engage in manipulative behavior rather than expressing themselves directly and assertively. All of these factors contribute to persistent problems in relationships and contribute to feelings of depression, hopelessness, and suicidality.

In addition, individuals with borderline personality disorder tend to engage in dichotomous thinking. This dichotomous thinking adds to the intensity of the emotional reactions, the interpersonal interactions, and the conclusions they draw in the situations discussed above.

This conceptualization of borderline personality disorder has clear implications for intervention (see Table 14.7). Clients with this usually enter therapy at a time of crisis, and therapy usually needs to start by working on dealing with these crises. As the therapist does so, the problems that Linehan (1993) terms "therapy-interfering behaviors" are likely to arise. Clients with borderline personality disorder are typically ambivalent about relying on others; anticipate rejection; and tend toward intense, unstable relationships. Behaviors ranging from noncompliance, to intense emotional reactions during the session, to suicidality and self-mutilation must be addressed promptly so that they do not disrupt therapy. Once these hurdles have been cleared, a therapist can work to increase a client's ability to cope with intense emotion, to help the client to shift to more adaptive interpersonal behavior, and eventually to modify the client's dysfunctional beliefs. Finally, therapy will end by working explicitly on relapse prevention.

This treatment approach makes use of many of the interventions commonly used in cognitive therapy, such as using thought records to identify dysfunctional thoughts and working to modify core beliefs (see J. S. Beck, 1995). However, it is also important to address issues that may not be a focus of therapy for the average client with an Axis I disorder, such as increasing af-

TABLE 14.7. Proposed Intervention Strategy for Borderline Personality Disorder

Establish a collaborative relationship.

Improve client's day-to-day coping and increase self-efficacy.

Decrease "therapy-interfering behaviors."

Increase client's ability to tolerate and modulate emotion (this includes identifying and testing automatic thoughts).

Help client shift to more adaptive interpersonal behavior.

Modify underlying assumptions.

Work on relapse prevention and prepare for termination.

fect tolerance and working on skills for coping with intense emotions (Farrell & Shaw, 1994). Therapists also need to pay more than the usual amount of attention to the therapeutic relationship and their own emotional responses. They may need to use cognitive therapy skills themselves to maintain empathy and commitment while working with clients whose dysfunctional behaviors and extreme emotionality can be quite challenging.

Please note that the discussion above applies specifically to borderline personality disorder. Each of the personality disorders is conceptualized differently, and intervention strategies vary among the personality disorders. A discussion of each of the personality disorders is beyond the scope of this chapter. Interested readers can find discussions of each Axis II disorder in Freeman et al. (1990) and in Beck et al. (2004).

THE EMPIRICAL STATUS OF COGNITIVE THERAPY AS A TREATMENT FOR PERSONALITY DISORDERS

One of the strengths of cognitive therapy is the extensive body of research supporting both the theory and the therapy. The research base for cognitive therapy with personality disorders is much smaller than is the case with many Axis I disorders, and in the past, some commentators expressed concern that the rapid expansion of theory and practice was outstripping the empirical research (Dobson & Pusch, 1993). Fortunately, a growing body of research supports cognitive therapy as an approach to understanding and treating personality disorders. A detailed review of empirical findings regarding cognitive therapy of personality disorders is beyond the scope of this chapter. Readers who wish a more comprehensive review should see Pretzer (1998) or Beck et al. (2004).

Research has produced a number of findings relevant to the cognitive understanding of personality disorders. For example, individuals diagnosed with personality disorders show elevated levels of dysfunctional attitudes (O'Leary et al., 1991; Illardi & Craighead, 1999); the endorsement of personality-disorder-relevant beliefs predicts the level of personality disorder traits (Arntz, Dietzel, & Dreessen, 1999; Ball & Cecero, 2001); and individuals with specific personality disorders endorse the particular beliefs hypothesized to play a role in those disorders (Arntz et al., 1999; Beck et al., 2001). Looking specifically at borderline personality disorder, Arntz and his colleagues found an elevated level of dichotomous thinking (Veen & Arntz, 2000), as predicted; they also found that dysfunctional beliefs mediate the relationship between traumatic experiences and borderline symptomatology (Arntz et al., 1999).

Table 14.8 provides an overview of the available research on the effectiveness of cognitive therapy or CBT as a treatment for individuals with personality disorders. Many clinical reports assert that cognitive therapy or CBT can provide effective treatment for these individuals, but there are fewer well-controlled outcome studies. Fortunately, the studies that are available provide findings that are quite encouraging. Single-case-design studies have shown that individualized CBT was effective for some clients with personality disorders; but only partially effective or ineffective for others (Turkat & Maisto, 1985; Nelson-Gray, Johnson, Foyle, Daniel, & Harmon, 1996). Studies of the effects of comorbid Axis II disorders on the outcome of CBT for Axis I disorders have produced a complex pattern of results: Sometimes the presence of an Axis II disorder decreases the effectiveness of treatment; sometimes it has no negative impact; and sometimes treatment for an Axis I disorder produces improvement in the Axis II disorder as well (see Pretzer, 1998, or Beck et al., 2004).

TABLE 14.8. The Effectiveness of Cognitive Therapy or CBT with Personality Disorders

Personality Disorder	Uncontrolled Clinical Reports	Single-case design studies	Studies of the effects of personality disorders on treatment outcome	Controlled outcome studies
Antisocial	+	−	+	[a]
Avoidant	+	+	±	+
Borderline	±	−	+	±
Dependent	+	+	+	
Histrionic	+		−	
Narcissistic	+	+		
Obsessive–compulsive	+	−		
Paranoid	+	+		
Passive–aggressive	+		+	
Schizoid	+			
Schizotypal				

Note. See Pretzer (1998) and Beck et al. (2004) for reviews of the research. +, cognitive-behavioral interventions found to be effective; −, cognitive-behavioral interventions found not to be effective; ±, mixed findings; [a]cognitive-behavioral interventions were effective with antisocial personality disorder subjects only when the individual was depressed at pretest.

Controlled outcome studies of CBT approaches have only been conducted for three personality disorders: antisocial (Woody, McLellan,
Luborsky, & O'Brien, 1985), avoidant (Stravynski, Marks, & Yule, 1982;
Greenberg & Stravynski, 1985), and borderline personality disorders.
Woody et al. (1985) found that subjects with antisocial personality disorder
and comorbid major depression responded well both to cognitive therapy
and to supportive–expressive therapy. These subjects showed significant
improvement on 11 of 22 outcome variables, including decreases in objective measures of antisocial behavior (such as drug use and other illegal activity). However, subjects with antisocial personality disorder who were not
depressed did not respond to either treatment, apparently due to a lack of
motivation for change.

Subjects with avoidant personality disorder were found to respond
both to social skills training and to social skills training combined with cognitive interventions (Stravynski et al., 1982); they showed significant decreases in social anxiety and avoidance, as well as improvement in interpersonal relationships. This finding was initially interpreted as showing that
cognitive interventions added little to treatment, even though the two treatment approaches were equally effective. However, in a subsequent study,
Greenberg and Stravynski (1985) observed that the clients' fear of ridicule
contributed to premature termination in many cases, and suggested that interventions to modify clients' cognitions could add substantially to the
effectiveness of treatment.

Research in using dialectical behavior therapy (DBT) for the treatment
of borderline personality disorder (Linehan, Armstrong, Suarez, Allmon, &
Heard, 1991; Linehan, Tutek, & Heard, 1992; Linehan, Heard &
Armstrong, 1993) has provided evidence that a cognitive-behavioral intervention can be effective with clients who have a severe personality disorder.
One year of DBT intervention produced significant improvement in clients
who met diagnostic criteria for borderline personality disorder and also
had histories of multiple psychiatric hospitalizations, were chronically
parasuicidal, and were unable to maintain employment. Subjects who received DBT showed significant decreases in suicide attempts, self-
mutilation, and rehospitalization, but continued to show elevated levels of
depression, anxiety, and interpersonal problems. The investigators
concluded that more than 1 year of treatment was needed to obtain
maximum benefits from DBT.

Controlled outcome research is sometimes criticized as not reflecting
the realities of clinical practice. Evidence regarding the effectiveness of cognitive therapy as a treatment for personality disorders in clinical practice is
provided by a study of the effectiveness of cognitive therapy for depression
in a real-life private practice setting conducted by Persons, Burns, and
Perloff (1988). When the investigators examined the impact of personality

disorders on treatment outcome, they found that clients with personality disorders were at higher risk of dropping out of treatment prematurely. However, when they were able to retain such clients in therapy, the eventual improvement in depression scores was similar for clients with or without a personality disorder diagnosis.

Obviously, much more research is needed to test cognitive or cognitive-behavioral conceptualizations of personality disorders, and to test the effectiveness of contemporary approaches to cognitive therapy for each personality disorder. The quality of this research can be improved in several ways. First, a number of studies have used the American Psychiatric Association's three clusters of personality disorders as the units of analysis, rather than looking at personality disorders individually. However, cognitive approaches conceptualize each personality disorder differently and propose somewhat different treatment approaches for each one. Although it can be difficult to obtain an adequate sample size with some of the less common personality disorders, combining disparate disorders into clusters for research purposes is not useful unless there is a clear theoretical rationale for doing so. Second, much of the existing cognitive-behavioral research relies on simple self-report measures of dysfunctional beliefs. Use of this methodology assumes that individuals can reliably rate the strength of their dysfunctional beliefs or schemas. Yet, according to cognitive theory, dysfunctional schemas often operate outside of awareness, and in clinical practice it often takes significant time and effort to identify clients' dysfunctional beliefs. Clear evidence is needed that these measures actually assess dysfunctional beliefs, not more superficial attitudes. Alternative methods for assessing dysfunctional beliefs and other relevant cognitions are available and should be used more widely. These include thought-sampling or experience sampling methodology (Hurlburt, Leach, & Saltman, 1984); laboratory tasks that provide a more direct method for assessing schemas (e.g., McNally, Reimann, & Kim, 1990); and content analysis of responses to schema-relevant stimuli.

The past two decades have seen rapid advances in theory, practice, and empirical research into the application of cognitive therapy to the treatment of personality disorders. Although there are grounds for legitimate concern that clinical innovation may outstrip the empirical research (Dobson & Pusch, 1993), a growing body of research supports cognitive therapy as an approach to understanding and treating personality disorders. Given the complexity of clients with personality disorders and the difficulties encountered in therapy with these individuals, it is encouraging that the past two decades have seen the evolution of more effective approaches to understanding and treating personality disorders. As research and innovation continue, we should see continued advances in theory and practice.

REFERENCES

American Psychiatric Association. (2000). *Diagnostic and statistical manual of mental disorders* (4th ed., text rev.). Washington, DC: Author.

Arntz, A., Dietzel, R., & Dreessen, L. (1999). Assumptions in borderline personality disorder: Specificity, stability and relationship with etiological factors. *Behaviour Research and Therapy, 37,* 545–557.

Ball, S. A., & Cecero, J. (2001). Addicted patients with personality disorders: Traits, schemas, and presenting problems. *Journal of Personality Disorders, 15,* 72–83.

Beck, A. T., Freeman, A., & Associates. (1990). *Cognitive therapy of personality disorders.* New York: Guilford Press.

Beck, A. T., Freeman, A., Davis, D., & Associates. (2004). *Cognitive therapy of personality disorders* (2nd ed.). New York: Guilford Press.

Beck, A. T., Rush, A. J., Shaw, B. F., & Emery, G. (1979). *Cognitive therapy of depression.* New York: Guilford Press.

Beck, A. T., Butler, A. C., Brown, G. K., Dahlsgaard, K. K., Newman, C. F., & Beck, J. S. (2001). Dysfunctional beliefs discriminate personality disorders. *Behaviour Research and Therapy, 39,* 1213–1225.

Beck, J. S. (1995). *Cognitive therapy: Basics and beyond.* New York: Guilford Press.

Beck, J. S. (1997). Personality disorders: Cognitive approaches. In L. J. Dickstein, M. B. Riba, & J. M. Oldham (Eds.), *American Psychiatric Press review of psychiatry* (Vol. 16). Washington, DC: American Psychiatric Press.

Beck, J. S. (1998). Complex cognitive therapy treatment for personality disorder patients. *Bulletin of the Menninger Clinic, 62,* 170–194.

Dobson, K. S., & Pusch, D. (1993). Toward a definition of the conceptual and empirical boundaries of cognitive therapy. *Australian Psychologist, 28,* 137–144.

Farrell, J. M., & Shaw, I. A. (1994). Emotion awareness training: A prerequisite to effective cognitive-behavioral treatment of borderline personality disorder. *Cognitive and Behavioral Practice, 1,* 71–91.

Fleming, B. (1983, August). *Cognitive therapy with histrionic patients: Resolving a conflict in styles.* Paper presented at the annual meeting of the American Psychological Association, Anaheim, CA.

Freeman, A., Pretzer, J. L., Fleming, B., & Simon, K. M. (1990). *Clinical applications of cognitive therapy.* New York: Plenum Press.

Giles, T. R., Young, R. R., & Young, D. E. (1985). Behavioral treatment of severe bulimia. *Behavior Therapy, 16,* 393–405.

Greenberg, D., & Stravynski, A. (1985). Patients who complain of social dysfunction: I. Clinical and demographic features. *Canadian Journal of Psychiatry, 30,* 206–211.

Hardy, G. E., Barkham, M., Shapiro, D. A., Stiles, W. B., Rees, A., & Reynolds, S. (1995). Impact of Cluster C personality disorders on outcomes of contrasting brief therapies for depression. *Journal of Consulting and Clinical Psychology, 63,* 997–1004.

Hurlburt, R. T., Leach, B.C., & Saltman, S. (1984). Random sampling of thought and mood. *Cognitive Therapy and Research, 8,* 263–276.

Illardi, S. S., & Craighead, W. E. (1999). The relationship between personality pathology and dsyfunctional cognitions in previously depressed adults. *Journal of Abnormal Psychology, 108,* 51–57.

Linehan, M. M. (1993). *Cognitive-behavioral treatment of borderline personality disorder.* New York: Guilford Press.

Linehan, M. M., Armstrong, H. E., Suarez, A., Allmon, D. J., & Heard, H. L. (1991). Cognitive-behavioral treatment of chronically suicidal borderline patients. *Archives of General Psychiatry, 48,* 1060–1064.

Linehan, M. M., Heard, H. L., & Armstrong, H. E. (1993). Naturalistic follow-up of a behavioral treatment for chronically parasuicidal borderline patients. *Archives of General Psychiatry, 50,* 971–974.

Linehan, M. M., Tutek, D. A., & Heard, H. L. (1992, November). *Interpersonal and social treatment outcomes in borderline personality disorder.* Paper presented at the 26th Annual Conference of the Association for Advancement of Behavior Therapy, Boston.

McNally, R. J., Reimann, B. C., & Kim, E. (1990). Selective processing of threat cues in panic disorder. *Behaviour Research and Therapy, 28,* 407–412.

Nelson-Gray, R. O., Johnson, D. Foyle. L. W., Daniel, S. S., & Harmon, R. (1996). The effectiveness of cognitive therapy tailored to depressives with personality disorders. *Journal of Personality Disorders, 10,* 132–152.

O'Leary, K. M., Cowdry, R. W., Gardner, D. L., Leibenluft, E., Lucas, P. B., & deJong-Meyer, R. (1991). Dysfunctional attitudes in borderline personality disorder. *Journal of Personality Disorders, 5,* 233–242.

Persons, J. B., Burns, B. D., & Perloff, J. M. (1988). Predictors of drop-out and outcome in cognitive therapy for depression in a private practice setting. *Cognitive Therapy and Research, 12,* 557–575.

Pretzer, J. (1998). Cognitive-behavioral approaches to the treatment of personality disorders. In C. Perris & P. D. McGorry (Eds.), *Cognitive psychotherapy of psychotic and personality disorders: Handbook of theory and practice.* New York: Wiley.

Pretzer, J., & Beck, A. T. (1996). A cognitive theory of personality disorders. In J. F. Clarkin & M. F. Lenzenweger (Eds.), *Major theories of personality disorder.* New York: Guilford Press.

Pretzer, J. L. (1983, August). *Borderline personality disorder: Too complex for cognitive behavioral approaches?* Paper presented at the annual meeting of the American Psychological Association, Anaheim, CA. (ERIC Document Reproduction Service No. ED 243 007)

Rothstein, M. M., & Vallis, T. M. (1991). The application of cognitive therapy to patients with personality disorders. In T. M. Vallis, J. L. Howes, & P. C. Miller (Eds.), *The challenge of cognitive therapy: Applications to nontraditional populations.* New York: Plenum Press.

Rush, A. J., & Shaw, B. F. (1983). Failures in treating depression by cognitive therapy. In E. B. Foa & P. G. M. Emmelkamp (Eds.), *Failures in behavior therapy.* New York: Wiley.

Safran, J. D., & McMain, S. (1992). A cognitive-interpersonal approach to the treatment of personality disorders. *Journal of Cognitive Psychotherapy: An International Quarterly, 6*, 59–68.

Simon, K. M. (1983, August). *Cognitive therapy with compulsive patients: Replacing rigidity with structure*. Paper presented at the annual meeting of the American Psychological Association, Anaheim, CA.

Stravynski, A., Marks, I., & Yule, W. (1982). Social skills problems in neurotic outpatients: Social skills training with and without cognitive modification. *Archives of General Psychiatry, 39*, 1378–1385.

Stephens, J. H., & Parks, S. L. (1981). Behavior therapy of personality disorders. In J. R. Lion (Ed.), *Personality disorders: Diagnosis and management* (2nd ed.). Baltimore: Williams & Wilkins.

Turkat, I. D., & Maisto, S. A. (1985). Personality disorders: Application of the experimental method to the formulation and modification of personality disorders. In D. H. Barlow (Ed.), *Clinical handbook of psychological disorders: A step by step treatment manual*. New York: Guilford Press.

Vallis, T. M., Howes, J. L., & Standage, K. (2000). Is cognitive therapy suitable for treating individuals with personality dysfunction? *Cognitive Therapy and Research, 24*, 595–606.

Veen, G., & Arntz, A. (2000). Multidimensional dichotomous thinking characterizes borderline personality disorder. *Cognitive Therapy and Research, 24*, 23–45.

Woody, G. E., McLellan, A. T., Luborsky, L., & O'Brien, C. P. (1985) Sociopathy and psychotherapy outcome. *Archives of General Psychiatry, 42*, 1081–1086.

Young, J. (1990). *Cognitive therapy for personality disorders: A schema-focused approach*. Sarasota, FL: Professional Resource Exchange.

Young, J., Klosko, J., & Weishaar, M. (2003). *Schema therapy: A practitioner's guide*. New York: Guilford Press.

Young, J., & Lindemann, M. D. (1992). An integrative schema-focused model for personality disorders. *Journal of Cognitive Psychotherapy: An International Quarterly, 6*, 11–24.

Young, J. E. (1983, August). *Borderline personality: Cognitive theory and treatment*. Paper presented at the annual meeting of the American Psychological Association, Anaheim, CA.

Chapter 15

Cognitive-Behavioral Treatment of Personality Disorders in Childhood and Adolescence

ARTHUR FREEMAN

The very title of this chapter raises discomfort and disagreement among clinicians. Can a child or adolescent have a personality disorder? What qualifies a child for a diagnosis of a personality disorder? Clinicians are often left in a confusing position. Child psychologists, child psychiatrists, classroom teachers, pediatricians, child care workers, and clinicians working in acute treatment and residential settings regularly see children and adolescents who meet criteria for personality disorders (Beren, 1998; Bleiberg, 2001; Kernberg, Weiner, & Bardenstein, 2001; Shapiro, 1997; Vela, Gottlieb, & Gottlieb, 1997; Freeman & Rigby, 2003). But can clinicians apply these "adult" diagnoses to this small, but visible group of children? What are the advantages and disadvantages of using these diagnoses for children and adolescents? What are the ramifications (in terms of placement, treatment, and politics) of using personality disorder diagnoses for children and adolescents? And, finally, does using these "adult" diagnoses have the effect of creating a "trash can" category that will be used for the most troubling and troubled of children or adolescents?

Bearing these questions in mind, I contend in this chapter that personality disorders can be manifested and identified among youth prior to age 18. These disorders can be diagnosed with the same criteria used for adults. Rather than trying to find euphemistic terms, titles, or diagnoses,

319

or seeing the identified patterns as clinical precursors to the adult disorders, I believe that the clinical reality of personality disorders in childhood must be appropriately assessed, diagnosed, and treated. Although many would agree that some youngsters have certain traits that may be precursors to later personality disorders, most contemporary clinicians are loath to diagnose a child as having a personality disorder (Paris, 2003). Some reasons for this hesitance are theoretical, some conceptual, and some "legal."

The goal of this chapter is to extend Aaron T. Beck's pioneering work in applying cognitive therapy to the treatment of personality disorders (Beck, Freeman, & Associates, 1990; Beck, Freeman, Davis, & Associates, 2004) and to examine the premise and the diagnosis of personality disorders in children and adolescents. I hope to do this by raising and discussing the conceptual, theoretical, and "legal" issues. These are followed by a discussion of the cognitive-behavioral conceptualization and directions for future study.

Several questions emerge. At what point are the behaviors of children or adolescents seen and diagnosed as personality-disordered? At what point do they move from "precursor" or antecedent behaviors (Paris, 2003) to being diagnosable as fully meeting the criteria for personality disorders? When do traits and styles of responding become diagnosed as pathology? At what point should the mental health community step in and attempt to challenge or to modify the noted behaviors? Are there issues present that require the inclusion of the criminal justice system or the child protective systems into the treatment plan? At what point do troubled or troubling children get diagnosed as having personality disorders?

The most frequent answer to these questions is that children cannot be "legally" diagnosed as having a personality disorder, according to the fourth edition (text revision) of the *Diagnostic and Statistical Manual of Mental Disorders* (DSM-IV-TR; American Psychiatric Association, 2000). The rationale for this position comes from an interpretation of the prototypical DSM-IV TR (APA, 2000) introduction in to all of the criteria sets for the personality disorders. The introduction states that each personality disorder involves "a pervasive pattern of [descriptive statements], beginning by early adulthood and present in a variety of contexts, as indicated by [a number] or more of the following [criteria listing]." Without any further reading, this repeated statement gives the impression that personality disorders are manifestations of behavior, affect, and cognition that arise and can only be diagnosed beginning in the early adult years (which generally mean 18 years and up).

Clearly, however, the introduction states that the disorders are in place "by early adulthood" rather than "in early adulthood." The reader might be inclined to see this as a piece of Talmudic *pilpul*.[1] Nevertheless, the term "personality disorder" implies an enduring pattern whose beginnings can, at the very least, be traced back to adolescence, and often to childhood. The one exception noted in DSM-IV-TR is the diagnosis of antisocial personality disorder, where a history of conduct disorder in childhood and adolescence is required (APA, 2000, p. 706). DSM-IV-TR states, "The features of a personality disorder usually become recognizable during *adolescence* or early adult life" (APA, 2000, p. 688; emphasis added).

DSM-IV TR (APA, 2000) also offers six broad criteria for defining a personality disorder. These six essential features of a personality disorder are as follows:

> An enduring pattern of inner experience and behavior that deviates markedly from the expectations of the individual's culture and is manifested in at least two of the following areas: cognition, affectivity, interpersonal functioning, or impulse control (Criterion A). This enduring pattern is inflexible and pervasive across a broad range of personal and social situations (Criterion B) and leads to clinically significant distress or impairment in social, occupational, or other important areas of functioning (Criterion C). The pattern is stable and of long duration, and its onset can be traced back at least to adolescence or early adulthood (Criterion D). The pattern is not better accounted for as a manifestation or consequence of another mental disorder (Criterion E) and is not due to the direct physiological effects of a substance (e.g., a drug of abuse, a medication, exposure to a toxin) or a general medical condition (e.g., head trauma) (Criterion F). (p. 686)

According to these criteria, children can easily be diagnosed as having personality disorders. The patterns of behavioral disorders described in children are exhibited in a wide range of social, school, and interpersonal contexts. They are not better accounted for by another disorder on Axis I, III, or IV, or by some developmental stage. An arguable point is that a personality pattern must be stable and of long duration. If the pattern has been in place for 2 or 3 years, does that qualify as accounting for a "significant duration"? If we think of a 10-year-old child, then 2 years is 20% of his or her life, and therefore can be quite significant in terms of its chronic impact on the child's life. Finally, the patterns are not the result of some chemical or toxic reaction. Furthermore, DSM-IV-TR states:

> Personality Disorder categories may be applied to children or adolescents in those relatively unusual instances in which the individual's particular

[1] *Pilpul* describes a method of reasoning and text understanding that involves the careful reading and interpretation of content, context, placement, order, and choice of language.

maladaptive personality traits appear to be pervasive, persistent, and unlikely to be limited to a particular developmental stage or an episode of an Axis I disorder. It should be recognized that the traits of a Personality Disorder that appear in childhood will often not persist unchanged into adult life. To diagnose a Personality Disorder in an individual under age 18 years, the features must have been present for at least 1 year. The one exception to this is Antisocial Personality Disorder, which cannot be diagnosed in individuals under age 18 years. (APA, 2000, p. 687).

Probably the easiest markers for understanding and identifying personality disorders are that the behaviors are inflexible (i.e., the individual seems to have little choice in his or her response style), compulsive (i.e., the individual will almost always respond in the same idiosyncratic way, even when he or she sees and understands that the behavioral choice may have negative consequences), and maladaptive (i.e., the behaviors may serve to get the individual into trouble), and that they cause significant functional impairment (i.e., the individual's adaptive function is limited or impaired) and subjective distress (i.e., the individual experiences marked and frequent discomfort).

Ideally, be mounted for maximizing the value of therapy by addressing behaviors before they have become more powerfully and frequently reinforced and habituated. For instance, I think that would be far better to address a clearly identified case of early borderline personality disorder in a 12-year-old child than when the same individual seeks therapy as a 25-year-old adult. The 13 years in which the problem is not treated, treated tangentially, or treated as some euphemistic precursor to borderline personality disorder will not serve the child. The behavioral, cognitive, and affective style will, in the 13-year period, become more firmly entrenched and habituated. It would make much better sense to treat the disorder as the disorder. Essentially, if it looks like a duck, walks like a duck, and quacks like a duck, it would make sense to call the animal a duck.

The behavioral characteristics that are used to define personality disorders in adults must also be distinguished from characteristics that are part of normal and predictable developmental patterns for children. Or behavioral patterns may emerge in response to specific situational or developmental factors. For example, the clinging and dependent behavior seen in a 3- or 4-year-old may be developmentally appropriate and should not then be used as diagnostic signs of a dependent personality. I am not suggesting that every behavioral pattern seen in childhood is fully, or even in part, a personality disorder. Nor am I positing that every pattern in childhood will persist into the adult years and eventually become a personality disorder.

MALADAPTIVE VISIBILITY

Behaviors may be seen by an objective observer to be strange or unusual when those behaviors are judged by the standards of the larger community or group. Of course, the characteristics that may meet criteria for a personality disorder may not be considered problematic by the identified child or the child's family, despite these behaviors' appearing to an objective observer to be self-defeating, self-injurious, or self- or other-punitive. The observed individual, or the members of that individual's family group or cultural subgroup, may be unperturbed by, sanguine about, or nonobservant of those same behaviors. For the family or cultural subgroup, the identified behaviors may be seen as acceptable and even laudable. Obviously, judgments about personality functioning must take into account the individual's cultural and psychosocial background. When clinicians are evaluating children from a background different from their own, it would be essential to obtain additional information from informants who are familiar with the children's sociocultural history, background, and experience.

Making the diagnostic process even more complex is the fact that under some circumstances, the behaviors that are diagnosed as a personality disorder in an adult individual may have been quite functional and strongly reinforced during that individual's childhood or adolescence. The patterns that are later used to establish a diagnosis of personality disorder may, during the childhood years, have had value and purpose that began to wear away as the child moved into the adult years. A personality style may move to disorder or be exacerbated following the loss of significant supporting persons (e.g., the death of a parent) or previously stabilizing social situations (e.g., changing schools, moving homes). It is not always the case that children with unusual behaviors go through school unnoticed. Olin et al. (1997) found that teacher ratings of adolescents subsequently diagnosed as having schizotypal personality disorder indicated observable analogues of the adult disorder in late childhood or early adolescence. Wolff, Townshend, McGuire, and Weeks (1991) found that of 32 children described as having schizoid personality in childhood, three-quarters later met DSM criteria for schizotypal personality disorder. In fact, some of these patterns may be apparent by the end of preschool, between ages 4 and 6 (National Advisory Mental Health Council, 1995).

For example, the child who is diagnosed by teachers as having a conduct disorder, and who resists authorities and terrorizes his peers, may be seen by his parents or others in their culture as a "real boy" or a "kid who doesn't take shit from anyone." The question is whether the aggression is isolated, occasional, and episodic, or whether it meets DSM-IV-TR criteria and is part of a pervasive pattern. If it is not pervasive, the DSM code V71.02 ("child or adolescent antisocial behavior") might be used.

ARGUMENTS AGAINST DIAGNOSING PERSONALITY DISORDERS IN CHILDHOOD

The argument can be made that children below the age of 18 years cannot, by definition, have a personality disorder. This argument posits that in childhood the personality is still forming, and that to label it as "disordered" gives the impression that the personality of the child is fully formed, fixed, and encased in stone. I would respond to this argument by pointing out that the age of 18 as the entry point to adulthood is not typical of all cultures. In certain cultures, the age at which children reach their majority may be as low as 13. It is at that point that the child may be married, begin bearing children, and have adult responsibilities

A second argument against diagnosing personality disorders in childhood is that personality is in a constant and rapid state of an individual's development throughout the developmental years. To take a "snapshot" of behavior at any point in those years and use that picture to draw conclusions gives an inaccurate view of the individual. These patterns may (and probably will) change. My response to this criticism is that *all* diagnoses are conditional, and can and should be revised as clinicians obtain additional data.

A third argument against using personality disorder diagnoses for children and adolescents has to do with the diagnosis or label "personality disorder."

Simply stated, the diagnosis of a personality disorder for a child may have the effect of therapists' and teachers' quickly giving up on the child without trying to help. An extension of this point is that the diagnosis will follow that child throughout his or her school years and may be used as an excuse for limiting or even withholding treatment. I would in fact agree with this argument, inasmuch as diagnoses in a child's record will be viewed, for good or ill, throughout the child's school career and possibly beyond. Indeed, I am very concerned that the acceptance of the present thesis of childhood personality disorders will result in malpractice among therapists, teachers, and institutions.

A fourth concern, and an extension of the point noted above, is that the personality disorder diagnosis will be applied inappropriately to socially or culturally different groups. It would then become an easy way for individual therapists or entire systems and institutions not to treat minority group children. Here again, I am very concerned that the diagnosis will be too quickly and inappropriately applied. If adults choose to "give up" on a child because the child has been diagnosed with a personality disorder, we will all have a very serious problem. In point of fact, however, the children who do qualify for such diagnoses are the ones who need to be identified, so that they can receive the best and most appropriate care. If doing this becomes a "copout" for therapists, then it is more a problem of the mental health system than it is of the need for, or the validity of, the diagnosis. The system is truly broken if it avoids treating those who clearly most need treatment.

ARGUMENTS FOR DIAGNOSING PERSONALITY DISORDERS IN CHILDHOOD AND ADOLESCENCE

It is generally agreed that personality pathology originates in childhood and adolescence. I believe that it makes sense to diagnose the problems at the earliest possible opportunity, not only for the sake of the affected individuals, but also for their families. Early detection and intervention may limit pervasiveness and chronicity. Identification and prevention become essential ingredients in the treatment (Harrington, 2001).

Since most adults with personality disorders can identify childhood and adolescent manifestations of their disorders, the therapy for children can include extensive parental involvement. This might serve to limit some of the damage that is consequent to impaired parenting. For example, youngsters abused in early childhood are four times more likely than nonabused children to be diagnosed with a personality disorder by early adulthood (Johnson, Cohen, Brown, Smailes, & Bernstein, 1999; Johnson et al., 2001; Johnson, Smailes, Cohen, Brown, & Bernstein, 2000). If the patterns of behavior and the abuse could be identified earlier, possibly intervention could be implemented. If necessary, child protective services could be brought into the case management along with intensive home-based services, as needed. The school could be involved as an agency that identifies children and could then participate in the treatment. There may be the need for agency intervention, and opportunities for postvention, over several years.

BIOLOGICAL, PHYSIOLOGICAL, AND NEUROCHEMICAL PERSPECTIVES

Various theorists have pointed to neurological disturbances that may be implicated in the onset of personality disorders. The occurrence of childhood abuse (verbal, physical, and/or sexual) experienced by many patients with personality disorders may precipitate neurological changes. Teicher, Ito, Glod, Schiffer, and Gelbard (1994) have suggested that childhood abuse agitates the limbic system in a way that produces impulsivity, aggression, affective instability, and dissociative states. Goleman (1995) posits that continual emotional distress can create deficits in a child's intellectual abilities and damage the ability to learn in such a way that as the child develops, subsequent rational decision-making abilities are impaired.

DEVELOPMENTAL PERSPECTIVES

One explanation for the emergence of personality disorders in childhood centers on the mother–child relationship as described by object relations theorists (Kernberg, Weiner, & Bardenstein, 2000). According to this view, the child's intrapsychic structure develops through differentiation of self from object, with interrelated maturation of ego defenses (Masterson, 2000). Mahler (as discussed in Kramer & Akhtar, 1994) described four stages of development: autistic, symbiotic, separation–individuation, and object constancy. Problems encountered by the child in the separation–individuation phase in particular are implicated in the etiology of borderline personality disorder, for example. Kohut (as discussed in Kramer & Akhtar, 1994) examined the distortions of "self-object" that he believed to arise from narcissistic injury to the child at a particularly vulnerable moment or developmental stage. This injury was thought to lead to the formation of personality disorders.

Beck et al. (1990, 2004) have pointed out that certain behaviors observed in children, such as clinging, shyness, or rebelliousness, tend to persist throughout various developmental periods into adulthood—at which point they are given personality disorder labels, such as dependent, avoidant, and antisocial. There is evidence that certain relatively stable temperaments and behavioral patterns are present at birth. These innate tendencies may be reinforced by significant others during infancy, or modeled as appropriate and sought-after behaviors during early childhood. For example, the infant or toddler who clings and cries is much more likely to be singled out for attention by caregivers, which in turn reinforces the care-eliciting behavior. The difficulty arises when these patterns persist long after the developmental period in which they may be adaptive.

Kernberg et al. (2000) comment that enduring patterns of personality are increasingly being described in preschoolers. These include patterns of aggressive behavior, inflexible coping strategies, and insecure attachment. Adult manifestations of these patterns may include depression, drug use, and criminal behavior. The progression of childhood conduct disorder to antisocial personality disorder suggests that personality disorders have their origins in earlier developmental stages (Kasen et al,, 1999). Impulsivity and empathy are both apparent in children as young as age 2, and deviations in both impulsivity and empathy are components of certain personality disorders. The presence of concrete operational thinking in middle childhood makes it possible to discern thought disorders and impaired reality testing in school-age children.

FAMILY SYSTEM PERSPECTIVES

Problems in the family environment are important contributing factors in the development of personality disorders in childhood. The disruption of a child's attachment to primary caregivers through death, divorce, severe parental pathology, or otherwise chaotic family environments may elicit maladaptive personality patterns in the child.

Family and systemic factors contribute to the development of personality disorders in children by providing learning experiences that lead to the formation of maladaptive schemas, which persist throughout the developmental phases. These factors include the following:

1. *Parents' failure to teach frustration tolerance.* Even well-intentioned parents may fail to provide optimal training for dealing with frustrating experiences early in a child's life. This training would include the setting and maintaining of clear and consistent boundaries.

2. *Inappropriate child rearing and ignorance regarding child management skills.* Overly punitive or overly permissive parenting may initiate disturbances in the child's sense of boundaries and self-regulation.

3. *Skewed parental value systems.* For example, a highly achieving, perfectionistic child may be pushed by parents to excel, and reinforced by the parents' own need to succeed. Parents' beliefs are reflected in their choice of socialization strategies for their children, which in turn determine whether a child exhibits socially appropriate or socially deviant behavior (Rubin, Hymel, Mills, & Rose-Krasner, 1989). Cultural factors will also come into play (Harkness & Super, 2000).

4. *Parental psychopathology.* The relationship between parental psychopathology and childhood oppositional defiant disorder is quite strong. Hanish and Tolan (2001) and Hanish, Tolan, and Guerra (1996) have suggested that a parent with antisocial personality disorder, through the use of modeling and reinforcement, may transmit the idea to the child that it is acceptable to defy authority. As the child internalizes this belief, he or she begins to oppose the parent, and eventually other authority figures.

5. *Severe and persistent psychosocial stressors in the child's life.* Such stressors may include financial problems, displacement of the home, discord between the parents/parental figures, or stressors with the community. Hanish et al. (1996) found that marital/couple discord is a predictor of

childhood behavior problems—specifically noncompliant, disruptive behavior.

6. *Parental neglect and rejection*. Parental neglect and rejection may lead to the development of schemas suggesting to the child that he or she is disconnected from primary attachment figures, and thus may lead to a more pervasive sense of isolation.

7. *Difficult child temperament*. Children who are difficult infants may elicit responses from caregivers that contribute to the formation of maladaptive schemas. A crying, whining child may experience harsh punishment and more rejection, as well as excess attention from frequent attempts on the part of the parents to soothe the child themselves rather than fostering the infant's ability to self-soothe.

8. *Frequent and severe boundary violations*. These violations can occur on the part of both the child and the parent. For example, if the child is forced into a dependent role at the expense of normal development of autonomy because of a parent's own need for dependence, then the child will have difficulty with individuation. A child who is inclined to introversion may delay or inhibit natural steps toward autonomy, and an overly punitive parenting style may thwart the child's first steps toward a clearly defined self. Instances of physical and sexual abuse are clear and severe boundary violations that have been linked with the development of several personality disorders.

ASSESSMENT AND DIAGNOSTIC PERSPECTIVES

The clinician who suspects that the behavior of a child or adolescent may warrant an Axis II personality disorder diagnosis must thoroughly assess the child's behaviors, affect, and cognition across a variety of situations, as well as obtaining a thorough family and developmental history. The assessment should include contact or reports from the child's pediatrician and teachers in earlier grades. This is required to assess the chronicity and pervasiveness of the problem. Data can be collected through structured clinical interviews with the child and the child's parent(s); reports from teachers and other school personnel (administrators or counselors); psychological testing; behavioral observations at home and at school; repeated self-report measures when possible; symptom behavioral checklists; and school behavior report forms, family history, and the clinician's interview impressions.

Essential to making the diagnosis is a thorough grounding in developmental norms and an understanding of what is normative for that child, in that setting, at that time. For example, when one sees an adolescent who is contrary, argumentative, impulsive, antiauthority, and risk-taking, one can easily label this youth as normal. The assessment questions include the following:

Does a reported and/or observed behavior have a normal developmental explanation?

Does the behavior change over time or setting? Is it cyclical, variable, and unpredictable, or is the behavior constant, consistent, and predictable?

Could the observed/reported behavior be the result of discrepancies between the child's chronological age and the child's cognitive, emotional, social, and/or behavioral ages?

Does the child function similarly in different environments (e.g., does the behavior relate to the child's placement at home or in school)?

Is the observed/reported behavior culturally related?

Who has made the referral, and why was it made at this point?

Is there agreement between parents, or between parent(s) and teacher(s), on the cause, need, or purpose of the referral?

What are the expectations that are being made of the clinician in responding to the referral?

How does the child's behavior compare or contrast with the behavior of other children in that family, that socioeconomic or sociocultural setting, or that age group?

What is the history of the child's behavior in terms of length of existence; duration when stimulated; and the child's ability to control, contain, or withdraw from the behavior?

Does the child have insight into the behavioral cues that trigger the behavior, or into the consequences of the behavior?

Does the child see the behavior as something he or she would be interested in modifying?

What are the differing views of the child's behavior? Are the clinician's sources of data reliable?

The parent report is important in terms of the child's behavior at home. How does the child relate to siblings, neighborhood friends, clubs, sports, organizations, church activities, adult relatives, pets, and self-care (activities of daily living)?

Has there been recurrent physical, emotional, sexual, or verbal abuse? The parental view of what constitutes discipline versus child abuse is a key element to be considered.

Within societal norms, is the parental behavior inappropriately sexual or seductive? Is incest suspected?

What is the parental view of privacy for the child?

Are the parents inappropriately, unreasonably, or unjustifiably interfering with the child's relationships with other children?

Within societal norms, are the parents inappropriately involved with the child's personal hygiene beyond the child's necessity?

Kernberg et al. (2000) suggest a number of specific factors to be considered in the assessment. These include an evaluation of the child's temperament. This is probably based on biogenetic factors constituting a "disposition" that will influence the child's interactions with his or her world. This temperamental filter will influence the nature, style, frequency, "volume," and content of the child's approach to the world. Other factors to be considered include the following:

The child's internal, persistent, and developing internal mental construction of selfhood (identity) will need to be assessed.

Gender plays a role, inasmuch as gender carries with it both self- and other-expectations that are based in the culture. While certainly a component of identity, gender also carries with it significant societal norms and demands.

It is critical to be able to identify any neuropsychological deficits related to cognitive functioning. It is especially important to identify any problems in the manner in which the child organizes, processes, and recalls information.

The child's level, content, range, and repertoire of affect need to be assessed.

What is the child's characteristic mode of coping with internal and external stressors in his or her life? How does the child respond initially, and how do the attempts at coping increase or decrease as the stressors persist?

The clinician must assess the child's environment, which includes the child's family system, school experience, religious environment, and the stability of all of these. It will be important to assess the reactivity and reciprocal behavior of others within the systems.

The child's motivation and attempts to meet intrinsic and extrinsic needs are important. This will reflect the "why" of the child's actions. What is the goal of the child's drives and actions?

The child's social facility and repertoire of social interaction skills will assist the child in relating to, and coping with, significant others within his or her environment.

It is in light of the child's level of cognitive development and integration that his or her actions can be best understood. A child at preoperational levels cannot be expected to process information in the same manner as a child at the level of concrete or formal operations.

What are the most active and compelling schemas that the child uses to understand and organize his or her world?

Frequently, the euphemisms used to describe the child are suggestive of a particular personality disorder and can be added to the diagnostic mix. To give a few examples, a child described as "isolated and withdrawn" may have schizoid personality disorder; a child termed "chronically suspicious" may have paranoid personality disorder; a child called "excessively self-focused" may have narcissistic personality disorder; a child termed "very needy" may have dependent personality disorder; or a child described as "always conscientious and careful" may have obsessive–compulsive personality disorder.

Finally, there are a number of factors that can (and often do) complicate the differential diagnosis of personality disorder in adolescents:

First and foremost is the typical adolescent "neurosis." Adolescents are exploring new roles, shedding old roles, and confronting new challenges, all while trying to maintain a semblance of safety and stability. This describes much of adolescent behavior. Their actions are often responded to by parents' or other authorities' stating, "You should know better."

There are significant hormonal surges that will serve to influence the adolescent's behavior, cognitive processing, and affect. The significant mood shifts typical of adolescents are rooted in their physiology. These mood shifts may be similar to those seen in individuals with bipolar illness, or other disorders involving rapid alternation and shifting of mood.

Adolescence presents everyone with a Kafkaesque experience of metamorphosis. There are rapid (and often significant) changes in size, weight, and height, as well as in the development of secondary sex characteristics and therefore in body shape. These changes are usually expected and often taken in stride, with far greater equanimity than would be the case if an adult experienced these same physical changes in the same brief period of time. However, this is not always the case.

There are rapid alterations of identity, in which an adolescent moves from child to adult. The late Hank Ketcham, the cartoonist responsible for *Dennis the Menace*, once had Dennis state, "How come when I have to go to the doctor I am supposed to be a big boy, but when it's time for bed, I am still a little boy?" The adolescent tries out many identities in terms of dress, attitude, social circle, or relationship with family members. This shifting of identity could be mistaken as meeting criteria for a personality disorder.

Adolescents end up in conflicts with parents, school authority, or the justice system. Adolescence is filled with rebellion alternating with dependence. The push–pull of the relationship with parents is capsuled by an adolescent's wanting greater freedom while asking for financial or social support. This dichotomizing is also indicative of certain personality disorders.

The adolescent may rebel by joining an apparently neurotic or antisocial group. Parents may be concerned that the adolescent is hanging out with the "wrong group." In fact, the adolescent may make a very normal and appropriate adjustment to the group by how he or she acts, dresses, talks, responds to authorities, and responds to parents. The problem will be that the child or adolescent is not so much troubled as troubling to others.

The emergence of sexual behavior serves as another confounding variable. The onset of this new behavior has implications for adolescents' interpersonal action, responsibility for their safety, and adherence to parental demands and expectations. The dividing line between societally approved and disapproved sexuality as demonstrated by dress and action seems increasingly to be blurred. The adolescent icons seen on MTV or in advertisements for clothing, music, foods, or recreation are overtly sexual.

Finally, there is a normal body dysmorphia during adolescence that relates how one's body appears to oneself or may be viewed by others. A skin eruption at the time of a date or important school function may be viewed as more than a pimple. It may be perceived as a cause for cloistering oneself and not appearing in public.

COGNITIVE-BEHAVIORAL
TREATMENT CONCEPTUALIZATION

The clinician must work to identify the schemas that are driving the child's cognitions, affect, and behavior (Freeman, 1983; Freeman & Leaf, 1989; Freeman, Pretzer, Fleming, & Simon, 2004; Beck et al., 1990, 2004). Since these schemas evolve through assimilation and accommodation, the clinician must assess the schemas that are being used to address life problems.. The range of schemas can encompass personal, family, gender, cultural, age group, and religious schemas, with varying degrees of power and credibility for the child. For example, religious schemas may have more credibility and power for the child in a devoutly religious family than for the child whose family has no religious affiliation. The more powerful the reinforcers are for schemas, and the more frequently they are reinforced, the more likely strong bonds will exist for those schemas. It is important to determine how early in life schemas are acquired, for the earliest-acquired schemas are the most powerful. The clinician needs to be aware that schemas can be acquired through multifaceted, multisensory learning—through cognitive, behavioral, motor/kinesthetic, visual, olfactory, and gustatory modes, for example. This means that even infants have the capacity to acquire schemas; hence the ensuing difficulty in attempting to modify early-entrenched but maladaptive schemas.

Behaviors and beliefs can also be the result of modeling. The child observes significant others and learns that certain patterns of behavior are reinforced. The nature of a behavior may be adaptive or maladaptive, depending on the level of pathology present in parents. The child also gains reinforcement for a particular pattern of behaviors. Family environment and genetic predisposition may interact in a unique ways, resulting in the development of a child who manifests a pattern of behaviors.

TREATMENT COSTS

Is there a possibility or even a probability that the identified behavior pattern will spontaneously remit if treatment recommendations are refused, and treatment is not initiated? If there is a minimal environmental shift, will the behaviors then remit? Basically, the clinician must assess the "treatment costs" (financial and otherwise) to the child and family. For example, if the child and family are referred to therapy, is it possible that things may get worse for the child, the family, or both? Who in the family can be called upon and trusted to participate in the therapy? What supports can be offered or provided for the child and for the family? Who will fund the supports? For what period of time? In what context?

SELECTING THE OPTIMAL FOCUS FOR TREATMENT

The decision to engage the child in some form of psychological treatment is one that is ideally made in conjunction with, and with input from, a number of sources. At this point, it may be tempting to consider the child as the sole focus for treatment. However, such a singular emphasis on the child negates the reality that other forces have an impact on the child and are influencing the noted referral problem. If the referral problem is a result of a parent's lack of knowledge regarding normal development and norms of behavior in children and adolescents, then one aspect of treatment must include parenting information and education. The child's behavior may relate to parental behavior and expectations or to the parent's skills at parenting.

Given that a child spends half of his or her waking hours in school, it will be essential to engage not only the parents or other caretakers in the treatment plan, but also the school. The child likewise must be included in the treatment planning. The "problem" will need to be explained to the child, along with the reasons for intervention and the goals of treatment. Trying to treat a child who may have no idea why treatment is indicated may be a lost cause. The child may have little or no motivation to change, and may be frightened of and violently opposed to any changes in his or her behavior or world.

Depending on the child's age and level of cognitive development, treatment may have to be modified. For example, the child's developmental stage may not be adequate for verbal/abstract therapy, or an older child may have limited verbal skills and ability to generalize (an important factor in therapy). Most children will have great difficulty in being able to sit still, listen, concentrate, focus, and integrate the diverse pieces that arise in typical psychotherapy. Even spending an extended amount of time alone with an adult may be viewed as somewhere between strange and frightening by the child. Session length may have to be limited, based on the child's ability to attend for a prescribed length of time.

THE THERAPY PROCESS

Once therapy has been agreed to, the actual therapy session is a small part of what must be viewed as an integrated whole. On a regular basis, the clinician needs to review the occurrence of target behaviors since the last session (based on parent and/or teacher report). Goals of therapy include expanding the child's "emotional vocabulary" to describe positive and negative feelings, helping the child to identify and dispute dysfunctional ideas, teaching self-instructional techniques, teaching problem-solving skills (including consequential thinking and finding alternatives), and role-playing specific skills. When possible, significant others can act as therapy assistants by reinforcing learned skills in the child's home and/or school environment. Continued monitoring by parents and school personnel is encouraged for the purposes of collecting data, as well as fostering a sense of involvement and efficacy in those closest to the child.

It is assumed that the clinician has made a decision concerning the use of therapy to treat the child, one or both parents, the family, or the family system. The judicious use of time is essential. The clinician will want to set the agenda to allow the child and his or her parents to be alert to the goals of the session. When possible, both the child and the parents can suggest agenda items for discussion. Parents and teachers may be involved in assisting the child with homework assignments given in session, or providing additional reinforcement of skills learned in session. The amount of time that is allocated to child work, parent work, or family work will depend on the clinician's assessment of where the focus must be at any particular point in the treatment..

The clinician will ascertain the child's capacity to "uncover" or "process" experience, based on the child's cognitive level and response to therapy. For example, a child who is at the concrete operational level of thinking may respond best to therapeutic interventions that provide a limited range of choices for behavior. The focus of therapy should be on the change process itself. The therapist must develop the working alliance with the child by assessing the child's ability and willingness to connect both cognitively and emotionally. The therapist will be aided by an understanding of the basics of neuropsychology, the effects of anxiety on performance, and the impact on adaptive functioning of learning problems, as well as of developmental psychology.

DISCUSSION AND CONCLUSIONS

"Cognitive therapy with children, as is work with adults, is founded upon the assumption that behavior is adaptive, and that there is an interaction between the individual's thoughts, feelings, and behaviors" (Reinecke, Dattilio, & Freeman, 2003, p. 2). Cognitive-behavioral treatments are of benefit to children because they can be modified and tailored to meet their specific needs. Therapeutic interventions focus on such concrete concepts as misinterpretation of information, reality testing, adaptive responses along a continuum, and basic problem-solving skills, rather than emphasizing insight. Everyday problems at school or home are addressed with the goal of developing a wider and better repertoire of coping skills. Within this basic framework, various cognitive-behavioral interventions can be utilized: time management skills training, assertiveness training, problem-solving training, relaxation training, social skills training, self-management training, behavior analysis skill training, activity scheduling, self-monitoring, and developing adaptive self-talk.

Cognitive-behavioral therapy with children emphasizes the effects of maladaptive or dysfunctional beliefs and attitudes on current behavior. The presumption is made that a child's reaction to an event is influenced by the meanings he or she attaches to the event (Reinecke et al., 2003). When a child's behavioral and emotional responses to an event are maladaptive, it may be because the child lacks more appropriate behavioral skills, or because his or her beliefs or problem-solving capacities are in some way disturbed (the cognitive elements). With this framework in mind, cognitive-behavioral therapists attempt to enable children to acquire new behavioral skills and provide children with experiences that foster cognitive change.

There is a great need for protocols and research on each of the personality disorders in children and adolescents. We must develop new and more effective diagnostic tools, and sharpen our experience with existing tools. We also have to evaluate "best practices" for treatment. What works best, with whom, in what time frame, and under what circumstances? We will need to evaluate what are the idealistic goals for treatment, and what are the more realistic goals. Finally, we will have to be ready to pay the price in staff time, clinician effort, and economic cost to treat these children.

Choosing to ignore the reality of personality disorders among children and adolescents, to downplay the problem, or to search for euphemistic terms is to disregard the severity and impact of these disorders. The sooner that we can accept their reality, the sooner we will focus our efforts on treatment, and the sooner we can relieve the suffering of these children.

REFERENCES

American Psychiatric Association (APA). (2000). *Diagnostic and statistical manual of mental disorders* (4th ed., text rev.). Washington, DC: Author.

Beck, A. T., Freeman, A., & Associates (1990). *Cognitive therapy of personality disorders.* New York: Guilford Press.

Beck, A. T., Freeman, A., Davis, D. D., & Associates. (2004). *Cognitive therapy of personality disorders* (2nd ed.). New York: Guilford Press.

Beren, P. (1998). *Narcissistic disorders in children and adolescents.* Northvale, NJ: Aronson.

Bleiberg, E. (2001). *Treating personality disorders in children and adolescents: A relational approach.* New York: Guilford Press.

Freeman, A. (1983). Cognitive therapy: An overview. In A. Freeman (Ed.), *Cognitive therapy with couples and groups* (pp. 1–10). New York: Plenum Press.

Freeman, A., & Leaf, R. (1989). Cognitive therapy of personality disorders. In A. Freeman, K. M. Simon, L. Beutler, & H. Arkowitz (Eds.), *Comprehensive handbook of cognitive therapy* (pp. 403–434). New York: Plenum Press.

Freeman, A., Pretzer, J., Fleming, B., & Simon, K. M. (2004). *Clinical applications of cognitive therapy* (2nd ed.). New York: Kluwer Academic.

Freeman, A., Rigby, A. (2003). Personality disorders among children and adolescents: Is it an unlikely diagnosis? In M. A. Reinecke, F. M. Dattilio, & A. Freeman (Eds.), *Cognitive therapy with children and adolescents* (2nd ed.). New York: Guilford Press.

Goleman, D. (1995). *Emotional intelligence.* New York: Bantam Books.

Hanish, L. D., Tolan, P. H., & Guerra, N. G. (1996). Treatment of oppositional defiant disorder. In M. A. Reinecke, F. M. Dattilio, & A. Freeman (Eds.), *Cognitive therapy with children and adolescents* (pp. 62–78). New York: Guilford Press.

Hanish, L. D., & Tolan, P. H. (2001). Antisocial behaviors in children and adolescents: Expanding the cognitive model. In W. J. Lyddon & J. V. Jones, Jr. (Eds.), *Empirically supported cognitive therapies: Current and future applications* (pp. 182–199). New York: Springer.

Harkness, S., & Super, C. M. (2000). Culture and psychopathology. In A. J. Sameroff, M. Lewis, & S. M. Miller (Eds.), *Handbook of developmental psychopathology* (pp. 197–214). New York: Kluwer Academic/Plenum.

Harrington, R. C. (2001). Childhood depression and conduct disorder: Different routes to the same outcome? *Archives of General Psychiatry, 58*(3), 237–238.

Johnson, J. G., Cohen, P., Brown, J., Smailes, E. M., & Bernstein, D. P. (1999). Childhood maltreatment increases risk for personality disorders during early adulthood. *Archives of General Psychiatry, 56*(7), 600–606.

Johnson, J. G., Cohen, P., Smailes, E. M., Skodol, A. E., Brown, J., & Oldham, J. M. (2001). Childhood verbal abuse and risk for personality disorders during adolescence and early adulthood. *Comprehensive Psychiatry, 42*(1), 16–23.

Johnson, J. G., Smailes, E. M., Cohen, P., Brown, J., & Bernstein, D. P. (2000). Associations between four types of childhood neglect and personality disorder symptoms during adolescence and early adulthood. Findings of a community-based study. *Journal of Personality Disorders, 14*(2), 171–187.

Kasen, S., Cohen, P., Skodol, A. E., Johnson, J. G., Smailes, E. M., & Brook, J. S. (2001). Childhood depression and adult personality disorder: Alternate pathways of continuity. *Archives of General Psychiatry, 58*(3), 231–236.

Kernberg, P. F., Weiner, A. S., & Bardenstein, K. K. (2000). *Personality disorders in children and adolescents.* New York: Basic Books.

Kramer, S., & Akhtar, S. (Eds.). (1994). *Mahler and Kohut: Perspectives on development, psychopathology, and technique.* Northvale, NJ: Aronson.

Masterson, J. (2000). *The personality disorders: A new look at the developmental self and object relations approach.* Phoenix, AZ: Zeig, Tucker.

National Advisory Mental Health Council. (1995). Basic behavioral science research for mental health, a national investment: Emotion and motivation. *American Psychologist, 50*(10), 838–845.

Olin, S. S., Raine, A., Cannon, T. D., Parnas, J., Schulsinger, F., & Mednick, S. A. (1997). Childhood precursors of schizotypal personality disorder. *Schizophrenia Bulletin, 23*(1), 93–103.

Paris, J. (2003). *Personality disorders over time: Precursors, course, and outcome.* Washington, DC: American Psychiatric Press.

Reinecke, M. A., Dattilio, F. M., & Freeman, A. (Eds.). (2003). *Cognitive therapy with children and adolescents* (2nd ed.). New York: Guilford Press.

Rubin, K. H., Hymel, S., Mills, R. S., & Rose-Krasner, L. (1989). Sociability and social withdrawal in childhood: Stability and outcomes. *Journal of Personality, 57,* 238–255.

Shapiro, T. (1997). The borderline syndrome in children. In K. S. Robson (Ed.). *The borderline child.* Northvale, NJ: Aronson.

Teicher, M. H., Ito, Y., Glod, C. A., Schiffer, F., & Gelbard, H. (1994). Early abuse, limbic system dysfunction, and borderline personality disorder. In K. R. Silk (Ed.), *Progress in psychiatry: No. 45. Biological and neurobehavioral studies of borderline personality disorder* (pp. 177–207). Washington, DC: American Psychiatric Association.

Vela, R., Gottlieb, H., & Gottlieb, E. (1997). Borderline syndromes in children: A critical review. In K. S. Robson (Ed.), *The borderline child.* Northvale, NJ: Aronson.

Wolff, S., Townshend, R., McGuire, R. J., & Weeks, D. J. (1991). Schizoid personality in childhood and adult life: II. Adult adjustment and the continuity with schizotypal personality disorder. *British Journal of Psychiatry, 159,* 620–629.

Part V

SPECIFIC APPLICATIONS

Chapter 16

Integrating
Cognitive-Behavioral Therapy
and Pharmacotherapy

JESSE H. WRIGHT

Pharmacotherapy and cognitive-behavioral therapy (CBT) are the two most heavily researched forms of treatment for Axis I disorders. Both treatments have been well established as effective therapies for depression, anxiety disorders, eating disorders, and other nonpsychotic illnesses (Marangell, Silver, Goff, & Yudsofsky, 2002, Dobson, 1989; Robinson, Berman, & Neimeyer, 1990; Wright, Beck, & Thase, 2002). Although psychopharmacology is generally accepted as the standard treatment for psychoses, CBT has recently been shown to have significant effects in reducing symptoms of schizophrenia (Drury, Birchwood, Cochrane, & Macmillan, 1996; Kuipers et al., 1997; Tarrier et al., 1998; Pinto, La Pia, Mannella, Domenico, & De Simone, 1999; Sensky et al., 2000; Rector & Beck, 2001).

Because both CBT and psychopharmacology are effective interventions for a wide range of disorders, there may be possible advantages to combining these empirically proven approaches in an integrated treatment package. Potential ways in which CBT may interact with pharmacotherapy are detailed here. Then studies of combined treatment for four groups of disorders—depression, anxiety disorders, bulimia nervosa, and psychoses— are reviewed for evidence of interaction effects. The chapter concludes with a discussion of methods for facilitating the combination of CBT and medication in clinical practice.

POTENTIAL INTERACTIONS BETWEEN CBT AND PHARMACOTHERAPY

The possibility that medication and psychotherapy could have significant influences on one another has intrigued investigators and clinicians from the time effective medications were introduced (Group for the Advancement of Psychiatry, 1975). When tricyclic antidepressants and other medications first became available in the 1950s, psychodynamically oriented clinicians feared that psychopharmacological treatment would prematurely reduce symptoms and thus undermine patients' motivation for therapy. Many concerns were registered about the potential pitfalls of using medication when patients were involved in psychotherapy (Group for the Advancement of Psychiatry, 1975). But others hoped that the advent of a new age of psychopharmacology would have a positive influence on psychotherapeutic practice, and that psychotherapy might have a role in facilitating medication response (Uhlenhuth, Lipman, & Covil, 1969; Group for the Advancement of Psychiatry, 1975).

Uhlenhuth et al. (1969) proposed several different scenarios for interactions between psychotherapy and pharmacotherapy, including (1) *addition*—treatments given together produce results that are greater than the action of either component alone; (2) *potentiation* (or "synergism")—a positive interaction which is larger than the sum of the effects of individual treatments; and (3) *inhibition* (or "subtraction")—results of treatment are impaired by combining therapies. Most of the research on treatment interaction in the subsequent three decades was designed to measure the effects of combining medication and psychotherapy on symptom measures at the end of treatment, and thus to determine whether the two treatments together were superior, equal, or inferior to the therapies given alone.

The cognitive–biological model (Wright & Thase, 1992; Wright, Thase, & Sensky, 1993) provides a useful vantage point from which to view possible interactions between therapies. This model specifies that there may be influences from multiple systems (e.g., biological, cognitive, behavioral, interpersonal, and social) on the development and expression of mental disorders. Numerous studies (reviewed later in this chapter) have confirmed significant relationships between elements of this model. Application of the cognitive–biological model to the study of combined therapy suggests that outcome could be improved by directing treatment at more than one system simultaneously, or by promoting interactions with possible favorable influences (Wright & Schrodt, 1989; Gabbard & Kay, 2001).

Table 16.1 contains a list of possible interactions between CBT and pharmacotherapy in the process of treatment (Group for the Advancement of Psychiatry, 1975; Wright & Schrodt, 1989). Most research studies have focused on comparing the outcome of treatment with medication versus psychotherapy or combined therapy, instead of evaluating possible mechanisms of interaction (see "Outcome Research," below, for a review of these studies). Thus only a few of the proposed interactions in Table 16.1 have been investigated in a systematic manner.

The effects of different types of medication on learning and memory functioning have been evaluated in a large number of pharmacological studies. For example, tricyclic antidepressants with strong anticholinergic properties (Curran, Sakulsriprong, & Lader, 1988; Knegtering, Eijck, & Huijsman, 1994; Richardson et al., 1994) and benzodiazepines (Hommer, 1991; Wagemans, Notebaert, & Boucart, 1998; Verster, Volkerts, & Verbaten, 2002) have typically been found to impair learning ability. In contrast, selective serotonin reuptake inhibitors (SSRIs; Hasbroucq, Rihet, Blin, & Possamai, 1997; Levkovitz, Caftori, Avital, & Richter-Levin, 2002; Harmer, Bhagwagar, Cowen, & Goodwin, 2002) and newer antipsychotic

TABLE 16.1. Combined CBT and Pharmacotherapy: Possible Mechanisms of Interaction

Positive interactions

- Medications improve concentration and thus facilitate CBT.
- Medications reduce painful affect and/or physiological arousal, thereby increasing accessibility to CBT.
- Medications can decrease distorted or irrational thinking, thus adding to the effect of CBT.
- CBT improves medication compliance.
- CBT helps patients better understand and manage illness.
- CBT can facilitate withdrawal from medication when desired.
- CBT has biological effects, and thus can work in concert with medication to influence biochemical abnormalities.

Negative interactions

- Medications interfere with learning and memory, and this interference negatively influences CBT.
- Medications cause dependency, which impairs the effectiveness of CBT.
- Medications lead to premature relief of symptoms, and thus undermine motivation to continue in therapy.
- CBT places stress on patients with biological illnesses, and thus adds a burden to those who should be treated with medication.

medications (Harvey et al., 2000; Stevens et al., 2002; Weiss, Bilder, & Fleischhacker, 2002) usually improve cognitive functioning. These studies have shown that cognitive effects of medications can vary widely, depending on the type of medication, dosage, psychological measures utilized, and other factors. Learning and memory functioning have rarely been examined as possible mechanisms of interaction between CBT and pharmacotherapy. One group of investigators determined that the benzodiazepine alprazolam interfered with performance on a word recall task, but not with implicit memory or digit span performance, in patients being treated with exposure therapy (Curran, 1994). However, the possible actions of other medications on cognitive functioning in patients receiving CBT remain largely unexplored.

Several investigations have documented positive effects for CBT in improving medication compliance (Cochran, 1984; Perris & Skagerlind, 1994; Lecompte, 1995; Basco & Rush, 1995; Kemp, Hayward, Applewhaite, Everitt, & David, 1996). Cochran (1984) found that patients taking lithium who received a CBT compliance intervention were more likely to adhere to the medication regimen than those who received standard care. Persons who received CBT also had significantly lower rates of stopping lithium against medical advice, rehospitalization, or noncompliance-precipitated episodes of illness. Perris and Skagerlind (1994) found that CBT enhanced medication adherence in patients with schizophrenia treated in group homes. Lecompte (1995) also described CBT methods for improving medication adherence in patients with schizophrenia, and observed that this intervention led to a decline in the frequency of rehospitalization.

A specific CBT compliance intervention for schizophrenia was developed and tested by Kemp et al. (1996). In a randomized controlled trial, these investigators demonstrated that a brief CBT intervention (four to six sessions lasting 10–60 minutes each) significantly improved attitudes toward drug therapy and compliance with the medication regimen. A follow-up study by Kemp, Kirov, Everitt, Hayward, and David (1998) of 74 inpatients treated with their compliance intervention found enduring positive effects, including significant advantages in treatment adherence, global social functioning, and prevention of rehospitalization.

CBT may also interact favorably with pharmacotherapy by assisting in managing problems associated with drug administration, such as dependency or side effects. Dependency can be observed with benzodiazepines, but is not a significant problem with antidepressants, mood stabilizers, or antipsychotic drugs. Two groups of investigators have described CBT interventions that improved success with benzodiazepine withdrawal. Spiegel, Bruce, Gregg, and Nuzzarello (1994) used a CBT protocol compared to treatment as usual (a slow taper off medication) for persons who had been made "panic-free" with alprazolam. At the end of treatment, both groups had very high rates of alprazolam discontinuation. Although there were no differences between therapies at the end of treatment, patients who received CBT were much less likely to resume use of alprazolam. Otto et al. (1993) also found evidence for a positive effect of CBT on benzodiazepine discontinuation. These investigators observed that group CBT was superior to a slow-taper condition alone in assisting patients with withdrawal from alprazolam or clonazepam. At the end of treatment, 76% of those receiving CBT were able to discontinue medication, compared to 25% of controls. In addition, CBT was effective in reducing the rate of relapse.

The potential role of CBT in helping patients manage or cope with side effects has received little attention. However, recent studies have shown that CBT can be very effective in treating insomnia (Edinger et al., 2002; Backhaus, Hohagen, Voderholzer, & Riemann, 2001; Rybarczyk et al., 2002). The results of these investigations suggest that CBT may be an effective treatment for SSRI-induced insomnia. Other side effects that may be responsive to a CBT approach include weight gain, anxiety, agitation, and the distress associated with extrapyramidal reactions to antipsychotic medication. The work of Vasterling, Jenkins, Tope, and Burish (1993) in using CBT to reduce side effects from cancer chemotherapy also suggests that cognitive and behavioral methods could help patients cope better with reactions to psychotropic drugs.

The possibility that psychotherapy has biological effects that could act independently of medication or enhance the actions of pharmacotherapy has attracted considerable interest (Wright & Thase, 1992; Gabbard & Kay, 2001). However, only a few studies have been completed on the biological activity of CBT. Baxter et al. (1992) and Schwartz et al. (1996) have reported that behavioral interventions for obsessive–compulsive disorder have the same effects on brain positron emission tomography (PET) scans as fluoxetine. In one study, successful treatment with either behavior therapy or fluoxetine was associated with a reversal of PET scan abnormalities in the caudate nucleus (Baxter et al., 1992). A later investigation by this group (Brody et al., 1998) revealed that the degree of normalization of orbitofrontal cortex metabolism on PET scans was a predictor of treatment response to behavior therapy and fluoxetine.

CBT effects on brain function have also been studied in the treatment of social phobia. Furmark et al. (2002) found that responders to CBT and citalopram shared common changes in PET scan activity: decreased regional cerebral blood flow in the amygdala, hippocampus, and surrounding brain areas that are involved with defense reactions to threat.

A neuroendocrine investigation was reported by Joffe, Segal, and Singer (1996) who investigated the influence of CBT on thyroid hormone levels. In this study, serum thyroxine levels decreased in the responders to

CBT, while thyroxine levels increased in nonresponders. Although research on central nervous system (CNS) and neuroendocrine actions of CBT is still at an early stage, there appear to be several lines of evidence that CBT has significant biological effects that might be used to advantage in combinations with pharmacotherapy.

The possible mechanisms for negative interactions between CBT and medication listed in Table 16.1 have received little attention in controlled research. Concerns about negative influences of medication on CBT (e.g., interference with learning and memory, dependency) have been primarily directed at treatment with benzodiazepines (Curran, 1994). A number of outcome studies have utilized symptom measures to search for possible subtractive results for combined therapy, but there is limited information available on processes by which negative actions may occur.

Clinicians who strongly favor CBT over pharmacotherapy may assume that medication has a blanket effect of undermining motivation for therapy or producing other negative outcomes. Conversely, staunch biological psychiatrists may believe that CBT places an unnecessary burden on persons who should be treated with pharmacotherapy alone. However, the outcome studies reviewed below have revealed little evidence to suggest that most types of medication impair participation in CBT, or that CBT has any adverse effects on biological treatments. Instead, the weight of evidence supports the concept that CBT and pharmacotherapy often complement one another in enhancing the response to therapy.

OUTCOME RESEARCH

Depression

Blackburn and coworkers (1981) performed the first controlled trial that compared CBT alone to pharmacotherapy (tricyclic antidepressants) and combined treatment for depression. Results differed, depending on the treatment setting. Combined treatment was superior to medication in both hospital and general practice patients and to CBT alone in the hospital outpatients. The overall results of this study support an additive effect for CBT and antidepressant therapy.

Another trial comparing CBT with a tricyclic antidepressant (Murphy, Simons, Wetzel, & Lustman, 1984) did not find a significant advantage for combined treatment. At the end of treatment, all therapies were found to be equally effective. However, the percentage of patients with the best outcome (Beck Depression Inventory [BDI] scores ≤ 9) was higher for combined therapy (78%) than for the other treatments (CBT plus placebo = 65%, CBT = 53%, pharmacotherapy = 56%). A later study by Hollon et al. (1992) tested the efficacy of CBT, imipramine, or combined therapy in the treatment of 107 nonpsychotic depressed outpatients. The rate of attrition in this study was high (40%), but there were no differences in dropout rates in the three treatment groups. This finding rules against the hypothesis that medication decreases motivation for treatment and thus leads to premature termination of therapy (Table 16.1). The overall treatment response in the Hollon et al. (1992) study was excellent for all conditions. Although there was no significant advantage found for combined treatment, there was a trend for superior outcome in those who received both CBT and pharmacotherapy. For example, mean posttreatment Hamilton Rating Scale for Depression (HRSD) scores were lowest for combined treatment (4.2) as compared to CBT (8.8) and pharmacotherapy (8.4; significance = .17). Mean Minnesota Multiphasic Personality Inventory Depression scores were significantly lower in patients treated with combined therapy (61.4) than with CBT (71.8) or pharmacotherapy (72.5; significance = .04).

A more recent study of combined therapy in depression focused on treatment of "double depression" (major depression plus dysthymia). Miller, Norman, and Keitner (1999) randomly assigned 26 inpatients with double depression to 20 weeks of treatment with pharmacotherapy or combined antidepressant and cognitive-behavioral therapy. At the end of treatment, those who received combined therapy had significantly greater improvement in depressive symptoms and higher social functioning. Differences between pharmacotherapy and combined treatment were quite large in this study. Mean posttreatment HRSD scores were 25.8 for pharmacotherapy and 13.1 for combined treatment.

The latest investigation of combined therapy in depression was reported by a large multicenter group headed by Keller and McCullough (Keller et al., 2000). This influential study had a particularly large sample size ($n = 662$). Patients with chronic major depression were randomly assigned to pharmacotherapy with nefazadone (an antidepressant with serotonin and norepinephrine agonist properties), treatment with the cognitive behavioral analysis system of psychotherapy (CBASP), or combined therapy. CBASP is a form of CBT with modifications for chronic depression (McCullough, 2000). Treatment response rates for study completers were 55% for nefazadone, 52% for CBASP, and 85% for combined treatment.

Anxiety Disorders

Studies comparing CBT for anxiety disorders to pharmacotherapy alone and to a combination of CBT and medications of various types have been the subject of three major reviews (Spiegel & Bruce, 1997; Westra & Stewart, 1998; Bakker, van Balkom, & van Dyck, 2000) and a meta-analysis (van Balkom et al., 1997). Most studies reviewed by these authors examined the efficacy of a benzodiazepine compared to a CBT intervention such as exposure therapy or a combined treatment approach. Spiegel and Bruce (1997) concluded that benzodiazepines alone can be highly effective for panic disorder, but relapse rates of 50% or more are typically encountered even if the medication is tapered slowly. Also, benzodiazepines can be associated with tolerance and dependency. Their review found no consistent evidence for an advantage for combined treatment with benzodiazepines, and no negative interactions during acute treatment, but a suggestion for impairment of the long-term efficacy of exposure therapy after withdrawal from the low-potency benzodiazepine alprazolam. Westra and Stewart (1998) came to the same conclusions regarding combined treatment with benzodiazepines. They noted that higher-potency benzodiazepines with longer half-lives, such as diazepam, did not appear to have the negative effects seen with alprazolam.

The major study finding a negative long-term influence of alprazolam on CBT was reported by Marks et al. (1993), who compared high-dose alprazolam (5 mg per day) plus exposure with alprazolam plus relaxation, placebo plus exposure, and placebo plus relaxation for panic disorder with agoraphobia. Treatment continued for 8 weeks, after which alprazolam was tapered and stopped by Week 16. Acute treatment effects favored exposure over alprazolam, but both treatments were effective. Follow-up ratings indicated that persons treated with combined exposure and medication did less well than those who received exposure alone. From a pharmacological perspective, the results of this study can be questioned because of the high dose of alprazolam and a short duration of treatment. Typically, patients would not be treated with high-dose alprazolam for only 8 weeks in clinical practice. However, this study suggests that alprazolam (if it is discontinued) may impair the effectiveness of exposure therapy for panic disorder with agoraphobia.

Westra and Stewart (1998) also reviewed studies of antidepressants for anxiety disorders and observed that combined therapy with tricyclic antidepressants was more effective for acute treatment than monotherapy with medication or CBT alone. However, follow-up ratings up to 2 years after treatment typically showed no advantage. Naturalistic follow-up evaluations of efficacy studies for combined therapy are very difficult to interpret because patients often discontinue medication when this is not recommended, or they seek out other forms of therapy. For example, Herceg-Baron et al. (1979) noted that patients who dropped out of their study of psychotherapy versus pharmacotherapy for depression, and then entered other treatment, most commonly sought out clinicians who would provide both therapies.

There have been few studies of SSRIs combined with CBT for anxiety disorders (de Beurs et al., 1995; Sharp et al, 1997; Westra & Stewart,

1998). It is too early to determine whether the results of studies with SSRIs for anxiety disorders will have any different results from those performed with tricyclic antidepressants. Nevertheless, a review of studies of SSRIs combined with CBT found that combination therapy led to the greatest treatment gains (Bakker et al., 2000). The positive effects of SSRIs in enhancing learning and memory (Levkovitz et al., 2002), as compared to negative actions of tricyclic antidepressants on cognitive functioning (Curran et al., 1988), suggest that SSRIs may have a more favorable interaction profile with CBT than older antidepressant medications.

The largest and most recent trial of combined therapy with a tricyclic antidepressant and CBT for panic disorder was conducted at multiple centers by Barlow, Gorman, Shear, and Woods (2000). Patients with panic disorder with or without mild agoraphobia were randomly assigned to treatment with CBT alone, imipramine, placebo, CBT plus imipramine, or CBT plus placebo. The acute treatment phase lasted 3 months. Responders were seen monthly for 6 months in the maintenance phase of therapy, and then were followed for an additional 6 months after maintenance therapy was discontinued. At the end of acute treatment, all active treatments were effective and were superior to placebo. After 6 months of maintenance therapy, CBT plus imipramine was clearly superior to the other active treatments (57.1% response rate for combined treatment, compared to 39.5% for CBT and 37.8% for imipramine). However, this advantage disappeared by the end of the 6-month follow-up interval.

A meta-analysis of studies of pharmacotherapy, CBT, and combined treatment for panic disorder, including a total of 5,011 patients, was conducted by van Balkom et al. (1997). The results of this meta-analysis are consistent with the conclusions of Westra and Stewart (1998). The combination of antidepressants plus exposure therapy was found to be the most effective treatment for panic disorder. The mean effect size for combined treatment of agoraphobia was 2.47, as compared to 1.00 for benzodiazepines, 1.02 for antidepressants, 1.38 for exposure alone, and 0.32 for control conditions.

Bulimia Nervosa

Most research on combined therapy for bulimia nervosa has found advantages for using CBT and an antidepressant together (Bacaltchuk et al., 2000). For example, Agras et al. (1992) found that desipramine and CBT given for 24 weeks gave the broadest therapeutic benefit. Patients with bulimia nervosa were randomly assigned to CBT, desipramine, or both treatments. At 16 weeks, CBT and combined therapy were superior to pharmacotherapy, but at 32 weeks, only the combined approach was more efficacious than medication alone. Abstinence rates from binge eating were significantly higher in those treated for 24 weeks with combined therapy (70%) than with CBT (55%) or desipramine (42%). At the 1-year follow-up evaluation, 78% of patients who received combined treatment were free of binge eating and purging, compared to only 18% of those receiving desipramine (Agras et al., 1994).

Goldbloom et al. (1997) found responses similar to those of Agras et al. (1992) in a study of bulimia nervosa treated with CBT, fluoxetine, and combined therapy. However, in contrast to the Agras et al. investigation, treatment did not continue beyond 16 weeks. Goldbloom and coworkers observed that combined therapy was superior to fluoxetine on some measures. However, after 16 weeks of treatment, there were no clear advantages for combined treatment over CBT. The study design did not allow for comparisons beyond 16 weeks, such as those reported by Agras et al. (1992) which showed superiority for combined treatment over all other approaches.

The largest study of combined therapy for bulimia nervosa was performed by Walsh et al. (1997), who randomly assigned 120 women to treatment with CBT plus medication, CBT plus placebo, psychodynamic therapy plus medication, psychodynamic therapy plus placebo, or medication alone. The pharmacotherapy regimen included an initial trial with desipramine, with a switch to fluoxetine after 8 weeks if the response was not satisfactory or if there were significant side effects. Thus the research design was geared toward providing optimal pharmacotherapy. A significant advantage was found for combined therapy over psychotherapy plus placebo. Also, CBT plus medication was superior to medication alone.

The results of seven studies of psychological treatments given in combination with pharmacotherapy for bulimia nervosa were examined in a meta-analysis by Bacaltchuk et al. (2000). Five of the seven trials in this analysis included a CBT treatment condition. Although this meta-analysis is confounded by including different forms of psychotherapy, the overall results favored combined treatment over medication or psychotherapy alone. Bacaltchuk et al. (2000) noted that the remission rate (100% reduction in binge episodes) was 42% for combined treatment, as compared to 23% for medication alone in these studies. Remission also was more likely for combined treatment than for psychotherapy alone.

Psychosis

Several ground-breaking studies have been completed on the impact of adding CBT to medication for psychotic illnesses. Most patients in these studies have suffered from schizophrenia or related disorders. Because of the severity of the illness and strong evidence for effectiveness of antipsychotic medication, there have been no trials that have examined the efficacy of combined treatment compared to CBT alone. Instead, investigators have focused on determining whether CBT adds to the effect of medication plus treatment as usual. All studies completed to date have demonstrated a positive benefit for combined therapy.

The first randomized controlled trial was performed by Drury et al. (1996), who added individual and group CBT to treatment as usual in hospitalized patients with nonaffective psychoses. The control group received a matched number of hours of supportive therapist contact. Both groups were continued on antipsychotic medication. After completion of treatment, ratings of positive symptoms on the Psychiatric Assessment Scale strongly favored combined therapy. Highly significant differences were observed by the seventh week of treatment, and the advantage for combined treatment was maintained for the entire 9 months of observation. At the 9-month follow-up examination, 95% of the combined group reported no or minor hallucinations and delusions. Only 44% of the control group reached this level of improvement.

Other randomized controlled trials that found positive effects for combined treatment of psychosis were reported by Kuipers et al. (1997), Tarrier et al. (1998), Pinto et al. (1999), and Sensky et al. (2000). The Sensky et al. (2000) study is particularly notable because of the relatively large number of patients ($n = 90$), use of treatment manuals, careful supervision of therapists, inclusion of a credible psychotherapy for the control condition, general equivalence of antipsychotic medication use in treatment groups, and inclusion of measures for positive and negative symptoms. Patients with schizophrenia were treated for up to 9 months with antipsychotic medication plus CBT or medication plus "befriending" (empathic and nondirective contact with the therapist). At the end of the 9-month treatment period, both groups showed substantial improvement in positive and negative symptoms. Although there were no significant differences found between groups at the end of therapy, a marked advantage for combined treatment was observed at the 9-month follow-up evaluation. Patients treated with befriending lost some of their earlier gains, while those treated with CBT continued to improve.

A meta-analysis of controlled research on combined CBT and medication for psychosis (Rector & Beck, 2001) found significant advantages for using CBT and medication together. The mean effect sizes for positive symptoms were 1.31 for CBT plus medication and routine care, 0.04 for medication and routine care, and 0.63 for supportive therapy plus medication and routine care. Similar findings were observed for negative symptoms. Taken together, the results of the studies of CBT reviewed here indicate that CBT and medication for psychosis have significant additive effects. These research findings have led to treatment guidelines for including CBT in the clinical management of schizophrenia in the United Kingdom.

INTERPRETING RESULTS OF OUTCOME RESEARCH ON COMBINED THERAPY

After more than two decades of research on combined therapy for depression, questions still remain about the relative merits of using CBT and medication together as compared to using either treatment alone. Although combined therapy has been shown to be superior to monotherapy for severe and chronic depression, there have been mixed results of investigations of mild to moderate depression. Hollon, Shelton, and Loosen (1991) have noted that problems with study design and inadequate statistical power have plagued most of this research. Small sample sizes are a particular difficulty. Because both antidepressants and CBT typically work quite well, there may be a "ceiling effect." If the mean response is excellent in all conditions, there is little room at the top to show superior results for any therapy (see, e.g., Hollon et al., 1992). Very large sample sizes would be required to have the statistical power to demonstrate a true difference. Alternatively, a population with treatment-resistant or severe illness (as in the Keller et al. [2000] investigation), in which there is more room to observe differences between treatments, would need to be studied.

Entsuah, Huang, and Thase (2001) have recognized this problem in outcome research and have recommended a "mega-analysis" technique, in which data from studies of comparable design or from the same treatment center are pooled to test hypotheses. Using this technique, Entsuah et al. (2001) discovered a significant advantage for venlafaxine over other antidepressants in reaching remission from depression. This superiority was not detected in the individual studies used in the mega-analysis.

Most of the studies of combined therapy for depression were initiated before the introduction of newer antidepressants, such as SSRIs, venlafaxine, nefazadone, and others. Earlier investigations utilized tricyclic antidepressants, which are rarely prescribed in current pharmacotherapy practice. Because tricyclic antidepressants have much higher rates of unpleasant side effects and can impair learning and memory functioning (Curran et al., 1988; Knegtering et al., 1994; Richardson et al., 1994), these drugs would appear to be less well suited than SSRIs or other nontricyclic antidepressants for combination therapy with CBT—a treatment based on learning new ways of thinking and behaving. More recent studies with newer antidepressants have demonstrated a distinct advantage for combined therapy (Miller et al., 1999; Keller et al., 2000).

There are several other reasons why caution is needed in interpreting results of investigations on combined therapy of depression and of the other conditions (anxiety disorders, bulimia nervosa, and psychosis) reviewed in this chapter (Wright & Schrodt, 1989). The form of combined treatment used in research studies typically does not present the therapy as an integrated model or method. The therapies are delivered separately by two different clinicians, who may not communicate regularly or develop a team approach to treatment. Thus combined therapy may not have been performed at an optimal level in traditional outcome studies. The design requirements of efficacy studies also may lead to conditions that are dissimilar from those encountered in clinical practice. Outside the strict confines of a randomized controlled trial, clinicians are free to develop a flexible approach that creatively blends the contributions of biological treatments and CBT.

One of the research groups that conducted an early efficacy study performed a later investigation that raised an important issue about treatment with pharmacotherapy "alone" (Murphy, Carney, Knesevitch, Wetzel, & Whitworth, 1995). It is often assumed in studies of combined therapy that CBT plus pharmacotherapy is being compared to medication without psychotherapy. However, many psychiatrists may utilize psychotherapy methods, including cognitive and behavioral interventions, in "medication management" sessions. In a unique study, Murphy et al. (1995) gave specific instructions to the psychiatrist doing medication management *not* to do psychotherapy. Although a combined treatment condition was not used in this investigation, pharmacotherapy was significantly impaired by removing the psychotherapy component of medication management treatment. Subjects who received CBT were significantly more likely to improve to the predetermined criteria (BDI < 9) than those who received pharmacotherapy alone (CBT = 82% response, antidepressant = 29% response).

Another problem with interpreting results of efficacy studies is the use of inclusion and exclusion criteria that produce homogeneous groups of subjects. Many of the challenging patients seen in clinical practice who may be particularly suitable for combined therapy may be screened out of these studies. For example, a severely depressed patient with suicidal intent would not qualify for most of the studies reviewed above. But combined treatment with medication and psychotherapy would be chosen by many clinicians as the preferred treatment approach for this condition.

Efficacy studies also may obscure or miss interaction effects because they do not examine the processes or mechanisms of interaction (Table 16.1). Lack of significant differences between combined treatment and monotherapy does not conclusively prove that no interactions occurred. It is possible that there are positive interactions in some subjects and negative interactions in others (or even positive and negative interactions in the same subject) that are not detected when pooled data and mean scores are reported for results at the end of therapy. In the case of studies of depression, one patient may have side effects from an antidepressant (e.g., insomnia, agitation, or sedation) that may interfere with concentration, but another may experience enhanced learning and memory after being started on pharmacotherapy.

Despite the limitations of traditional, controlled efficacy studies, the investigations reviewed here have made major contributions to our understanding of the relative usefulness of different therapies for depression. The results of controlled research on combined therapy for depression, anxiety disorders, bulimia nervosa, and psychosis are summarized in Table 16.2.

COMBINING CBT AND PHARMACOTHERAPY IN CLINICAL PRACTICE

Although the overall results of outcome studies have supported additive effects between therapies, combined therapy may have been somewhat handicapped in these investigations. Most studies have been designed to pit one therapy against the other, thus creating a competitive instead of a cooperative environment. Combined therapy could have the greatest chance of being effective in real-world, clinical practice settings if it is offered in a uni-

TABLE 16.2. Combined CBT and Pharmacotherapy: Summary of Results of Outcome Research

Condition	Additive effects	Subtractive effects
Major depression	+	0
Chronic or severe major depression	+++	0
Anxiety disorders (alprazolam therapy)	0	++
Anxiety disorders (other benzodiazepines)	+/0	0
Anxiety disorders (antidepressant therapy)	++	0
Bulimia nervosa	++	0
Psychosis	+++	0

Note. 0, no consistent evidence for interaction; +, mild interaction effects; ++, moderate interaction effects; +++, large interaction effects.

fied package by clinicians who understand and endorse a fully integrated approach to treatment.

A comprehensive cognitive–biological model for combined therapy has been detailed elsewhere (Wright & Thase, 1992). This model (diagrammed in Figure 16.1) assumes the following:

1. Cognitive processes modulate the effects of the external environment (e.g., stressful life events, interpersonal relationships, social forces) on the CNS substrate (e.g., neurotransmitter function, activation of CNS pathways, autonomic and neuroendocrine responses) for emotion and behavior.
2. Dysfunctional cognitions can be produced by both psychological and biological influences.
3. Biological treatments can alter cognitions.
4. Cognitive and behavioral interventions can change biological processes.
5. Environmental, cognitive, biological, emotional, and behavioral processes should be conceptualized as part of the same system.
6. It is valuable to search for ways of integrating or combining cognitive and biological interventions to enhance treatment outcome.

The first assumption is a component of the basic cognitive model (Wright, Beck, & Thase, 2002). Assumptions 2–5 are supported by research reviewed earlier in this chapter on the effects of CBT on CNS function (see, e.g., Baxter et al., 1992; Furmark et al., 2002); by studies of the influence of pharmacotherapy on maladaptive cognitions (Blackburn &

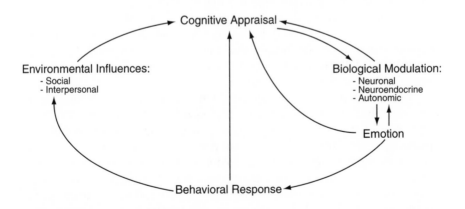

FIGURE 16.1. The cognitive-biological model for combined pharmacotherapy and psychotherapy.

Bishop, 1983; Simons, Garfield, & Murphy, 1984); and by the integrative formulations of Akiskal and McKinney (1975), Kandel (2001), and others. Assumption 6 is supported by the generally favorable results of outcome studies on combining treatment strategies.

The cognitive–biological model can be implemented in clinical practice in two major ways: (1) by a psychiatrist who is trained in both CBT and pharmacotherapy, or (2) by teams of physicians and nonmedical therapists. The most common approach is a team approach to integrated therapy. But growing numbers of psychiatrists are skilled cognitive therapists and may deliver all of the treatment (medication and CBT) in a comprehensive package and/or work with nonmedical cognitive therapists for the delivery of integrated care. The recent mandate in the United States for psychiatry residents to achieve competency in CBT may increase the likelihood that psychiatrists will provide combined CBT and biological therapy by themselves and also be effective members of cognitive–biological treatment teams.

When CBT and medication are administered by different clinicians, several steps can be taken to promote collaboration and strengthen the impact of combining treatments (Wright, 1987; Wright & Thase, 1992). First, the clinicians should work together regularly if possible. The ideal arrangement is for the therapist providing CT and the pharmacotherapist to be part of the same practice group or clinic. The clinicians should agree on a general formulation for combined treatment, such as the cognitive–biological model described above. They also should discuss what will be told to the patient about using the two treatments together, and should present a knowledgeable and generally favorable opinion of integrated therapy. It can help a great deal if a nonmedical therapist is conversant with the mechanisms of action, indications, and side effects of medication. Thus the therapist providing CBT can help educate the patient about pharmacotherapy, answer general questions, and promote compliance with the medication regimen. In a similar manner, the pharmacotherapist who knows the basics of CBT can support the work of the nonmedical therapist, reinforce homework adherence, and encourage the use of CBT skills to manage symptoms.

Specific methods for integrating CBT and pharmacotherapy have been described previously (Wright & Schrodt, 1989; Wright & Thase, 1992; Wright et al., 1993). The structure of therapy provides an excellent opportunity for uniting the different treatment approaches. Structuring techniques, such as agenda setting, feedback, and homework assignments, are core elements of CBT. In a similar manner, pharmacotherapy is organized around symptom assessments, side effect monitoring, directions for taking medication, and the writing of prescriptions. If one therapist is providing both pharmacotherapy and CBT, the agenda for the session should contain one or more items from each approach (e.g., side effects, drug interactions, homework assignments, improving self-esteem, coping with an environmental problem). The two treatments should be valued equally, but the time devoted to each will vary from session to session. In my own experience with combined therapy, sessions are usually weighted more heavily to CBT interventions than to discussions about pharmacotherapy.

If there are dual therapists, agenda setting can be used to link the therapies. For example, the pharmacotherapist can place items such as "progress in using CBT" and "How is the homework going?" on the agenda; the therapist providing CBT can help the patient address such topics as "attitudes about taking medication." In this manner, the two therapists can convey the importance of a combined approach to the patient and use a similar agenda setting method to help bring together the different elements of therapy.

Psychoeducation, another important shared feature of CBT and pharmacotherapy, can be used to forge an integrated treatment method. CBT is well known for using psychoeducational procedures to assist patients with learning new patterns of thinking and behaving. Typical educational methods include explanations in sessions, reading assignments, audio- and videotapes, computer-assisted instruction, modeling, homework, and cognitive and behavioral rehearsal (Wright, Thase, & Beck, 2002).

Pharmacotherapists employ psychoeducational methods to help patients acquire knowledge about psychiatric disorders, the biological model, medications, and side effects. Commonly used techniques include minididactic presentations in treatment sessions, videos, and readings in books or pamphlets. To combine therapies effectively, clinicians should carefully review educational materials provided to patients in order to minimize presentation of contradictory or strongly biased information (e.g., pharmaceutical company pamphlets that extol the value of their product instead of giving a balanced and comprehensive view of treatment).

There are several books for the general public that discuss both CBT and pharmacotherapy in a favorable light and can help readers understand how both treatments can be used effectively in psychiatric treatment. *Getting Your Life Back: The Complete Guide to Recovery from Depression* (Wright & Basco, 2002) presents a fully integrated cognitive–biological treatment method. *Feeling Good* (Burns, 1999) includes a section on medications. A newly developed technology, computer-assisted CBT, is now available for teaching patients CBT skills. Empirically tested programs such as *Good Days Ahead: The Multimedia Program for Cognitive Therapy* (Wright, Wright, Salmon, et al., 2002; Wright, Wright, & Beck, 2002) and *Fear Fighter* (Kenwright, Liness, & Marks, 2001) can assist clinicians in helping patients understand and use CBT methods.

Adherence to treatment recommendations is a critical element for implementation of both CBT and pharmacotherapy. In CBT, attendance at therapy sessions and homework are important for success. In pharmacotherapy, medication compliance, accurate reporting of side effects, and sticking with maintenance therapy regimens are key components of effective treatment. CBT interventions for improving treatment compliance are particularly well suited for integrating therapies and promoting adherence to all components of the treatment plan (Cochran, 1984; Wright & Thase, 1992; Basco & Rush, 1995; Kemp et al., 1996).

Simple behavioral interventions—such as using reminder systems, pairing medication taking with routine activities (e.g., brushing teeth, meals), and developing behavioral contracts—can be integrated into pharmacotherapy sessions in a time-efficient manner and can be utilized by nonmedical therapists to improve medication compliance. More detailed interventions, such as reinforcement programs and behavioral analyses of barriers to pharmacotherapy adherence, also can be employed when needed.

Maladaptive cognitions about medication or medical treatment are other potential targets for combined CBT and pharmacotherapy. Treatment compliance can be undermined by dysfunctional cognitions related to schematic themes, such as (1) personal weakness (e.g., "Taking a medication means that I am weak," "I should be able to do this on my own"); (2) distrust in the therapeutic relationship (e.g., "Doctors just try to push medication instead of understanding people," "You can't trust doctors"); (3) fears of dependency (e.g., "I'll be dependent on the medication," "I won't be in control"); and (4) fears of medication effects (e.g., "I'm always the one to get side effects," "These drugs are dangerous") (Wright & Schrodt, 1989; Wright & Thase, 1992). Negative automatic thoughts and core beliefs such as these can go unrecognized if the clinician does not inquire about the patient's reactions to medication prescription. When maladaptive responses to pharmacotherapy are uncovered, therapists can use CBT methods, such as thought recording and examining the evidence, to develop realistic cognitions that will support medication adherence.

A flexible, customized approach to the "dosing" and timing of interventions for individual patients can provide an additional opportunity for enhancing the effects of combined therapy. In most outcome studies, all patients receive essentially the same dose of medication and psychotherapy along a strictly controlled time course. However, in clinical practice, therapists can capitalize on the specific attributes of various medications and CBT interventions to arrange a sequence and dosing regimen to help meet treatment goals. For example, in my own work with highly suicidal inpatients, I target hopelessness and suicidal ideation with CBT interventions on the day of admission to reduce suicidal risk and dysphoria rapidly. Although antidepressants are also started immediately, these medications are unlikely to exert positive effects until several days have elapsed. A different clinical situation may be encountered with patients in the midst of severe manic or psychotic episodes, who may require stabilization with medication before meaningful psychotherapy can begin.

The response, or lack of response, to treatment also may call for adjustments in the combined therapy approach. Psychopharmacological considerations may include increasing the dose of medication if there is inadequate relief of symptoms, utilizing augmentation strategies for treatment resistance, or adding an antipsychotic medication if psychotic features are detected. In a parallel manner, CBT interventions can be intensified, reformulated, or modified in other ways to meet the specific problems and needs of each patient. When a fully integrated therapy approach is used, these adjustments are part of a comprehensive treatment plan that seeks to draw the best from both CBT and pharmacotherapy to maximize the chances of response.

SUMMARY

Outcome studies of combined CBT and medication have focused on testing for superiority of therapies at the end of treatment and thus have not helped elucidate possible mechanisms of interaction and have not encouraged the development of integrative treatment models. Nevertheless, the overall results of outcome research support additive effects between treatments for most disorders and combinations of treatment interventions. Strong evidence has been collected for enhanced treatment response for combinations of antidepressants and CBT for severe or chronic depression, anxiety disorders, and bulimia nervosa. The newest area of research, combined treatment for psychosis, has consistently documented advantages for adding CBT to treatment with antipsychotic medication. The only form of combined treatment that may show negative interactions is short-term alprazolam use in patients receiving CBT.

Possible future research directions for combined CBT and pharmacotherapy could include designs with larger sample sizes and/or "megaanalyses" (Entsuah et al., 2001) to detect effects that may be obscured in smaller studies; investigations of combined therapy for severe and treatment-resistant symptoms; and explorations of ways for making combined therapy more efficient or effective. Also, research directed at the processes of interaction could help in the development of more refined and more specific treatment methods for utilizing a combined therapy approach. Examples of such refinements might include titration of medication dose to ideal levels that would enhance learning and memory function or reduce other barriers to effective psychotherapy, or the development of CBT methods targeted directly at facilitating the CNS effects of pharmacotherapy. Research on the biological actions of CBT offers a significant opportunity to understand how cognitive and behavioral interventions might work in concert with medication to augment treatment response.

Clinical implementation of the combined therapy approach may vary widely, depending on the theoretical orientation of clinicians and the degree of communication between therapists. It is recommended that clinicians adopt an integrated cognitive–biological model, develop a unified and comprehensive therapy plan for each patient, and draw from the advantages of both CBT and pharmacotherapy in selecting interventions.

Although CBT and biological psychiatry have evolved from different theoretical and scientific backgrounds, these two important treatment approaches have many things in common. They share a strong empirical basis, an emphasis on structure and psychoeducation, a pragmatic view of therapy, and the common objective of reducing psychiatric symptoms to the greatest extent possible. Both treatments influence thoughts, emotions, and the biological substrate for human behavior. A partnership between CBT and pharmacotherapy offers potential for advancing the treatment of mental disorders.

DISCLOSURE STATEMENT

I may receive a portion of profits from sales of *Good Days Ahead*, a computer program described in this chapter. A portion of profits from sales of *Good Days Ahead* is donated to the Foundation for Cognitive Therapy and Research and the Norton Foundation.

REFERENCES

Agras, W. S., Rossiter, E. M., Arnow, B., Schneider, J. A., Telch, C. F., Raeburn, S. D., et al. (1992). Pharmacologic and cognitive-behavioral treatment for bulimia nervosa: A controlled comparison. *American Journal of Psychiatry, 149*, 82–87.

Agras, W. S., Rossiter, E. M., Arnow, B., Telch, C. F., Raeburn, S. D., Bruce, B., et al. (1994). One-year follow-up of psychosocial and pharmacologic treatments for bulimia nervosa. *Journal of Clinical Psychiatry, 55*, 179–183.

Akiskal, H. A., & McKinney, W. T. (1975). Overview of recent research in depression: Integration of ten conceptual models into a comprehensive clinical frame. *Archives of General Psychiatry, 32*, 285–305.

Bacaltchuk, J., Trefiglio, R. P., Oliveira, I. R., Hay, P., Lima, M. S., & Mari, J. J., et al. (2000), Combination of antidepressants and psychological treatments for bulimia nervosa: A systematic review. *Acta Psychiatrica Scandinavica, 101*, 256–264.

Backhaus, J., Hohagen, F., Voderholzer, U., & Riemann, D. (2001). Long-term effectiveness of a short-term cognitive-behavioral group treatment for primary insomnia. *European Archives of Psychiatry and Clinical Neuroscience, 251,* 35–41.

Bakker, A., van Balkom, A. J., & van Dyck, R. (2000). Selective serotonin reuptake inhibitors in the treatment of panic disorder and agoraphobia. *International Clinical Psychopharmacology, 15*(Suppl, 2), 25–30.

Barlow, D. H., Gorman, J. M., Shear, M. K., & Woods, S. W. (2000). Cognitive-behavioral therapy, Imipramine, or their combination for panic disorder: A randomized controlled trial. *Journal of the American Medical Association, 283,* 2529–2536.

Basco, M. R., & Rush, A. J. (1995). Compliance with pharmacotherapy in mood disorders. *Psychiatric Annals, 25,* 269–279.

Baxter, L. R., Jr., Schwartz, J. M., Bergman, K. S., Szuba, M. P., Guze, B. H., Mazziotta, J. C., et al. (1992). Caudate glucose metabolic rate changes with both drug and behavior therapy for obsessive–compulsive disorder. *Archives of General Psychiatry, 49,* 681–689.

Blackburn, I. M., & Bishop, S. (1983). Changes in cognition with pharmacotherapy and cognitive therapy. *British Journal of Psychiatry, 143,* 609–617.

Blackburn, I. M., Bishop, S., Glen, A. I. M., Whalley, L. J., & Christie, J. E. (1981). The efficiency of cognitive therapy in depression: A treatment using cognitive therapy and pharmacotherapy, each alone and in combination. British Journal of Psychiatry, *139,* 181–189.

Brody, A. L., Saxena, S., Schwartz, J. M., Stoessel, P. W., Maidment, K., Phelps, M. E., et al. (1998). FDG-PET predictors of response to behavioral therapy and pharmacotherapy in obsessive compulsive disorder. *Psychiatric Research, 84,* 1–6.

Burns, D. D. (1999). *Feeling good: The new mood therapy* (rev. ed.). New York: Avon Books.

Cochran, S. D. (1984). Preventing medical noncompliance in the outpatient treatment of bipolar affective disorders. *Journal of Consulting and Clinical Psychology, 52,* 873–878.

Curran, H. V. (1994). Memory functions, alprazolam and exposure therapy:A controlled longitudinal study of agoraphobia with panic disorder. *Psychological Medicine, 24,* 969–976.

Curran, H. V., Sakulsriprong, M., & Lader, M. (1988). Antidepressants and human memory: An investigation of four drugs with different sedative and anticholinergic profiles. *Psychopharmacology, 95,* 520–527.

de Beurs, E., van Balkom, A. J. L. M., Lange, A., Koele, P., & van Dyck, R. (1995). Treatment of panic disorder with agoraphobia: Comparison of fluvoxamine, placebo, and psychological panic management combined with exposure and of exposure *in vivo* alone. *American Journal of Psychiatry, 152,* 683–691.

Dobson, K. S. (1989). A meta-analysis of the efficacy of cognitive therapy for depression. *Journal of Consulting and Clinical Psychology, 57,* 414–419.

Drury, V., Birchwood, M., Cochrane, R., & Macmillan, F. (1996). Cognitive therapy and recovery from acute psychosis: A controlled trial. I. Impact on psychotic symptoms. *British Journal of Psychiatry, 169,* 593–601.

Edinger, J. D., Wohlgemuth, W. K., Radtke, R. A., Marsh, G. R., & Quillian, R. E., et al. (2001). Cognitive behavioral therapy for treatment of chronic primary insomnia: A randomized controlled study. *Journal of the American Medical Association, 285,* 1856–1864.

Entsuah, R. A., Huang, H., & Thase, M. E. (2001). Response and remission rates in different subpopulations with major depressive disorder administered venlafaxine, selective serotonin reuptake inhibitors, or placebo. *Journal of Clinical Psychiatry, 62,* 869–877.

Furmark, T., Tillfors, M., Marteinsdottir, I., Fischer, H., Pissiota, A., Langstrom, B., et al. (2002). Common changes in cerebral blood flow in patients with social phobia treated with citalopram or cognitive-behavioral therapy. *Archives of General Psychiatry, 59,* 425–433.

Gabbard, G. O., & Kay, J. (2001). The fate of integrated treatment: Whatever happened to the biopsychosocial psychiatrist? *American Journal of Psychiatry, 158*(12), 1956–1963.

Goldbloom, D. S., Olmsted, M., Davis, R., Clewes, J., Heinmaa, M., Rockert, W., et al. (1997). A randomized controlled trial of fluoxetine and cognitive behavioral therapy for bulimia nervosa: Short-term outcome. *Behaviour Research and Therapy, 35,* 803–811.

Group for the Advancement of Psychiatry. (1975). *Pharmacotherapy and psychotherapy: Paradoxes, problems, and progress* (Vol. 9, Report No. 93). New York: Mental Health Materials Center.

Harmer, C. J., Bhagwagar, Z., Cowen, P. J., & Goodwin, G. M. (2002). Acute administration of citalopram facilitates memory consolidation in healthy volunteers. *Psychopharmacology, 163,* 106–110.

Harvey, P. D., Moriarty, P. J., Serper, M. R., Schnur, E., & Lieber, D. (2000). Practice-related improvement in information processing with novel antipsychotic treatment. *Schizophrenia Research, 46,* 139–148.

Hasbroucq, T., Rihet, P., Blin., O., & Possamai, C. A. (1997). Serotonin and human information processing: Fluvoxamine can improve reaction time performance. *Neuroscience Letters, 229,* 204–208.

Herceg-Baron, R. L., Prusoff, B. A., Weissman, M. M., DiMascio, A., Neu, C., & Klerman, G. L. (1979). Pharmacotherapy and psychotherapy in acutely depressed patients: A study of attrition patterns in a clinical trial. *Comprehensive Psychiatry, 20*(4), 315–325.

Hollon, S. D., DeRubeis, R. J., Evans, M. D., Wiemer, M. J., Garvey, M. J., Grove, W. M., et al. (1992). Cognitive therapy and pharmacotherapy for depression: Singly and in combination. *Archives of General Psychiatry, 49,* 774–781.

Hollon, S. D., Shelton, R. C., & Loosen, P. T. (1991). Cognitive therapy and pharmacotherapy for depression. *Journal of Consulting and Clinical Psychology, 59,* 88–99.

Hommer, D. W. (1991). Benzodiazepines: Cognitive and psychomotor effects. In P. P. Roy-Byrne & D. S. Cowley (Eds.), *Benzodiazepines in clinical practice: Risks and benefits* (pp. 111–130). Washington DC: American Psychiatric Press.

Joffe, R., Sega, Z., & Singer, W. (1996). Change in thyroid hormone levels following response to cognitive therapy for major depression. *American Journal of Psychiatry, 153*(3), 411–413.

Kandel, E. R. (2001). Psychotherapy and the single synapse: The impact of psychiatric thought on neurobiological research. *New England Journal of Medicine, 301,* 1028–1037.

Keller, M. B., McCullough, J. P., Klein, D. N., Arnow, B., Dunner, D. L., Gelenberg, A. J., et al. (2000). A comparison of nefazodone, the cognitive behavioral-analysis system of psychotherapy, and their combination for the treatment of chronic depression. *New England Journal of Medicine, 342,* 1462–1470.

Kemp, R., Hayward, P., Applewhaite, G., Everitt, B., & David, A. (1996). Compliance therapy in psychotic patients: randomized controlled trial. *British Medical Journal, 312,* 345–349.

Kemp, R., Kirov, G., Everitt, B., Hayward, P., & David, A. (1998). randomized controlled trial of compliance therapy: 18–month follow-up. *British Journal of Psychiatry, 172,* 413–419.

Kenwright, M., Liness, S., & Marks, I. (2001). Reducing demands on clinicians by offering computer-aided self-help for phobia–panic: Feasibility study. *British Journal of Psychiatry, 181,* 456–459.

Knegtering, H., Eijck, M., & Huijsman, A. (1994). Effects of antidepressants on cognitive functioning of elderly patients. A review. *Drugs and Aging, 5,* 192–199.

Kuipers, E., Garety, P., Fowler, D., Dunn, G., Beggington, P., Freeman, D., et al. (1997). London–East Anglia randomized controlled trial of cognitive-behavioural therapy for psychosis: I. Effects of the treatment phase. *The British Journal of Psychiatry, 171,* 319–327.

Lecompte, D. (1995). Drug compliance and cognitive-behavioral therapy in schizophrenia. *Acta Psychiatrica Belgica, 95,* 91–100.

Levkovitz, Y., Caftori, R., Avital, A., & Richter-Levin, G. (2002). The SSRIs drug fluoxetine, but not the noradrenergic tricyclic drug desipramine, improves memory performance during acute major depression. *Brain Research Bulletin, 58,* 345–350.

Marrangell, L. B., Silver, J. M., Goff, D. C., & Yudofsky, S. C. (2002). Psychopharmacology and electroconvulsive therapy. In R. E. Hales, S. C. Yudofsky, & J. A. Talbott (Eds.), *Textbook of clinical psychiatry* (4th ed., pp. 1245–1284). Washington, DC: American Psychiatric Press.

Marks, I. M., Swinson, R. P., Basoglu, M., Kuch, K., Noshirvsni, H., O'Sullivan, G., et al. (1993). Alprazolam and exposure alone and combined in panic disorder with agoraphobia: A controlled study in London and Toronto. *British Journal of Psychiatry, 162,* 776–787.

McCullough, J. P., Jr. (2000). *Treatment for chronic depression: Cognitive behavioral analysis system of psychotherapy.* New York: Guilford Press.

Miller, I. W., Norman, W. H., & Keitner, G. I. (1999). Combined treatment for patients with double depression. *Psychotherapy and Psychosomatics, 68,* 180–185.

Murphy, G. E., Carney, R. M., Knesevich, M. A., Wetzel, R. D., & Whitworth, P. (1995). Cognitive behavior therapy, relaxation training, and tricyclic antidepressant medication in the treatment of depression. *Psychological Reports, 77,* 403–420.

Murphy, G. E., Simons, A. D., Wetzel, R. D., & Lustman, P. J. (1984). Cognitive therapy and pharmacotherapy: Singly and together in the treatment of depression. *Archives of General Psychiatry, 41*, 33–41.

Otto, M. W., Pollack, M. H., Sachs, G. S., Reiter, S. R., Meltzer-Brody, S., & Rosenbaum, J. F. (1993). Discontinuation of benzodiazepine treatment: Efficacy of cognitive-behavioral therapy for patients with panic disorder. *American Journal of Psychiatry, 150*, 1485–1490.

Perris, C., & Skagerlind, L. (1994). Cognitive therapy with schizophrenic patients. *Acta Psychiatrica Scandinavica, 89*(Suppl. 382), 65–70.

Pinto, A., La Pia, S., Mennella, R., Domenico, G., & De Simone, L. (1999). Cognitive-behavioral therapy and clozapine for clients with treatment-refractory schizophrenia. *Psychiatric Services, 50*, 901–904.

Rector, N. A., & Beck, A. T. (2001). Cognitive behavioral therapy for schizophrenia: An empirical review. *Journal of Nervous and Mental Disease, 189*, 278–287.

Richardson, J. S., Keegan, D. L., Bowen, R. C., Blackshaw, S. L., Cebrian-Perez, S., Dayal, N., Saleh, S., et al. (1994). Verbal learning by major depressive disorder patients during treatment with fluoxetine or amitriptyline. *International Clinical Psychopharmacology, 9*, 35–40.

Robinson, L. A., Berman, J. S., & Neimeyer, R. A. (1990). Psychotherapy for the treatment of depression: A comprehensive review of controlled outcome research. *Psychological Bulletin, 108*, 30–49.

Rybarczyk, B., Lopez, M., Benson, R., et al. (2002). Efficacy of two behavioral treatment programs for comorbid geriatric insomnia. *Psychology and Aging, 17*, 288–298.

Schwartz, J. M., Stoessel, P. W., Baxter, L. R. Jr., Martin, K. M., & Phelps, M. E. (1996). Systematic changes in cerebral glucose metabolic rate after successful behavior modification treatment of obsessive–compulsive disorder. *Archives of General Psychiatry, 53*, 109–113.

Sensky, T., Turkington, D., Kingdon, D., Scott, J. L., Scott, J., Siddle, R., et al. (2000). A randomized controlled trial of cognitive-behavioral therapy for persistent symptoms in schizophrenia resistant to medication. *Archives of General Psychiatry, 57*, 165–172.

Sharp, D. M., Power, K. G., Simpson, R. J., Swanson, V., & Anstee, J. A. (1997). Global measures of outcome in a controlled comparison of pharmacological and psychological treatment of panic disorder and agoraphobia in primary care. *British Journal of General Practice, 47*, 150–155.

Simons, A. D., Garfield, S. L., & Murphy, G. E. (1984). The process of change in cognitive therapy and pharmacotherapy for depression. *Archives of General Psychiatry, 41*, 45–51.

Spiegel, D. A., & Bruce, T. J. (1997). Benzodiazepines and exposure-based cognitive behavior therapies for panic disorder: Conclusions from combined treatment trials. *American Journal of Psychiatry, 154*, 773–781.

Spiegel, D. A., Bruce, T. J., Gregg, S. F., & Nuzzarello, A. (1994). Does cognitive behavior therapy assist slow-taper alprazolam discontinuation in panic disorder? *American Journal of Psychiatry, 151*, 876–881.

Stevens, A., Schwarz, J., Schwarz, B., Ruf, I., Kolter, T., & Czekalla, J. (2002). Implicit and explicit learning in schizophrenics treated with olanzapine and with classic neuroleptics. *Psychopharmacology, 160,* 299–306.

Tarrier, N., Yusupoff, L., Kinney, C., McCarthy, E., Gledhill, A., Haddock, G., et al. (1998). randomized controlled trial of intensive cognitive behaviour therapy for patients with chronic schizophrenia. *British Medical Journal, 317,* 303–307.

Ulenhuth, E. H., Lipman, R. S., & Covil, L (1969). Combined pharmacotherapy and psychotherapy. *Journal of Nervous and Mental Disease, 148,* 52–64.

van Balkom, A. J. L. M., Bakker, A., Spinhoven, P., Blaauw, B. M., Smeenk, S., & Ruesink, B. (1997). A meta-analysis of the treatment of panic disorder with or without agoraphobia: A comparison of psychopharmacological, cognitive-behavioral, and combination treatments. *Journal of Nervous and Mental Disease, 185,* 510–516.

Vasterling, J., Jenkins, R. A., Tope, D. M., & Burish, T. G. (1993). Cognitive distraction and relaxation training for the control of side effects due to cancer chemotherapy. *Journal of Behavioral Medicine, 16,* 65–80.

Verster, J. C., Volkerts, E. R., & Verbaten, M. N. (2002). Effects of alprazolam on driving ability, memory functioning and psychomotor performance: A randomized, placebo-controlled study. *Neuropsychopharmacology, 27*(2), 260–269.

Wagemans, J., Notebaert, W., & Boucart, M. (1998). Lorazepam but not diazepam impairs identification of pictures on the basis of specific contour fragments. *Psychopharmacology, 138,* 326–323.

Walsh, B. T., Wilson, G. T., Loeb, K. L., Delvin, M. J., Pike, K. M., Roose, S. P., et al. (1997). Medication and psychotherapy in the treatment of bulimia nervosa. *American Journal of Psychiatry, 154,* 523–531.

Weiss, E. M., Bilder, R. M., & Fleischhacker, W. W. (2002). The effects of second-generation antipsychotics on cognitive functioning and psychosocial outcome in schizophrenia. *Psychopharmacology, 162,* 11–17.

Westra, H. A., & Stewart, S. H. (1998). Cognitive behavioural therapy and pharmacotherapy: Complementary or contradictory approaches to the treatment of anxiety? *Clinical Psychology Review, 18,* 307–340.

Wright, J. H. (1987). Cognitive therapy and medication as combined treatment. In A. Freeman & V. Greenwood (Eds.), *Cognitive therapy: Applications in psychiatric and medical settings* (pp. 36–50). New York: Human Sciences Press.

Wright, J. H., & Basco, M. R. (2002). *Getting your life back: The complete guide to recovery from depression.* New York: Touchstone.

Wright, J. H., Beck, A. T., & Thase, M. E. (2002). Cognitive therapy. In R. E. Hales, S. C. Yudofsky, & J. A. Talbott (Eds.), *Textbook of clinical psychiatry* (4th ed., pp. 1245–1284). Washington, DC: American Psychiatric Press.

Wright, J. H., & Schrodt, G. R., Jr. (1989). Combined cognitive therapy and pharmacotherapy. In A. Freeman, K. M. Simon, L. E. Beutler, & H. Arkowitz (Eds.), *Comprehensive handbook of cognitive therapy* (pp. 267–282). New York: Plenum Press.

Wright, J. H., & Thase, M. E. (1992). Cognitive and biological therapies: A synthesis. *Psychiatric Annals*, 22(9), 451–458.

Wright, J. H., Thase, M. E., & Sensky, T. (1993). Cognitive and biological therapies: A combined approach. In J. H. Wright, M. E. Thase, A. T. Beck, & J. W. Ludgate (Eds.), *Cognitive therapy with inpatients: Developing a cognitive milieu* (pp. 193–218). New York: Guilford Press.

Wright, J. H., Wright, A. S., & Beck, A. T. (2002). *Good days ahead: The multimedia program for cognitive therapy*. Louisville, KY: Mindstreet.

Wright, J. H., Wright, A. S., Salmon, P., Beck, A. T., Kuykendall, J., Goldsmith, L. J., et al. (2002). Development and initial testing of a multimedia program for computer-assisted cognitive therapy. *American Journal of Psychotherapy*, 56, 76–86.

Chapter 17

Cognitive-Behavioral Therapy with Couples

Theoretical and Empirical Status

NORMAN B. EPSTEIN

Although cognitive therapy principles and procedures were initially developed for the individual treatment of psychopathology, during the past two decades there has been a rapid growth in conjoint cognitive-behavioral approaches to assessment and intervention with distressed couples and families. The article "Cognitive Therapy with Couples" (Epstein, 1982) which appeared in the *American Journal of Family Therapy*, was one of the first publications identifying how therapists could use cognitive restructuring approaches during joint sessions with distressed couples. On the one hand, for years cognitive therapists had used individual therapy to help people modify their own cognitions, emotional responses, and behavior toward significant others, just as they addressed clients' dysfunctional responses to other types of life events. As is common in individual therapy, the relevant life events for which a person's responses were to be changed did not occur during treatment sessions. For example, a therapist was not able to observe directly an individual's tendency to make negative arbitrary inferences about a spouse's actions. Neither could the therapist observe the spouse's behavior *in vivo* to judge the degree to which that behavior and not the other's interpretation of it was the problem. On the other hand, marital and family therapists who used behavioral and other theoretical orientations to intervene directly in the process of moment-to-moment interactions had made limited overt use of established cognitive restructuring interventions. Structural and strategic family therapists acknowledged the importance of subjective interpretations in their use of "relabeling," in which they proposed more benign alternative explanations than those that family members had formulated about each other's upsetting actions (Todd, 1986). Those who used a behavioral approach to marital therapy (e.g., Jacobson & Margolin, 1979; Stuart, 1980) noted the impact that negative cognitions such as attributions and unrealistic expectations could have on partners' distress with their relationship; however, their clinical writings presented few systematic guidelines for assessing and intervening with inappropriate or distorted cognitions during conjoint sessions. Thus cognitive-behavioral therapy and conjoint marital and family therapy were two major approaches to the treatment of human problems that until the early 1980s had intersected minimally.

Until the 1980s, researchers' and clinicians' abilities to assess and intervene with individuals' subjective cognitions and emotions during couple interactions were also limited by the absence of measures to assess cognitions and emotional responses regarding intimate relationships. A colleague and I (Eidelson & Epstein, 1982; Epstein & Eidelson, 1981) initiated the development of measures of relationship cognitions by constructing the Relationship Belief Inventory (RBI). The RBI assesses five types of beliefs that clinical literature and experienced marital therapists identified as potentially unrealistic, and therefore as possible risk factors for partners' distress and conflict: (1) Disagreement between partners is destructive; (2) partners should be able to mind-read each other's thoughts and emotions; (3) partners cannot change their relationship; (4) innate differences between females and males are a cause of relationship problems; and (5) one must be a perfect sexual partner. Publication of the RBI provided a self-report measure of relationship cognitions for use in research (including treatment outcome studies evaluating cognitive interventions for couples) and in clinical practice. In spite of the limited range of beliefs assessed by the RBI, and some limitations in validity of some subscales (Bradbury & Fincham, 1993), the measure has generally performed well in empirical studies and has drawn attention to forms of cognition that influence couples' relationships.

When I joined the staff of the Center for Cognitive Therapy in Philadelphia in 1981, my work there with individuals experiencing clinical depression, anxiety, and other problems enhanced my understanding of the cognitive model and the range of techniques available for intervention with distressed individuals. During this period, I further developed an integration of the cognitive model and the concepts and methods of traditional behavioral marital therapy. During this period, Aaron Beck was developing a focus on cognitive processes involved in intimate conflict, and Beck's interest in my work with couples provided an environment that supported further development of clinical methods and research initiatives. Some of us (Epstein, Pretzer, & Fleming, 1982) conducted a pilot test at the Center for Cognitive Therapy, comparing the impacts of cognitive-behavioral interventions and communication training with distressed client couples. We also began the development of the Marital Attitude Survey (Pretzer, Epstein, & Fleming, 1991), which assesses partners' attributions and expectancies concerning relationship problems. Beck's growing interest in applying cognitive therapy to distressed relationships resulted in the publication of his book *Love Is Never Enough* (Beck, 1988), which increased the public's awareness of this important approach to alleviating conflict in close relationships.

The precursors to cognitive-behavioral treatments for couples were behavioral models of relationship distress (e.g., Jacobson & Margolin, 1979; Stuart, 1980) that viewed partners' interactions as resulting from normal learning experiences. According to this view, members of a couple behave maladaptively with each other because they learned to do so in past relationships, because they lack the skills to behave appropriately, or because they receive reinforcement (e.g., attention from the partner) for acting that way in the current relationship. Although there has not been much in the way of direct empirical evidence that such learning processes have led to couples' current negative interactions, there has been substantial evidence that members of unhappy couples exhibit more negative and fewer positive acts toward each other than members of happy couples (Weiss & Heyman, 1990, 1997). In addition to behaving more negatively overall than happy couples, members of distressed couples are more likely to *escalate* their reciprocal criticism, threats, and so forth, during conflicts than are happy couples. Furthermore, research has identified particular *sequences* of negative behavior (demand by one partner → withdrawal by the other; criticism by one partner → defensiveness by the other) that predict deterioration in couples' relationships over time (Christensen & Shenk, 1991; Gottman, 1994). Microanalytic (i.e., act-by-act) coding of couples' discussions of issues in their relationships has indicated that, compared to nondistressed couples, distressed couples indeed tend to have skill deficits in communicating (Notarius & Markman, 1993; Weiss & Heyman, 1997). Consequently, behavioral marital therapists focused on interventions designed to teach distressed couples constructive communication skills, problem-solving skills, and the use of behavioral contracts or agreements for mutual positive changes.

Overall, the results of treatment outcome studies have indicated that behavioral marital therapy that includes combinations of behavioral contracting, communication training, and problem-solving training has produced improvements in couples' levels of relationship distress, compared to couples who were in waiting-list control conditions (Baucom, Shoham, Mueser, Daiuto, & Stickle, 1998). However, the results of outcome studies also have demonstrated that in many instances, increases in communication skills and problem solving have had limited impact on couples' subjective distress (Halford, Sanders, & Behrens, 1993; Iverson & Baucom, 1990). In other words, changing partners' behavior toward each other does not necessarily improve their feelings about each other. Also, when behavioral marital therapy has been compared to other approaches that do not involve teaching behavioral skills, the various interventions have generally been equally efficacious in reducing overall relationship distress (Baucom et al., 1998). For example, insight-oriented marital therapy that focuses on partners' exploration of thoughts, emotions, and personal needs (including those that have been beyond awareness) that contribute to their relationship distress has been found to be as effective as behavioral marital therapy in increasing self-reported marital adjustment at a posttherapy assessment (Snyder & Wills, 1989). Furthermore, the insight-oriented treatment produced greater marital adjustment and a lower rate of divorce than the behavioral approach at a 4-year follow-up (Snyder, Wills, & Grady-Fletcher, 1991). Emotionally focused marital therapy (Greenberg & Johnson, 1988; Johnson & Denton, 2002), which is based on individuals' attachment needs and the role of emotional responses associated with insecure attachment, has been found to be superior to behavioral marital therapy and a waiting-list control condition in increasing marital adjustment (Johnson & Greenberg, 1985). Thus behavioral interventions do not seem to be sufficient for all distressed couples, and some couples benefit from interventions that emphasize insight rather than behavioral skills training.

As a result of such findings and the "cognitive revolution" in the behavior therapy field in the 1980s, theorists, researchers, and clinicians who focused on couple relationships sought to enhance behavioral models of marital therapy, targeting partners' cognitions and emotional responses that contribute to relationship problems. The types of cognitions that might contribute to couples' relationship problems were "borrowed" by couple specialists from basic cognitive psychology and social psychology research, as well as literature on cognitive variables in individual psychopathology. For example, Doherty (1981a, 1981b) drew on research regarding individuals' attributions and expectancies associated with depression (i.e., attributing negative life events to global, stable, internal causes; low efficacy expectancies associated with learned helplessness responses) in identifying types of negative attributions and expectancies that may be associated with couples' relationship distress and inadequate problem-solving efforts. I (Epstein, 1982) described the use of traditional cognitive therapy interventions to modify distressed partners' inappropriate attributions, expectancies, and unrealistic beliefs about their relationships.

In the early 1980s, Donald Baucom and I discovered each other's work on behavioral and cognitive factors in couple relationships at conventions of the Association for Advancement of Behavior Therapy, and we developed a collaborative program of research and writing that has focused on understanding cognitive, affective, and behavioral variables that influence the quality of couples' relationships. This collaboration has continued for over 20 years and has focused on the development of cognitive-behavioral assessment and treatment methods for distressed couples (e.g., Baucom & Epstein, 1990; Baucom, Epstein, Rankin & Burnett, 1996; Epstein & Baucom, 1993, 2002). For example, we developed the Inventory of Specific Relationship Standards (ISRS; Baucom et al., 1996) to assess partners' personal standards concerning the characteristics that they believe their couple relationship should have. The ISRS assesses standards along the dimensions of (1) "boundaries" (the degree to which partners should function autonomously vs. share various aspects of their lives; (2) "power/control" (the degree to which partners should share decision making vs. one person's having greater influence); and (3) "investment" (how much time and energy partners should invest in instrumental and expressive acts for the benefit of the relationship). ISRS items assess these major dimensions in 12 areas of the relationship, such as finances, household tasks, relationships with friends, and communication of negatives. Research on the ISRS indicates that partners' satisfaction with the ways in which their standards are met in their relationship is associated with their level of relationship satisfaction and the quality of their communication (Baucom et al., 1996).

The Baucom and Epstein (1990) volume *Cognitive-Behavioral Marital Therapy* was the first comprehensive clinical description of cognitive-behavioral assessment and intervention methods with distressed couples, based on empirical findings in the field regarding cognitive, affective, and behavioral factors that influence relationship quality. A growing number of clinicians (e.g., Dattilio & Padesky, 1990; Ellis, Sichel, Yeager, DiMattia, & DiGiuseppe, 1989; Jacobson, 1984; Rathus & Sanderson, 1999) have worked to integrate cognitive restructuring strategies with behavioral marital therapy interventions to modify negative interaction patterns in distressed relationships. Also, preventive premarital programs such as Markman, Stanley, and Blumberg's (1994) Prevention and Relationship Enhancement Program combine components of communication skill training and modification of problematic cognitions such as unrealistic expectations about marriage (Halford & Moore, 2002). These cognitive-behavioral approaches focus on identifying and modifying problematic aspects of the moment-to-moment processes that occur as members of a couple interact. Our (Epstein & Baucom, 2002) recent book *Enhanced Cognitive-Behavioral Therapy for*

Couples: A Contextual Approach builds on traditional concepts and methods, but it expands the scope of the cognitive-behavioral model to encompass developmental changes in relationships as the partners attempt to adapt to demands from the partners' individual characteristics, the couple's dyadic patterns, and their physical and interpersonal environment. This model and its implications for clinical assessment and treatment are described later in this chapter.

Cognitive-behavioral assessment and treatment methods have been influenced by rapid growth in research on types of behavior, cognitions, and affect that may influence couples' levels of conflict and subjective distress. An extensive description of the research findings is beyond the scope of this chapter, but there are a number of published reviews available (Baucom & Epstein, 1990; Epstein & Baucom, 1993, 2002; Fincham, Bradbury, & Scott, 1990; Weiss & Heyman, 1990, 1997). Behavioral responses that have traditionally been foci of behavioral couple therapy and continue to be central in a cognitive-behavioral approach include (1) deficits in positive acts such as validation, affection, clear expression of thoughts and emotions, responses reflecting empathic listening, and positive problem solving; and (2) excesses of negative acts, such as blame, criticism, contempt, defensiveness, and withdrawal (Epstein & Baucom, 2002; Gottman, 1994; Weiss & Heyman, 1990, 1997). Concerning cognitive factors, we (Baucom, Epstein, Sayers, & Sher, 1989) identified five major types of cognition that have been implicated in relationship quality: (1) "selective perceptions" (in which the individual notices only a subset of the information available during couple interactions), (2) "attributions" (inferences about the causes of relationship events), (3) "expectancies" (predictions about future events in couple interactions), (4) "assumptions" (beliefs about the nature of relationships and the two partners), and (5) "standards" (beliefs about the characteristics that the relationship "should" have). Finally, aspects of emotion that have the potential to influence the quality of couple relationships include (1) awareness of one's emotional states and their relation to events in one's life, (2) ability to express feelings to one's partner effectively, and (3) ability to regulate the experience and expression of strong emotions (Epstein & Baucom, 2002). These types of behavior, cognition, and affect have become foci of cognitive-behavioral couple therapy (Epstein & Baucom, 2002; Rathus & Sanderson, 1999).

The remainder of this chapter describes typical components of cognitive-behavioral couple therapy, summarizes its empirical status, and describes recent theoretical and clinical developments. For greater detail, the reader is referred to publications that provide more extensive clinical descriptions and empirical evidence regarding cognitive-behavioral couple assessment and therapy (Baucom & Epstein, 1990; Baucom, Epstein, & LaTaillade, 2002; Baucom et al., 1998; Epstein & Baucom, 1998, 2002).

TRADITIONAL COGNITIVE-BEHAVIORAL TREATMENTS

A central premise of a cognitive-behavioral model of relationship dysfunction is that partners' satisfaction commonly depends on their actual positive versus negative behavior toward each other, their cognitions about each other and the relationship, and their emotional responses to each other. Theory and research on couples have identified particular types of behavior, cognition, and affect that can contribute to the development of distress and the dissolution of intimate relationships. Based on this theoretical and research foundation, cognitive-behavioral couple therapy includes interventions intended to modify behaviors, cognitions, and emotions that are contributing to a couple's problems. The following are brief summaries of typical types of interventions.

Interventions for Modifying Behavior

We (Epstein & Baucom, 2002) have divided the standard types of interventions used for modifying partners' behavioral interactions into two major categories: (1) "guided behavior change" and (2) "skills-based interventions." Guided behavior change involves the therapist's helping the couple to identify and to implement changes in excesses of negative behavior and deficits of positive behavior in their interactions through structured efforts during daily life. Based on social exchange theory (Thibaut & Kelley, 1959) and research supporting it (Weiss & Heyman 1990, 1997), relationship satisfaction is a function of the ratio of pleasing to displeasing acts occurring between partners. A number of interventions developed by behavioral marital therapists (e.g., Jacobson & Margolin, 1979; Liberman, Levine, Wheeler, Sanders, & Wallace, 1976; Stuart, 1980) can be used to increase the proportion of positive to negative acts that partners direct toward each other.

Behavioral contracting involves the two partners' making specific agreements, often in writing, to exchange particular positive acts that each person desires from the other. Whereas earlier versions of behavioral contracts involved a quid pro quo agreement in which each person's positive changes were contingent on the other person's making his or her own positive changes, behavioral therapists moved toward the use of contracts in which each partner made a commitment to change regardless of what the other person did (Jacobson & Margolin, 1979). The procedure of "love days" (Weiss, Hops, & Patterson, 1973) or "caring days" (Stuart, 1980) involves a person's agreeing to take responsibility for behaving during a particular day in a variety of ways intended to please his or her partner, without any prior specification of what those positive acts will be or exactly when they will occur. We (Baucom & Epstein, 1990) also described procedures for coaching couples who engage in relatively few mutually pleasing joint activities toward greater involvement in such activities. In some cases, over time a couple has stopped engaging in mutually satisfying activities that the partners shared earlier in their relationship, often due to competing demands on their time from their jobs and child rearing. In other cases, joint activities that contributed to intimacy in the past have lost their reinforcing quality, and there is a need for the couple to find new activities. In either case, if a couple has difficulty generating new "bonding" experiences, a therapist can provide a list of various activities that the partners may share (e.g., going for walks together, viewing a movie together) and coach them in selecting some to try. Finally, members of distressed couples often fail to provide each other with forms of social support, and therapists can assist them in identifying the types of support that they would find helpful when facing personal problems, and in communicating those needs to each other (Epstein & Baucom, 2002). Then the partners can focus on giving each other the desired types of support, such as sympathetic listening, physical comfort and affection, or direct assistance in solving a problem. As with the other forms of guided behavior change, these planned supportive actions do not involve training in any specific skills, but they address deficits in pleasing behavior exchanged by the members of a couple.

The major forms of skills-based interventions are training in communication skills and in problem-solving skills. Most often couple therapists teach partners specific skills for expressing their thoughts and emotions, as well as skills for empathic listening (Baucom & Epstein, 1990; Epstein & Baucom, 1989, 2002; Jacobson & Margolin, 1979; Stuart, 1980). The major steps that a therapist uses in skills training are (1) educating the couple about problematic and constructive behavior involved in the particular skill, (2) modeling the behavioral skills for the partners, (3) coaching the partners and giving them corrective feedback as they practice the skills during therapy sessions, and (4) having the couple practice the skills in daily life. Although behavioral marital therapists sometimes assumed that distressed couples had skill deficits in these areas that required remediation, it is recognized that some individuals possess the skills and exhibit them with people other than their intimate partners. Sometimes partners fail to exhibit effective communication and problem-solving skills due to other circumstances, such as a conscious decision to behave aversively in order to punish a partner. The Epstein and Baucom (2002) book includes strategies that therapists can use to address the cognitive and affective factors interfering with couples' use of constructive communication and problem-solving skills.

Interventions for Modifying Cognitions

For the most part, the interventions that are used to modify inappropriate or distorted cognitions in couple therapy are similar to those used in individual cognitive therapy (Beck, Rush, Shaw, & Emery, 1979; J. S. Beck, 1995; Leahy, 1996). Some involve Socratic questioning, in which the therapist directs the partners in examining the logic or evidence bearing on the validity of their thoughts regarding each other and their relationship; others involve "guided discovery," in which the therapist sets up experiences for the partners that provide new data for them to consider, which may support or be inconsistent with their prevailing views. A fundamental difference between cognitive restructuring efforts with a couple and those with an individual is the effect that the presence of an individual's partner has on the person's openness to considering alternatives to his or her existing cognitions. As we (Epstein & Baucom, 2002) have described, members of distressed couples have commonly accused each other of holding distorted views, so they are both likely to become defensive if a therapist challenges their thinking in a conjoint session. Consequently, couple therapists must walk a fine line between guiding each person in examining the validity or appropriateness of his or her thinking and providing support and validation for both individuals.

Several interventions are used by couple therapists to modify partners' problematic cognitions. For detailed descriptions of these and other interventions, the reader can consult the Epstein and Baucom (2002) text. Much as in individual cognitive therapy, a therapist can coach each partner in evaluating personal experiences and logic that may support or contradict a particular distressing cognition. As an example of evaluating personal experiences, when an individual states that his or her partner "never shows any appreciation for the things I do," and the partner protests that this is untrue, the therapist can point out that the term "never" means "not ever, in any form, in any situation" and can ask the individual to think about any possible exceptions to that absolute statement. The person's partner often will present examples of such exceptions, and the therapist can refer to this as "useful input" to consider in evaluating whether the original "never" descriptor is appropriate.

An intervention that focuses on the utility of thinking in a particular way involves weighing the advantages and disadvantages of a cognition. This approach is often used to increase partners' awareness of the consequences of trying to live according to standards that are unrealistic or inappropriate for the couple's real-life circumstances. For example, a therapist might coach an individual in listing advantages and disadvantages of his or her belief that the two partners should share in all of each other's personal interests in order to achieve intimacy.

When partners exhibit negative emotional and behavioral responses that appear to be based on negative expectancies regarding events that they anticipate will occur in their relationship, the therapist can coach them in considering the worst and best possible outcomes in those situations. Thus, if an individual predicts that his or her partner will reject any attempts that the person may make to provide emotional support (e.g., words of reassurance or caring, a hug, an offer to listen empathically), the therapist can encourage the individual to think of the worst possible consequences that could occur if he or she did offer the partner such support. The therapist then can challenge this catastrophizing with questions such as "Is it possible that your partner will accept your support?", "What is the worst thing that would happen to you if your partner did reject your offer of support?", or "How might it be useful to learn that you can tolerate it if your partner rejects your offer of support?" (Leahy, 1996). In addition, the therapist can coach the couple in setting up a behavioral experiment to test the individual's negative expectancy; for example, the couple might agree to observe how the partner responds if the individual offers the partner some form of emotional support the next time the partner reveals a personal problem (J. S. Beck, 1995).

We (Epstein & Baucom, 2002) also describe how a therapist may modify partners' cognitions through forms of psychoeducation, including "mini-lectures," readings, and videos. For example, when working with a couple who have formed a stepfamily and are in conflict about the role that each partner should play in disciplining the other's children, a therapist might ask the partners to read popular books on common stressors and coping in stepfamilies (e.g., Berman, 1986; Visher & Visher, 1982). The therapist also might present a brief "mini-lecture" on what is known from research on special adjustments that couples face in stepfamilies, and strategies that couples have used to resolve such issues.

The downward-arrow technique (Burns, 1980) can be used to identify the basic meanings that partners attach to events they find upsetting in their interactions. Thus, when an individual becomes angry when the partner forgets to pay some of the couple's bills on time, the therapist may ask questions with the theme "And if that occurs, what does it mean to you?" The person may respond with the thought "Then it would mean that she is irresponsible and I cannot rely on her for anything important." The therapist then can coach the individual in considering alternative explanations (attributions) for the partner's distressing actions.

Among the hallmarks of cognitive restructuring in couple therapy are interventions designed to increase partners' "relational thinking"—the tendency to notice and construe the circular process of mutual influence between the members of the couple (Epstein & Baucom, 2002). For example, in order to counteract the general tendency for distressed partners to blame each other for relationship problems, the therapist coaches them in thinking about alternative attributions, including ways in which each partner's own actions influence those of the other. The therapist also may point out sequences in the couple's interactions in which each person both responded to and elicited the other's actions. Videotape playback of the couple's interactions can vividly demonstrate dyadic patterns to the couple.

Finally, a therapist can help a couple identify macro-level patterns (such as boundary issues) that are sources of conflict and distress because the partners attach significant meanings to them. The couple can become aware of the macro-level patterns in the relationship as the therapist coaches them in observing cross-situational patterns. Thus a review of circumstances associated with several arguments may reveal that the members of a couple desire different degrees of sharing/togetherness versus independence, and awareness of this core theme can help the couple problem-solve about ways to achieve a mutually acceptable balance in this area.

Interventions for Modifying Deficits and Excesses in Experiencing and Expressing Emotions

Emotion is a key aspect of intimate relationships, and cognitive-behavioral couple therapists target both deficits and excesses in partners' tendencies to experience and express affect. The following are representative interventions, and the reader can find more extensive descriptions in the Epstein and Baucom (2002) text.

When an individual has difficulty noticing and expressing positive and negative emotions within the relationship, the therapist can use a variety of interventions for accessing and heightening emotional experience. These include normalizing emotional experience when an individual holds a belief that emotions are abnormal, a sign of weakness, or the like. For individuals who are aware of their thoughts but not their emotions, the therapist can coach them in clarifying their thoughts in particular situations (especially as they occur during sessions) and then relate automatic thoughts to emotions that occur at the moment. The therapist can also use questions, reflections, and interpretations to draw out unexpressed "primary" emotions that underlie expressed emotions—for example, hurt feelings that tend to be masked by expressions of anger. The therapist can track and discourage an individual's attempts to distract him- or herself from experiencing emotion during couple sessions. Furthermore, the therapist can encourage acceptance of an inhibited individual's experience by the partner.

In contrast, when partners have difficulty containing their experience and expression of intense negative emotions, the therapist can coach the couple in scheduling times to discuss emotions, using "time outs" or mutually agreed-upon breaks from each other as needed, engaging in self-soothing activities (e.g., exercise, a bath, listening to music), calming self-instruction, and exposure practice in tolerating distressing feelings. In addition, the therapist can coach the couple in constructive means for communicating emotions.

THEORETICAL AND CLINICAL DEVELOPMENTS

The Epstein and Baucom (2002) text describes an enhanced cognitive-behavioral couple therapy that expands the traditional foci on assessment and modification of forms of behavior, cognition, and affect that contribute to relationship problems. First, traditional cognitive-behavioral therapy has focused on couples' dyadic interaction patterns, but the enhanced model gives equal weighting to characteristics of the two individuals and of the physical and interpersonal environment that influence the couple's functioning. Characteristics of the individuals include their unique learning histories and unresolved issues from prior relationships, their communally and individually oriented needs, their interaction styles, and their psychopathology. The couple's dyadic characteristics include communication and other behavioral patterns (e.g., mutual attack, demand–withdraw, mutual withdrawal) that affect the couple's ability to resolve issues. Their physical environment (e.g., housing conditions, a violent neighborhood) and interpersonal environment (e.g., children, extended family, friends, larger community, social institutions such as schools) may place demands on the couple, but also may provide resources that can help the couple cope with life stressors.

The Epstein and Baucom (2002) enhanced cognitive-behavioral model for couple therapy also includes a developmental perspective, in which it is assumed that the two individuals and their relationship change over time, requiring them to adapt. This adaptation requires cognitive and behavioral flexibility, which some couples possess to a greater degree than others, but which therapy may enhance. For example, in the early stages of their relationship, the members of a young couple may have little difficulty fulfilling their personal standard that partners should demonstrate caring and commitment to each other by spending a great deal of leisure time together. However, as they have their first child and face increasing demands from their careers, resulting in far fewer intimate experiences as a couple, they may feel distant from each other and dissatisfied with their relationship. The more that they cling to their original standards regarding the qualities of a close relationship, the more distressed they are likely to become. Couple therapy not only can foster behavioral changes that can restore some intimate interaction; it also can involve cognitive restructuring to modify standards that have become unrealistic for the couple's current life, and to modify partners' negative attributions that their increased involvement in work and other competing activities is due to a lack of love for each other.

Enhanced cognitive-behavioral couple therapy also distinguishes between partners' micro-level responses versus macro-level patterns and themes. Micro-level responses are discrete distressing and pleasing acts, whereas macro-level patterns are repetitive and cross-situational, and have core meanings and significance for the partners. As described earlier, macro-level patterns such as boundaries, investment in the relationship, and distribution of power are typically reflected in partners' micro-level acts in various situations. We (Epstein & Baucom, 2002) propose that traditional interventions for modifying partners' micro-level behavior and cognitions have the most impact on a couple's satisfaction when they address the partners' macro-level concerns. For example, an individual who receives empathic listening from a partner regarding a personal problem is likely to experience it as pleasing and meaningful if he or she interprets it as a reflection of the partner's overall caring and investment in their relationship.

We (Epstein & Baucom, 2002) also distinguish between "primary distress" in a relationship due to unresolved core relationship issues, such as a difference in partners' needs for autonomy and togetherness, and "secondary distress" resulting from dyadic patterns (e.g., mutual attack) that the couple has developed in attempts to resolve the core issues. It is important to modify the negative interactions associated with secondary distress initially in therapy, in order to create the conditions that the partners need to find better solutions to their core unresolved issues.

Finally, the enhanced cognitive-behavioral model balances the traditional focus on relationship problems with an increased focus on strengths and positive experiences in the couple's relationship. Decreasing sources of partners' distress is crucial, but couples usually want to experience more than an absence of negatives in their relationship. A therapist can assess and build on a couple's existing strengths and resources, and can help the couple enrich the relationship. Interventions that traditionally have been considered to be within the domain of relationship education and enrichment (Halford & Moore, 2002; van Widenfelt, Markman, Guerney, Behrens, & Hosman, 1997) can be used by therapists in conjunction with interventions for problems to enhance distressed couples' relationships.

EVIDENCE OF THE EFFECTIVENESS OF COGNITIVE-BEHAVIORAL COUPLE THERAPY

To date, most of the outcome studies on cognitive-behavioral couple therapy have tested the effects of the behavioral components: training in communication skills for expression and listening, training in problem solving, and forms of behavioral contracts. Reviews of these studies have indicated that these behavioral interventions are more effective than either waiting-list control conditions or nonspecific or placebo treatments in increasing self-reported relationship satisfaction (e.g., Baucom et al., 1998; Dunn & Schwebel, 1995; Hahlweg & Markman, 1988; Shadish et al., 1993).

Following treatment, from one-third to two-thirds of couples score in the nondistressed range on self-report measures of relationship satisfaction. Unfortunately, only a limited number of studies have included follow-up assessments, and these have indicated that approximately a third of the treated couples exhibit relapses in their levels of distress.

Only a few studies—none recent and none investigating the recent theoretical and clinical developments described in the Epstein and Baucom (2002) book—have tested the effects of interventions focused on modifying couples' negative cognitions, and only two of the published studies (Emmelkamp et al., 1988; Huber & Milstein, 1985) tested cognitive restructuring interventions that were not combined with any behavioral interventions. In Huber and Milstein's (1985) study, 17 distressed community couples were randomly assigned either to six weekly sessions of cognitive restructuring that focused on modifying unrealistic beliefs about individual and relationship functioning, or to a waiting-list control condition. The cognitive restructuring involved didactic presentations on negative impacts of unrealistic beliefs, as well as exercises in which partners identified and challenged their own unrealistic beliefs. The results indicated that the couples in the cognitive restructuring group had a significantly greater increase in marital adjustment and a significantly greater decrease in adherence to unrealistic relationship beliefs than couples in the control group. The investigators did not conduct a follow-up assessment. In the Emmelkamp et al. (1988) study, behavioral marital therapy was compared with cognitive restructuring that was focused on modifying unrealistic relationship beliefs. No difference was found between the two treatments' effects on partners' self-reported levels of marital adjustment.

Three other studies have examined cognitive-behavioral treatments involving combinations of cognitive restructuring and behavioral interventions. All of these studies have found the combined interventions to be equivalent to solely behavioral interventions in decreasing couples' distress. However, because the sample sizes in the studies were fairly small, they had limited statistical power for detecting differences between the treatment conditions. The following are brief descriptions of the studies.

Baucom and Lester (1986) randomly assigned 24 distressed couples to (1) 12 weeks of behavioral interventions (problem-solving training, communication training, and behavioral contracting); (2) 6 weeks of cognitive restructuring followed by 6 weeks of the behavioral interventions; or (3) a waiting-list control condition. During cognitive restructuring sessions, the therapists gave didactic presentations about problems that occur when partners blame each other for relationship problems and attribute each other's negative behavior to global, stable causes. Therapists also described negative effects of applying unrealistic beliefs to one's relationship. Both during and between sessions, couples explored their own problematic attributions and potentially unrealistic beliefs concerning issues in their own relationships. In the Baucom, Sayers, and Sher (1990) study, 60 distressed couples were randomly assigned to (1) six sessions of problem-solving skill training plus six sessions of behavioral contracting; (2) six sessions of cognitive restructuring regarding negative attributions and unrealistic relationship standards, three sessions of problem-solving training, and three sessions of contracting; (3) three sessions of problem-solving training, three sessions of behavioral contracting, and six sessions of training in expressive and listening skills; or (4) three sessions of cognitive restructuring, three of problem-solving training, three of contracting, and three of expressive and listening skill training.

The overall findings from both studies by Baucom and his associates were that couples were most likely to improve on the factors (e.g., unrealistic beliefs, negative communication behavior) that were targeted in the interventions. Although all treated groups improved, no intervention combination was superior to the others in improving self-reported marital adjustment and coded communication behavior. In addition to conducting tests of statistical significance among group means on the outcome measures, Baucom et al. (1990) used criteria for clinical improvement on the Dyadic Adjustment Scale (DAS; Spanier, 1976) for each individual of (1) at least a 1.96 standard error improvement, and (2) movement into the accepted nondistressed range of scores on the DAS. Across the four treatment combinations (with no differences among treatments), 69% of the women and 56% of the men exhibited at least a 1.96 standard error improvement, and 54% of the women and 46% of the men were also nondistressed on the DAS at the end of therapy.

Taken together, the findings from these two studies sometimes have been interpreted as indicating that adding cognitive restructuring to traditional behavioral interventions does not improve the effectiveness of couple therapy. However, such a conclusion does not take into account the fact that in order to keep the total number of sessions constant across groups in the studies, the researchers had to reduce the numbers of sessions devoted to one type of intervention in order to add another type of intervention. For example, adding six sessions of cognitive restructuring required a reduction in the number of sessions of behavioral interventions. Consequently, it is questionable whether couples in the combined cognitive-behavioral condition received sufficient amounts of any of the cognitive and behavioral interventions. Thus it is unlikely that three sessions of intervention can have a substantial influence on partners' long-standing relationship beliefs. Another potential limitation of the cognitive restructuring used in the studies is that it involved standard skill-building modules administered to all couples at the same point, without consideration for their relevance for each couple's needs.

The findings of these studies are encouraging evidence that cognitive restructuring interventions provide effects that are comparable to those from behavioral interventions. However, the treatments that were compared differ substantially in amount and content from cognitive-behavioral interventions that clinicians typically tailor to the needs of individual couples.

In the only other published controlled outcome study comparing a combined cognitive-behavioral intervention with solely behavioral treatment, Halford et al. (1993) assigned 26 distressed couples to between 12 and 15 weekly sessions of either behavioral marital therapy or a combination treatment involving behavioral interventions, cognitive restructuring, exploration of affect, and generalization training. The cognitive restructuring was applied in a more flexible manner, more typical of clinical practice, than in the studies by Baucom and his associates. The therapist identified each couple's problematic relationship beliefs and attributions, and used Socratic questioning, techniques challenging the logic of partners' negative cognitions, and self-instructional training to modify those cognitions. In the combination treatment, the therapist also varied the sequence and amount of time devoted to each type of intervention for each couple, according to clinical assessment of the couple's needs. Both forms of treatment resulted in significant improvements on partners' self-reports of marital satisfaction, unrealistic relationship beliefs, and negative thoughts about their partners, as well as on coders' ratings of couples' negative behavior during discussions of conflictual issues in their relationships. Overall the two treatments produced minimal differences on the outcome measures, and they showed no difference in percentages of individuals who exhibited clinically significant change on the DAS as defined earlier. Across the treatments, 73% of the males and 65% of the females improved by at least 1.96 standard errors on the DAS, and 54% of the males and 42% of the females were in the nondistressed range on the DAS at the end of therapy. However, the purely behavioral treatment resulted in a significantly greater decrease in negative behavioral interactions between partners than the intervention that included cognitive restructuring, affect exploration, and generalization training. As in the studies by Baucom and associates, it appears that introducing multiple types of interventions while holding the total number of sessions relatively constant may dilute the effectiveness of each type of intervention.

According to the current criteria developed by Chambless and Hollon (1998) for judging the efficacy of therapeutic interventions, a treatment is labeled "possibly efficacious" if it has been found to be superior to a waiting-list control condition in a single study, or in more than one study by the same research team, but has not been found to be superior to an alternative active treatment. Because only one research team (Baucom and colleagues) included a waiting-list condition in the design, current research results suggest that cognitive-behavioral couple therapy is most appropriately viewed as "possibly efficacious." Unfortunately, this conclusion is based on a very small number of existing outcome studies, and at present there is no evidence that the body of outcome research in this area is increasing.

Concerning long-term effects of cognitive-behavioral couple therapy, few of the small number of existing studies have included follow-up assessments, and the results of those follow-ups have been mixed. Couples in Baucom et al.'s (1990) study exhibited no significant changes in self-reported marital adjustment from posttherapy to a 6–month follow-up (i.e., changes tended to be stable). Posttherapy gains in the Halford et al. (1993) study were maintained or enhanced on some outcome measures but not others at a 3–month follow-up. Specifically, stable or enhanced gains were found for marital satisfaction, positive feelings toward one's partner, and reduced requests for partner behavior change, for men but not for women. In addition, reductions in unrealistic beliefs continued for both sexes at follow-up. There were no differences between the pure behavioral treatment and the enhanced treatment at follow-up. Halford et al. found some relapse in clinically significant change, with 42% of the males and 39% of the females still reporting significant improvement on the DAS, and 31% of the males and 27% of the females still in the nondistressed range. Until more studies that include follow-up assessments are conducted on cognitive-behavioral couple therapy, no conclusion can be drawn about lasting treatment effects.

DIRECTIONS FOR FUTURE RESEARCH

Given the increasing popularity of cognitive-behavioral interventions with couples, the relative lack of outcome studies is problematic. In addition to the overall need for basic controlled outcome studies to test the impact of therapy on cognitive, affective, and behavioral aspects of couples' functioning, there is a need for studies that examine a number of more specific questions.

Although future studies should examine whether there are benefits to matching treatments to the types of deficits (e.g., poor communication skills) that couples present, Whisman and Snyder (1997) argue that interventions can also be matched to couples' areas of strength. Thus couples who already track and challenge their own thinking may make better use of cognitive restructuring interventions than those who are less introspective.

Whisman and Snyder (1997) note that outcome studies are generally limited by their reliance on measures that define success solely in terms of partners' staying together and feeling satisfied being together. There is evidence that partners who begin therapy more severely distressed or emotionally disengaged from each other have more negative therapy outcomes, in terms of posttherapy DAS scores and decisions to dissolve their relationships (Snyder, Mangrum, & Wills, 1993). Thus for some partners a more favorable outcome may be ending the relationship and being satisfied with the direction of one's individual life, rather than decreasing dissatisfaction with the relationship. Consequently, Whisman and Snyder recommend goal attainment scaling (Kiresuk, Smith, & Cardillo, 1994) to assess the degree to which partners' individual goals for therapy have been achieved.

There is also a need for research on characteristics of couples that might affect the effectiveness of cognitive-behavioral couple therapy. Studies that have tested for gender effects have found minimal differences, and those that have examined other demographic characteristics as predictors of couple therapy outcome have produced mixed findings for age, education, occupational status, socioeconomic status, length of marriage, number of previous marriages, and number of children (Snyder et al., 1993). In contrast, little is known about such characteristics as personal relationship standards, attributional styles, and forms of psychopathology (e.g., depression) as moderators of couple therapy impact.

Finally, the studies indicating that behavioral and cognitive-behavioral treatments are equally efficacious have been conducted only in Western cultures (Baucom et al., 1998). At present, nothing is known about the impact that cognitive-behavioral couple therapy may have on couples from different cultures, such as those that emphasize collectivist values, in contrast to the individualistic values of the Western cultures within which the treatment model has been developed. Cross-cultural treatment outcome research is clearly needed.

The practice of cognitive-behavioral couple therapy has outpaced empirical investigations of its efficacy. Further refinement of interventions and clinical decision making will require additional research evidence about what works, and for whom.

REFERENCES

Baucom, D. H., & Epstein, N. (1990). *Cognitive-behavioral marital therapy*. New York: Brunner/Mazel.

Baucom, D. H., Epstein, N., & LaTaillade, J. J. (2002). Cognitive-behavioral couple therapy. In A. S. Gurman & N. S. Jacobson (Eds.), *Clinical handbook of couple therapy* (3rd ed., pp. 26–58). New York: Guilford Press.

Baucom, D. H., Epstein, N., Rankin, L. A., & Burnett, C. K. (1996). Assessing relationship standards: The Inventory of Specific Relationship Standards. *Journal of Family Psychology, 10*, 72–88.

Baucom, D. H., Epstein, N., Sayers, S., & Sher, T. G. (1989). The role of cognitions in marital relationships: Definitional, methodological, and conceptual issues. *Journal of Consulting and Clinical Psychology, 57,* 31–38.

Baucom, D. H., & Lester, G. W. (1986). The usefulness of cognitive restructuring as an adjunct to behavioral marital therapy. *Behavior Therapy, 17,* 385–403.

Baucom, D. H., Sayers, S. L., & Sher, T. G. (1990). Supplementing behavioral marital therapy with cognitive restructuring and emotional expressiveness training: An outcome investigation. *Journal of Consulting and Clinical Psychology, 58,* 636–645.

Baucom, D. H., Shoham, V., Mueser, K. T., Daiuto, A. D., & Stickle, T. R. (1998). Empirically supported couple and family interventions for marital distress and adult mental health problems. *Journal of Consulting and Clinical Psychology, 66,* 53–88.

Beck, A. T. (1988). *Love is never enough.* New York: Harper & Row.

Beck, A. T., Rush, A. J., Shaw, B. F., & Emery, G. (1979). *Cognitive therapy of depression.* New York: Guilford Press.

Beck, J. S. (1995). *Cognitive therapy: Basics and beyond.* New York: Guilford Press.

Berman, C. (1986). *Making it as a stepparent: New roles/new rules.* New York: Harper & Row.

Bradbury, T. N., & Fincham, F. D. (1993). Assessing dysfunctional cognition in marriage: A reconsideration of the Relationship Belief Inventory. *Psychological Assessment, 5,* 92–101.

Burns, D. D. (1980). *Feeling good: The new mood therapy.* New York: Morrow.

Chambless, D. L., & Hollon, S. D. (1998). Defining empirically supported therapies. *Journal of Consulting and Clinical Psychology, 66,* 7–18.

Christensen, A., & Shenk, J. L. (1991). Communication, conflict, and psychological distance in nondistressed, clinic, and divorcing couples. *Journal of Consulting and Clinical Psychology, 59,* 458–463.

Dattilio, F. M., & Padesky, C. A. (1990). *Cognitive therapy with couples.* Sarasota, FL: Professional Resource Exchange.

Doherty, W. J. (1981a). Cognitive processes in intimate conflict: I. Extending attribution theory. *American Journal of Family Therapy, 9*(1), 5–13.

Doherty, W. J. (1981b). Cognitive processes in intimate conflict: II. Efficacy and learned helplessness. *American Journal of Family Therapy, 9*(2), 35–44.

Dunn, R. L., & Schwebel, A. I. (1995). Meta-analytic review of marital therapy outcome research. *Journal of Family Psychology, 9,* 58–68.

Eidelson, R. J., & Epstein, N. (1982). Cognition and relationship maladjustment: Development of a measure of dysfunctional relationship beliefs. *Journal of Consulting and Clinical Psychology, 50,* 715–720.

Ellis, A., Sichel, J. L., Yeager, R. J., DiMattia, D. J., & DiGiuseppe, R. (1989). *Rational–emotive couples therapy.* New York: Pergamon Press.

Emmelkamp, P. M. G., van Linden van den Heuvell, C., Ruphan, M., Sanderman, R., Scholing, A., & Stroink, F. (1988). Cognitive and behavioral interventions: A comparative evaluation with clinically distressed couples. *Journal of Family Psychology, 1,* 365–377.

Epstein, N. (1982). Cognitive therapy with couples. *American Journal of Family Therapy, 10*(1), 5–16.

Epstein, N., & Baucom, D. H. (1989). Cognitive-behavioral marital therapy. In A. Freeman, K. M. Simon, H. Arkowitz, & L. Beutler (Eds.), *Comprehensive handbook of cognitive therapy* (pp. 491–513). New York: Plenum Press.

Epstein, N., & Baucom, D. H. (1993). Cognitive factors in marital disturbance. In K. S. Dobson & P. C. Kendall (Eds.), *Psychopathology and cognition* (pp. 351–385). San Diego, CA: Academic Press.

Epstein, N., & Baucom, D. H. (1998). Cognitive-behavioral couple therapy. In F. M. Dattilio (Ed.), *Case studies in couple and family therapy: Systemic and cognitive perspectives* (pp. 37–61). New York: Guilford Press.

Epstein, N., & Eidelson, R. J. (1981). Unrealistic beliefs of clinical couples: Their relationship to expectations, goals and satisfaction. *American Journal of Family Therapy, 9*(4), 13–22.

Epstein, N., Pretzer, J. L., & Fleming, B. (1982, November). *Cognitive therapy and communication training: Comparison of effects with distressed couples.* Paper presented at the annual meeting of the Association for Advancement of Behavior Therapy, Los Angeles.

Epstein, N. B., & Baucom, D. H. (2002). *Enhanced cognitive-behavioral therapy for couples: A contextual approach.* Washington, DC: American Psychological Association.

Fincham, F. D., Bradbury, T. N., & Scott, C. K. (1990). Cognition in marriage. In F. D. Fincham & T. N. Bradbury (Eds.), *The psychology of marriage: Basic issues and applications* (pp. 118–149). New York: Guilford Press.

Gottman, J. M. (1994). *What predicts divorce?: The relationship between marital processes and marital outcomes.* Hillsdale, NJ: Erlbaum.

Greenberg, L. S., & Johnson, S. M. (1988). *Emotionally focused therapy for couples.* New York: Guilford Press.

Hahlweg, K., & Markman, H. J. (1988). Effectiveness of behavioral marital therapy: Empirical status of behavioral techniques in preventing and alleviating marital distress. *Journal of Consulting and Clinical Psychology, 56,* 440–447.

Halford, W. K., & Moore, E. N. (2002). Relationship education and the prevention of couple relationship problems. In A. S. Gurman & N. S. Jacobson (Eds.), *Clinical handbook of couple therapy* (3rd ed., pp. 400–419). New York: Guilford Press.

Halford, W. K., Sanders, M. R., & Behrens, B. C. (1993). A comparison of the generalization of behavioral marital therapy and enhanced behavioral marital therapy. *Journal of Consulting and Clinical Psychology, 61,* 51–60.

Huber, C. H., & Milstein, B. (1985). Cognitive restructuring and a collaborative set in couples' work. *American Journal of Family Therapy, 13*(2), 17–27.

Iverson, A., & Baucom, D. H. (1990). Behavioral marital therapy outcomes: Alternate interpretations of the data. *Behavior Therapy, 21,* 129–138.

Jacobson, N. S. (1984). The modification of cognitive processes in behavioral marital therapy: Integrating cognitive and behavioral intervention strategies. In K. Hahlweg & N. S. Jacobson (Eds.), *Marital interaction: Analysis and modification* (pp. 285–308). New York: Guilford Press.

Jacobson, N. S., & Margolin, G. (1979). *Marital therapy: Strategies based on social learning and behavior exchange principles.* New York: Brunner/Mazel.

Johnson, S. M., & Denton, W. (2002). Emotionally focused couple therapy: Creating secure connections. In A. S. Gurman & N. S. Jacobson (Eds.), *Clinical handbook of couple therapy* (3rd ed., pp. 221–250). New York: Guilford Press.

Johnson, S. M., & Greenberg, L. S. (1985). Differential effects of experiential and problem-solving interventions in resolving marital conflict. *Journal of Consulting and Clinical Psychology, 53*, 175–184.

Kiresuk, T. J., Smith, A., & Cardillo, J. E. (1994). *Goal attainment scaling: Applications, theory, and measurement.* Hillsdale, NJ: Erlbaum.

Leahy, R. (1996). *Cognitive therapy: Basic principles and applications.* Northvale, NJ: Aronson.

Liberman, R., Levine, J., Wheeler, E., Sanders, N., & Wallace, C. J. (1976). Marital therapy in groups: A comparative evaluation of behavioral and interaction formats. *Acta Psychiatrica Scandinavica, 266*(Suppl.), 1–34.

Markman, H., Stanley, S., & Blumberg, S. L. (1994). *Fighting for your marriage.* San Francisco: Jossey-Bass.

Notarius, C. I., & Markman, H. J. (1993). *We can work it out: Making sense of marital conflict.* New York: Putnam.

Pretzer, J., Epstein, N., & Fleming, B. (1991). Marital Attitude Survey: A measure of dysfunctional attributions and expectancies. *Journal of Cognitive Psychotherapy: An International Quarterly, 5*, 131–148.

Rathus, J. H., & Sanderson, W. C. (1999). *Marital distress: Cognitive behavioral interventions for couples.* Northvale, NJ: Aronson.

Shadish, W. R., Montgomery, L. M., Wilson, P., Wilson, M. R., Bright, I., & Okwumabua, T. (1993). Effects of family and marital psychotherapies: A meta-analysis. *Journal of Consulting and Clinical Psychology, 61*, 992–1002.

Snyder, D. K., Mangrum, L. F., & Wills, R. M. (1993). Predicting couples' response to marital therapy: A comparison of short- and long-term predictors. *Journal of Consulting and Clinical Psychology, 61*, 61–69.

Snyder, D. K., & Wills, R. M. (1989). Behavioral versus insight-oriented marital therapy: Effects on individual and interspousal functioning. *Journal of Consulting and Clinical Psychology, 57*, 39–46.

Snyder, D. K., Wills, R. M., & Grady-Fletcher, A. (1991). Long-term effectiveness of behavioral versus insight-oriented marital therapy: A 4-year follow-up study. *Journal of Consulting and Clinical Psychology, 59*, 138–141.

Spanier, G. B. (1976). Measuring dyadic adjustment: New scales for assessing the quality of marriage and similar dyads. *Journal of Marriage and the Family, 38*, 15–28.

Stuart, R. B. (1980). *Helping couples change: A social learning approach to marital therapy.* New York: Guilford Press.

Thibaut, J. W., & Kelley, H. H. (1959). *The social psychology of groups.* New York: Wiley.

Todd, T. C. (1986). Structural–strategic marital therapy. In N. S. Jacobson & A. S. Gurman (Eds.), *Clinical handbook of marital therapy* (pp. 71–105). New York: Guilford Press.

van Widenfelt, B., Markman, H. J., Guerney, B., Behrens, B. C., & Hosman, C. (1997). Prevention of relationship problems. In W. K. Halford & H. J. Markman

(Eds.), *Clinical handbook of marriage and couples interventions* (pp. 651–675). Chichester, UK: Wiley.

Visher, E. B., & Visher, J. S. (1982). *How to win as a stepfamily*. New York: Dembner Books.

Weiss, R. L., & Heyman, R. E. (1990). Observation of marital interaction. In F. D. Fincham & T. N. Bradbury (Eds.), *The psychology of marriage: Basic issues and applications* (pp. 87–117). New York: Guilford Press.

Weiss, R. L., & Heyman, R. E. (1997). A clinical-research overview of couples interactions. In W. K. Halford & H. J. Markman (Eds.), *Clinical handbook of marriage and couples interventions* (pp. 13–41). Chichester, UK: Wiley.

Weiss, R. L., Hops, H., & Patterson, G. R. (1973). A framework for conceptualizing marital conflict, a technology for altering it, some data for evaluating it. In L. A. Hamerlynck, L. C. Handy, & E. J. Mash (Eds.), *Behavior change: Methodology, concepts and practice* (pp. 309–342). Champaign, IL: Research Press.

Whisman, M. A., & Snyder, D. K. (1997). Evaluating and improving the efficacy of conjoint couple therapy. In W. K. Halford & H. J. Markman (Eds.), *Clinical handbook of marriage and couples interventions* (pp. 679–693). New York: Wiley.

Chapter 18

Cognitive-Behavioral Family Therapy

A Coming-of-Age Story

FRANK M. DATTILIO

The use of cognitive-behavioral therapy (CBT) with families has met with especially harsh criticism in the past, particularly in the field of family therapy. In the early 1980s, I had an experience that really brought its rejection home. I had submitted my application for a special credential to the American Association for Marriage and Family Therapy (AAMFT), the primary association in the United States for qualifying marital (or, more recently, couple) and family therapists prior to the licensing laws that now exist in all but six states and the District of Columbia (Northey, 2002). Upon receiving my clinical membership, I applied for an additional credential known as "Approved Supervisor" status, which called for a sample of my work (a case study). Each applicant was required to declare a modality, and to provide a discussion of his or her experience as a supervisor in that modality. My work sample was rejected by the committee because of what was deemed to be "inadequate theory." When I wrote to the president of the organization in appeal, I received a telephone call from one of the board members, who informed me that my work sample was declined because the committee didn't feel that CBT, in and of itself, was very effective with families. It was the committee's decision that I should rewrite my case example, integrating CBT with one of the more "acceptable" models of family therapy, such as the systems theory. As I look back, I realize that the decision and the subsequent request for an amended case no doubt reflected a bias on the part of the committee; nevertheless, I grudgingly acquiesced and resubmitted my work. This time, it was approved. As fate would have it, the integration of these two modalities would eventually become a foundation for my work in family therapy, despite the fact that I firmly believe that CBT can hold its own as a sole modality when applied to certain families.

My experience was not uncommon. Early in the family therapy movement, the behavior and cognitive therapies were given little credence by classical systems theorists, who saw them as lacking the necessary depth to deal with underlying dynamics and family dysfunction (Dattilio, 1998a; 2001). Since that time, AAMFT and the couple and family therapy community have definitely warmed to the cognitive-behavioral theories. In fact, in a recent survey conducted by the AAMFT (Northey, 2002), participants were asked, "In a word or two, what is your primary treatment modality for intervention?" Of the 27 different modalities that were mentioned, CBT, multisystemic, eclectic, and solution-focused were the most frequently cited. CBT topped the list, which is quite a surprising change from what I experienced more than 20 years ago.

At the outset, however, behavioral family therapy was seen as useful only in cases involving children with behavioral disorders or family problems, where parenting issues were the focus. The subsequent addition of the cognitive component to the behavioral approach to couples and families failed to bring much more acceptance from the couple and family therapy community. In fact, some behavioral family therapists rejected this component outright and still do today, because they see it as hindering the process of behavioral interventions (Forgatch & Patterson, 1998).

Ironically, despite the sentiments on both sides, structural family therapy and Bowenian systems (which dominated the scene) actually folded many cognitive-behavioral techniques and interventions into the fabric of their approaches, although they employed different vocabularies to refer to them (Dattilio, 1998a). It has only been within the past decade that the field of couple and family therapy has begun to directly acknowledge the power and effectiveness of CBT—whether as a mode of integration with various forms of family therapy (Dattilio, 1998a; Dattilio & Epstein, 2003) or as an independent modality (Epstein & Baucom, 2002).

HISTORICAL OVERVIEW

In the early 1980s, cognitive-behavioral family therapy (CBFT) developed as an extension of its application to couples in conflict (Epstein, 1982). Although Albert Ellis (1977) has written that he adapted his model of rational–emotive therapy (RET) to work with couples as early as the late 1950s, little was written in marital and family therapy journals on this topic prior to 1980 (Ellis, 1977, 1978, 1986). It's not clear why Ellis (or anyone else, for that matter) never published more on the topic. However, it was most likely that the focus was placed more on individual issues. Also, the various forms of CBT were not well received in the family therapy arena during this decade. The later studies developed as offshoots of the behavioral approach, which first described interventions with couples and families in the late 1960s and early 1970s.

Principles of behavior modification were applied to interactional patterns of family members only after their successful application to couples in distress (Bandura, 1977; Patterson & Hops, 1972; Stuart, 1969, 1976). This work with couples was followed by several single-case studies involving the use of family interventions in treating children's behavior. For the first time, behaviorists recognized family members as having an impact on children's natural environment, and they were integrated into the treatment process (Falloon, 1991).

At about the same time, Patterson, McNeal, Hawkins, and Phelps (1967) and Patterson (1971) described a more refined and comprehensive style of intervention with the family unit. Since then, the professional literature has addressed the application of behavioral therapy to family systems, with a strong emphasis on contingency contracting and negotiation strategies (Gordon & Davidson, 1981; Jacobson & Margolin, 1979; Liberman, 1970; Patterson, 1982, 1985) as well as on environmental reprogramming (Patterson et al., 1967). Its reported applications remain oriented toward families with children who are diagnosed with specific behavioral problems (Sanders & Dadds, 1993).

Since its introduction almost 30 years ago, behavioral family therapy has received less attention from practitioners of couple and family therapy than have some of the other modalities. The lukewarm reception by the family therapy community to such an effective modality may be attributable to a combination of factors. For example, strategic, structural, and (more recently) postmodern approaches to family therapy have been promoted by such noted theorists as Minuchin (1974), Bowen (1978), Satir (1967), Madanes (1981), and White and Epston (1990), and many practitioners have been drawn to them. Furthermore, the behavioral approach may be seen by some as being too scientific to apply to families—that is, as too "wooden" or "sterile" to incorporate the art of treatment. It has also been criticized as failing to capture some of the commonly occurring dynamics of a family's interaction because of its staunch focus on thoughts and behaviors (Dattilio, 1998c). Finally, the behavioral approaches traditionally have been considered too linear in perspective and are viewed by many family therapists as inconsistent with systemic constructs (Nichols & Schwartz, 1998).

In truth, the strength of the pure behavioral approach is more in changing specific behavioral problems, such as poor communication or acting-out behaviors, than in understanding the comprehensive system of family dynamics (Sanders & Dadds, 1993; Goldenberg & Goldenberg, 1991). Clearly, the behavior therapies focus on observable behavior (symptoms) rather than on efforts to establish an intrapsychic or interpersonal causality. Certain targeted behaviors are directly manipulated through external means of reinforcement that undoubtedly reflect the rigor of behavior therapy (Dattilio, 2002). Families are also trained to monitor these reinforcements and to make modifications where necessary (Jacobson & Addis, 1993).

Regarding the focus on thinking in family therapy, a cognitive approach or cognitive component provided a viable supplement to traditional behaviorally oriented marital and family therapy (Margolin, Christensen, & Weiss, 1975). In addition to the work of Ellis (1977), an important study by Margolin and Weiss (1978), which suggested the effectiveness of a cognitive component to behavioral marital therapy, sparked further investigation into the use of cognitive techniques with dysfunctional couples (Baucom & Epstein, 1990; Baucom & Lester, 1986; Beck, 1988; Dattilio, 1989, 1990a, 1990b, 1992, 1993a, 1993b; Dattilio & Padesky, 1990; Doherty, 1981; Ellis, Sichel, Yeager, DiMattia, & DiGiuseppe, 1989; Epstein, 1992; Fincham, Bradbury, & Beach, 1990; Schindler & Vollmer, 1984; Weiss, 1984). Only a few studies have actually examined the impact of adding cognitive restructuring interventions to behavioral protocols (e.g., Baucom, Sayers, & Sher, 1990), typically by substituting some sessions of cognitive interventions for behaviorally oriented sessions in order to maintain equality across the treatments that were compared (Dattilio & Epstein, 2003). The results suggest that the combination of cognitive and behavioral interventions is as effective as the behavioral conditions, although cognitively focused interventions tend to produce more cognitive change, while behavioral interventions modify behavioral interactions (Baucom, Shoham, Mueser, Daiuto, & Stickle, 1998).

This interest in cognitive-behavioral approaches to couples also led behavioral family therapists to recognize that cognition plays a significant role in the events that mediate family interactions as well (Alexander & Parsons, 1982; Bedrosian, 1983). The important role of cognitive factors—not only in determining relationship distress, but also in mediating behavioral change—has become a popular topic among practitioners (Epstein, Schlesinger, & Dryden, 1988; Alexander, 1988; Dattilio, 1993a).

Although marital and family therapists began to realize decades ago that cognitive factors played a very important role in the alleviation of relationship dysfunction (Dicks, 1953), it took some time before cognition was formally included as a primary component of treatment (Munson, 1993). It also appears that traditional family therapists were guarded against becoming too "rationally oriented" in their work with families, preferring to be more of a "reflective instrument of change" (Minuchin, 1998). Even so, it appears that cognitive restructuring and the inclusion of behavioral change mechanisms are high on the list of what family therapists attempt to do, regardless of the modality they espouse (Bedrosian, 1993; Baucom & Lester, 1986; Dattilio, 1993a, 1994, 1998b; Dattilio & Bevilacqua, 2000). This has made for some interesting debate among theorists from a wide range of therapeutic modalities (Dattilio, 1998a).

A COGNITIVE-BEHAVIORAL MODEL
OF FAMILY THERAPY

The RET approach to family therapy, as proposed by Ellis (1978), places emphasis on each individual's perception and interpretation of the events that occur in the family environment. The theory assumes that "family members largely create their own world by the phenomenological view they take of what happens to them" (p. 310). The therapy focuses on how particular problems of the family members affect their well-being as a unit. During the process of treatment, family members are treated as individuals, each of whom subscribes to his or her own particular set of beliefs and expectations (Huber & Baruth, 1989; Russell & Morrill, 1989). The role of the family therapist is to help members make the connection that illogical beliefs and distortions serve as the foundation for their emotional distress.

Ellis's A-B-C theory maintains that family members blame their problems on certain activating events in the family environment (A). Members are taught to probe for irrational beliefs (B), which are then to be logically challenged by each family member and, finally, debated and disputed (C). The goal is to modify the beliefs and expectations to fit a more rational basis (Ellis, 1978). The role of the therapist, then, is to teach the family unit in an active and directive manner that the causes of emotional problems stem from irrational beliefs. By changing these self-defeating ideas, family members may improve the overall quality of the family relationship (Ellis, 1978, 1982). Unfortunately, RET does not place much emphasis on combining its principles with a systems approach, operating in a more linear fashion.

CBFT, while similar in some ways to the RET approach, assumes a different posture by focusing in greater depth on family interaction patterns and underlying dynamics. This is not to say that the RET theorists ignore underlying dynamics; however, CBFT appears to remain more consistent with elements derived from a systems perspective, while at the same time placing core emphasis on cognitive restructuring and behavioral change (Epstein et al., 1988; Leslie, 1988; Watts, 2001). In fact, CBFT in most cases is conducted against the backdrop of a systems approach. Within this framework, family relationships, cognitions, emotions, and behavior are viewed as exerting a mutual influence upon one another, so that a cognitive inference can evoke emotion and behavior, and emotion and behavior likewise can influence cognition. Once such a cycle among family members is initiated, a "system" of interaction occurs, yielding dysfunctional cognitions, behaviors, or emotions that can result in conflict. Teichman (1992) describes in detail the reciprocal model of family interaction, proposing that cognitions, feelings, behaviors, and environmental feedback are in constant reciprocal contact, and sometimes serve to maintain the dysfunction of the family unit. CBFT is grounded in cognitive mediation of individual functioning, which purports that an individual's emotional and behavioral reactions to life events are shaped by the particular interpretations that the individual makes of the events, rather than solely by objective characteristics of the events themselves (Beck, 1976; Ellis, 1978). Family members' behaviors are then viewed as constant life events that are interpreted and evaluated by other family members (Epstein & Schlesinger, 1996). (For a more detailed explanation of this concept, the reader is referred to Dattilio, 1998b, 1998c.)

Consistent and compatible with systems theory, the CBFT model includes the premise that members of a family simultaneously influence and are influenced by each other. Consequently, a behavior of one family member leads to behaviors, cognitions, and emotions in other members, which in turn elicit cognitions, behaviors, and emotions in response (Dattilio, Epstein, & Baucom, 1998). As the cycle continues, the volatility of the family dynamics escalates, rendering parts of the family unit vulnerable to a negative spiral of conflict. As the number of family members involved increases, so does the complexity of the dynamics, adding more fuel to the escalation process.

Cognitive therapy, as described by Beck (1976), places a heavy emphasis on schemas, or what have also been defined as core beliefs (Beck, Rush, Shaw, & Emery, 1979; DeRubeis & Beck, 1988). It was not until much later in his career that Beck applied his theories of schemas to couples. His book *Love Is Never Enough* (Beck, 1988) sparked my own interest in applying these concepts to my work with families. In this context, the therapeutic intervention draws on the assumptions of the family members as they interpret and evaluate one another, and on the emotions and behaviors that are generated in response to these cognitions. Although cognitive-behavioral theory does not hold that cognitive processes cause all family behavior, it does suggest that cognitive appraisal plays a significant role in the interrelationships among events, cognitions, emotions, and behaviors (Epstein et al., 1988; Wright & Beck, 1993). With the cognitive component of CBFT, restructuring distorted beliefs has a pivotal impact on changing dysfunctional behaviors, and vice versa. In fact, the use of CBT with families—as opposed to cognitive therapy or behavior therapy alone—has a number of advantages. I've come to view the therapies as being inseparable, like two sides of a coin, different but stronger together.

The Crucial Role of Schemas

Schemas are usually the backbone of CBFT. Just as people maintain basic schemas about themselves, their world, and their future, they also maintain schemas about their immediate families and families of origin. As I have stated in earlier writings, a heavier emphasis should be placed on examining cognitions among individual family members, as well as on what may be termed the "family schemas" (Dattilio, 1993b). These latter are jointly held beliefs of the family that have formed through years of integrated interactions among members of the family unit. It is suggested that individuals basically maintain two separate sets of schemas about families. These are family schemas related to the parents' families of origin and schemas related to families in general, or what Schwebel and Fine (1994) refer to as a personal theory of family life. The experiences and perceptions from the families of origin are what shape the schemas about both the immediate family and families in general. These schemas have a major impact on how each individual thinks, feels, and behaves in the family setting. A classic example involves parenting, especially disciplinary issues. Parents who may have come from families that maintained diametrically opposed values on discipline often experience conflict only after their own offspring are born. Hence one parent who was reared in an environment that was fairly strict may believe in following along the same line with his or her own offspring. However, if the other parent was raised in a different environment in which discipline was more relaxed, this may lead to conflict, especially if the couple cannot agree on a middle ground. The impact that this ultimately has on the children may vary, with the child potentially resenting the parent who espouses a more strict disciplinary regimen and allying with the parent who is more permissive. This dynamic may spawn certain schemas about loyalty and the balance of power in the family, which in turn will affect the offspring in his or her own relationships.

Schwebel and Fine (1992) elaborate on the term "family schemas" as used in their family model by describing these schemas as the cognitions that individuals hold about their immediate family life and about family life in general. They include attributions and beliefs about why events occur in the family, and beliefs about what should exist within the family unit (Baucom & Epstein, 1990). The family schemas also include ideas about how the spouses'/partners' relationships should work, what different types of problems should be expected in a couple relationship and how they should be handled, what is involved in building and maintaining a healthy family, what responsibilities each family member should have, what consequences should be associated with failure to meet responsibilities or to fulfill roles, and what costs and benefits each adult partner should expect to have as a consequence of being in a relationship. The late family therapy pioneer Virginia Satir wrote: "The marital relationship is the axis around which all of the family relationships are formed. The mates are the architects of the family" (Satir, 1967, p. 1). This suggests that the mates' core beliefs about life and family have a profound impact on the immediate family dynamics, including thoughts and behaviors.

Elsewhere (Dattilio, 1993a, 1998b), it has been suggested that the family of origin of each partner in a relationship plays a crucial role in the shaping of immediate family schemas. Beliefs funneled down from the family of origin may be both conscious and unconscious, and may contribute to joint schemas or blended schemas that lead to the development of the current family schemas.

These family schemas are subsequently disseminated and applied in the rearing of the children; when mixed with their individual thoughts and perceptions of their environment and life experiences, they contribute to the further development of the overall family schemas. The family schemas are subject to change as major events occur during the course of family life (e.g., death, divorce), and they also continue to evolve over the course of ordinary day-to-day experience.

Consequently, focusing on family schemas is the most essential aspect of treatment. Uncovering and identifying family schemas involve a series of cognitive and behavioral assessment procedures. From there, strategies used to restructure the basic or core beliefs of the family begin to take shape, and altering or modifying dysfunctional behavioral patterns becomes possible. The approach may encompass the use of inventories or questionnaires, such as the Family Beliefs Inventory (Vincent-Roehling & Robin, 1986) or the Family Inventory of Life Events and Changes (McCubbin, Patterson, & Wilson, 1985); or it may involve the extensive interviewing of family members. The behavioral component of CBFT focuses on several aspects of family members' actions, including (1) excess negative interactions and deficits in pleasing behaviors exchanged by family members, (2) expressive and listening skills used in communication, (3) problem-solving skills, and (4) negotiation and behavior changes skills. The theoretical models underlying behavioral approaches to family therapy are social learning theory (e.g., Bandura, 1977) and social exchange theory (e.g., Thibaut & Kelly, 1959).

The Role of Homework in the Restructuring Process

Among the many techniques in CBFT that are used to promote change, the use of homework assignments is probably given the least attention, even though it is cited as an integral part of a number of theoretical orientations. Homework assignments, or "out-of-session assignments," are usually utilized to help bolster the effects of the therapy process. Cognitive-behavioral therapists are recognized for the emphasis they place on homework assignments as a key component of treatment for a broad spectrum of disorders.

There are a number of benefits to using out-of-session assignments in the treatment of families. First, few situations are more volatile than that of a family in crisis, and the systematic use of such assignments helps to expand the therapeutic process beyond the therapy room. In other words, patients spend the majority of time outside the session, in the original environment from which the dysfunction often emanates, and homework keeps the therapeutic process alive as they move through their daily lives. This is particularly true in CBFT, which is predicated on structure and specific exercises. Homework also helps to move the family members into active involvement, signifying that they've already acknowledged the notion that change is beneficial (and possible) at both the personal and interpersonal levels (Dattilio, 2002b). A good example of this is a family whose members experience significant dysfunctional interaction with each other during the routine course of the day. Family members may develop negative schemas about their ability ever to get along with one another. As a result, assigning the family members to interact with one another in an enjoyable activity that is designed for success may be an initial step in helping them to restructure their thinking and promote optimism about their future relationship.

An additional benefit of homework is that the assignments provide the opportunity for patients to integrate insights and coping behaviors that have been discussed during the treatment process. The out-of-session work serves to heighten awareness of various issues that have been uncovered during the session and to expand this awareness at home. The very idea of homework assignments increases an atmosphere of positive expectation to follow through on *making* change, rather than simply considering the potential for change within the context of the therapy sessions. So, to continue with the example above, after the family has embarked on the assignment of interacting in an enjoyable activity, the subsequent therapy session may involve focusing on more positive feelings and having each family member view the others in a different light.

Various types of homework can be assigned at different stages of treatment. Bibliotherapy, for example, along with self-monitoring or other exercises that are designed to provide clinicians with valuable information about family interaction outside of the session, may be most efficacious early in treatment. Other types of homework may include behavioral tasks that enhance communication or problem-solving skills. Restructured self-talk and assignments that involve locating common bonds among family members, as well as other strategies, are often quite powerful in facilitating change.

Homework assignments are usually collaborative efforts involving both the family members and the therapist in their design and plans for implementation. Collaborative decisions may include the timing of an assignment, who will be involved, how often it will be carried out, and the length of time required to complete it. The advent of effective treatment and homework planners (Dattilio, 2000; Bevilacqua & Dattilio, 2001) has made out-of-session assignments an attractive and convenient option. Additional research will help to identify the long-term utility of such interventions.

RESEARCH IN CBFT: $N = 0$?

Faulkner, Klock, and Gale (2002) have recently conducted a content analysis on articles published in the marital/couple and family therapy literature from 1980 to 1999. The *American Journal of Family Therapy, Contemporary Family Therapy, Family Process*, and the *Journal of Marital and Family Therapy* were among the top journals from which 131 articles were examined that used quantitative research methodology. Of these 131 articles, fewer than half involved outcome studies. None of the studies reviewed considered CBFT, which is interesting, particularly since the 1990s witnessed a dramatic increase in the incidence rate of published studies using quantitative methodology. There has been some research conducted in the area of behavior therapy with families. For example, Patterson (1971) examined the effects of parent training during the course of family therapy. Falloon, Boyd, and McGill (1984) conducted one of the earlier studies addressing the treatment of schizophrenia during the process of using family behavior therapy. In an excellent article by Baucom et al. (1998), empirically supported couple and family interventions have been evaluated; however, most of the focus is on couple therapy rather than on actual family interventions. Few studies are presented that evaluate family intervention programs maintaining a strong behavioral orientation. The behavioral models are highlighted for their incorporation of traditional elements of CBT, such as functional assessment, teaching skills, homework, and time-limited treatment (Baucom et al., 1998, p. 79). The models typically combine education with training in communication and problem-solving skills. Attention is also given to the combination of education and stress management, relapse prevention, and goal attainment (Barrowclough & Tarrier, 1992). The curious paucity of material on CBFT in the literature may be traced to several unfortunate factors.

First, few family therapists actually limit their practice to CBFT (although quite a few employ psychoeducational methods that include providing information to change family members' view of problems, plus communication skills training). As a result, family therapists generally are not drawn to empirically comparing CBFT with some of the more popular modalities. And of those who do use CBFT exclusively, most are clinical practitioners rather than researchers. Second, conducting empirical research with families is a daunting prospect, particularly when one thinks about recruiting entire families for long-term outcome studies. Third, the trend in family therapy research has leaned more toward aspects of the therapeutic process (e.g., divorce and family relationships) than toward treatment outcome (Faulkner et al., 2002).

Still a youngster in the field of family therapy, albeit middle-aged in the developmental spectrum of psychotherapy, CBFT may not have gained the respect it deserves from family therapy researchers, despite its popularity in other domains. Add to these factors the limited funding for such research and the fact that less value is placed on family therapy in general by managed care organizations, and the lack of CBFT-specific research becomes less of a mystery.

There have been many more quantitative studies in cognitive-behavioral couple therapy than in family therapy (Baucom, Epstein, Sayers, & Sher, 1989; Baucom et al., 1998; Epstein, 2001), but it would be presumptive to fully apply the results of these studies to family dynamics. The dynamics underlying the family processes involve different and more complex interactional dynamics among multiple family members than in couples or dyadic relationships. Nevertheless, there is a place for studies that examine the cross-application of cognitive-behavioral interventions for families with those that have been used for individuals and couples. It would also be interesting to examine various characteristics of family members to determine what might constitute differential responses to treatment, as well as optimal sequences of behavior and the restructuring of schemas. For example, upon first determining the level of interfamily dependency that exists, we might look at the potential for such dependency to be equated with family members' tendencies to be more or less influenced by their interactions.

THE FUTURE OF CBFT

The trend in psychotherapy is toward effective short-term treatments, with many of the postmodern approaches to couple and family therapy promulgated by the strong influence of managed health care in the clinical sector. CBFT is likely to be more fully accepted by the family therapy community when it is integrated with other modalities that work from a systems perspective. Like other modalities, CBFT is effective itself, but its power is enhanced when it is combined with other paradigms. In this sense, the sum is greater than its parts—when the parts come together in the right combination. CBFT is particularly well positioned to join forces with other modalities to create treatment that is innovative, fresh, alive, and effective.

So where are we headed from here? Each year sees new texts, or revised versions of earlier texts, on family therapy theory and process. And with each new publication, more and better attention is devoted to CBT with couples and families (Nichols & Schwartz, 2001; Goldenberg & Goldenberg, 2003). The second edition of the *Handbook of Family Therapy,* edited by Sexton, Weeks, and Robbins (2003), includes an invited chapter by Dattilio and Epstein (2000) on CBT with couples and families. The first edition of this text, published in two volumes 10 years apart (1981 and 1991) and edited by Gurman and Kniskern, included one chapter on behavioral marital therapy by the late Neil Jacobson (1991) and one chapter on behavioral parenting training by Gordon and Davidson (1981). Very little mention was made in these chapters about the cognitive components of couple therapy, and there was nothing on the actual cognitive processes in family therapy. In a very short time, we have already come a long way.

REFERENCES

Alexander, P. (1988). The therapeutic implications of family cognitions and constructs. *Journal of Cognitive Psychotherapy, 2*(4), 219–236.

Alexander, J., & Parsons, B. V. (1982). *Functional family therapy.* Monterey, CA: Brooks/Cole.

Bandura, A. (1977). *Social learning theory.* Englewood Cliffs, NJ: Prentice-Hall.

Barrowclough, C., & Tarrier, N. (1992). *Families of schizophrenic patients: Cognitive-behavioral interventions.* London: Chapman & Hall.

Baucom, D. H., & Epstein, N. (1990). *Cognitive-behavioral marital therapy.* New York: Brunner/Mazel.

Baucom, D. H., Epstein, N., Sayers, S., & Sher, T. (1989). The role of cognition in marital relationships: Definitional, methodological, and conceptual issues. *Journal of Consulting and Clinical Psychology, 57,* 31–38.

Baucom, D. H., & Lester, G. W. (1986). The usefulness of cognitive restructuring as an adjunct to behavioral marital therapy. *Behavior Therapy, 17,* 385–403.

Baucom, D. H., Sayers, S. L., & Sher, T. G. (1990). Supplementing behavioral marital therapy with cognitive restructuring and emotional expressiveness training: An outcome investigation. *Journal of Consulting and Clinical Psychology, 58,* 636–645.

Baucom, D. H., Shoham, V., Mueser, K. T., Daiuto, A. D., & Stickle, T. R. (1998). Empirically supported couples and family therapy for adult problems. *Journal of Consulting and Clinical Psychology, 66*, 53–88.

Beck, A. T. (1967). *Depression: Clinical, experimental, and theoretical aspects.* New York: Harper & Row.

Beck, A. T. (1976). *Cognitive therapy and the emotional disorders.* New York: International Universities Press.

Beck, A. T. (1988). *Love is never enough.* New York: Harper & Row.

Beck, A. T., Rush, J. A., Shaw, B. F., & Emery, G. (1979). *Cognitive therapy of depression,* New York: Guilford Press.

Bedrosian, R. C. (1983). Cognitive therapy in the family system. In A. Freeman (Ed.), *Cognitive therapy with couples and groups* (pp. 95–106). New York: Plenum Press.

Bevilacqua, L. J., & Dattilio, F. M. (2001). *Brief family therapy homework planner.* New York: Wiley.

Bowen, M. (1978). *Family therapy in clinical practice.* New York: Aronson.

Dattilio, F. M. (1989). A guide to cognitive marital therapy. In P. A. Keller & S. R. Heyman (Eds.), *Innovations in clinical practice: A source book* (Vol. 8, pp. 27–42). Sarasota, FL: Professional Resource Exchange.

Dattilio, F. M. (1990a). Cognitive marital therapy: A case study. *Journal of Family Psychotherapy, 1*(1), 15–31.

Dattilio, F. M. (1990b). Una guida alla teràpia di coppia àd orientàsmente cognitivistà. *Terapia Familiare, 33*, 17–34.

Dattilio, F. M. (1992). Les therapies cognitives de couple. *Journal de Therapie Comportmentale et Cognitive, 2*(2), 17–29.

Dattilio, F. M. (1993a). Cognitive techniques with couples and families. *The Family Journal, 1*(1), 51–65.

Dattilio, F. M. (1993b). Un abordaje cognitivo en la terapia de parejas. *Revista Argentina de Clinica Psicologica, 2*(1), 45–57.

Dattilio, F. M. (1994). Videotape. *Cognitive therapy with couples: The initial phase of treatment,* Sarasota, FL: Professional Resource Press.

Dattilio, F. M. (1998a). (Ed.). *Case studies in couple and family therapy: Systemic and cognitive perspectives.* New York: Guilford Press.

Dattilio, F. M. (1998b). Cognitive-behavioral family therapy. In F. M. Dattilio (Ed.), *Case studies in couple and family therapy: Systemic and cognitive perspectives* (pp. 62–84). New York: Guilford Press.

Dattilio, F. M. (1998c). Finding the fit between cognitive-behavioral and family therapy. *The Family Therapy Networker, 22*(4), 63–73.

Dattilio, F. M. (2000). Families in crisis. In F. M. Dattilio & A. Freeman (Eds.), *Cognitive-behavioral strategies in crisis intervention* (2nd ed., pp. 316–338). New York: Guilford Press.

Dattilio, F. M. (2001). Cognitive-behavioral family therapy: Contemporary myths and misconceptions. *Contemporary Family Therapy, 23*(1), 3–18.

Dattilio, F. M. (2002a). Cognitive-behavior therapy comes of age: Grounding symptomatic treatment in an existential approach.. *The Psychotherapy Networker, 26*(1), 75–78.

Dattilio, F. M. (2002b). Homework assignments in couple and family therapy. *Journal of Clinical Psychology, 58*(5), 535–547.

Dattilio, F. M., & Bevilacqua, L. B. (Eds.). (2000). *Comparative treatment of couples relationships*. New York: Springer.

Dattilio, F. M., & Epstein, N. B. (2003). Cognitive-behavioral couple and family therapy. In T. Sexton, G. Weeks, & M. Robbins (Eds.), *Handbook of family therapy: The science and practice of working with families and couples* (pp. 147–173). New York: Brunner-Routledge.

Dattilio, F. M., Epstein, N. B., & Baucom, D. H. (1998). An introduction to cognitive-behavioral therapy with couples and families. In F. M. Dattilio (Ed.), *Case studies in couple and family therapy: Systemic and cognitive perspectives* (pp. 1–36). New York: Guilford Press.

Dattilio, F. M., & Padesky, C. A. (1990). *Cognitive therapy with couples*. Sarasota, FL: Professional Resource Exchange.

DeRubeis, R. J., & Beck, A. T. (1988). Cognitive therapy. In K. S. Dobson (Ed.) *Handbook of cognitive-behavioral therapies* (pp. 273–306). New York: Guilford Press.

Dicks, H. (1953). Experiences with marital tensions seen in the psychological clinic. *British Journal of Medical Psychology, 26*, 181–196.

Doherty, W. J. (1981). Cognitive processes in intimate conflict: 1. Extending attribution theory. *American Journal of Family Therapy, 9*, 5–13.

Ellis, A. (1977). The nature of disturbed marital interactions. In A. Ellis & R. Greiger (Eds.), *Handbook of rational–emotive therapy* (pp. 77–92). New York: Springer.

Ellis, A. (1978). Family therapy: A phenomenological and active-directive approach. *Journal of Marriage and Family Counseling, 4*(2), 43–50.

Ellis, A. (1982). Rational–emotive family therapy. In A. M. Horne & M. M. Ohlsen (Eds.), *Family counseling and therapy* (pp. 302–328). Itasca, IL: Peacock.

Ellis, A. (1986). Rational–emotive therapy applied to relationship therapy. *Journal of Rational–Emotive Therapy, 4*–21.

Ellis, A., Sichel, J. L., Yeager, R. J., DiMattia, D. J., & DiGiuseppe, R. (1989). *Rational–emotive couples therapy*. Needham Heights, MA: Allyn & Bacon.

Epstein, N. (1982). Cognitive therapy with couples. *American Journal of Family Therapy, 10*(1), 5–16.

Epstein, N. (1992). Marital therapy. In A. Freeman & F. M. Dattilio (Eds.), *Comprehensive casebook of cognitive therapy* (pp. 267–275), New York: Plenum Press.

Epstein, N. (2001). Cognitive-behavioral therapy with couples: Empirical status. *Journal of Cognitive Psychotherapy, 15*(2), 299–310.

Epstein, N., & Baucom, D. H. (2002). *Enhanced cognitive-behavioral therapy for couples: A contextual approach*. Washington, DC: American Psychological Association.

Epstein, N., & Schlesinger, S. E. (1996). Treatment of family problems. In M. Reinecke, F. M. Dattilio, & A. Freeman (Eds.), *Cognitive therapy with children and adolescents: A casebook for clinical practice* (pp. 299–326). New York: Guilford Press.

Epstein, N., Schlesinger, S., & Dryden, W. (1988). Concepts and methods of cognitive-behavioral family treatment. In N. Epstein, S. Schlesinger, & W. Dryden

(Eds.), *Cognitive-behavioral therapy with families* (pp. 5–48). New York: Brunner/Mazel.

Falloon, I. R. H. (1991). Behavioral family therapy. In A. S. Gurman & D. P. Kniskern (Eds.), *Handbook of family therapy* (Vol. 2, pp. 65–95), New York: Brunner/Mazel.

Falloon, I. R. H., Boyd, J. L., & McGill, C. W. (1984). *Family care of schizophrenia.* New York: Guilford Press.

Faulkner, R. A., Klock, K., & Gale, J. E. (2002). Qualitative research in family therapy: Publication trends from 1980 to 1999. *Journal of Marital and Family Therapy, 28*(1), 69–74.

Fincham, F. D., Bradbury, T. N., & Beach, S. R. H. (1990). To arrive where we began: A reappraisal of cognition in marriage and in marital therapy. *Journal of Family Psychology, 4*(2), 167–184.

Forgatch, M. S., & Patterson, G. R. (1998). Behavioral family therapy. In F. M. Dattilio (Ed.), *Case studies in couple and family therapy: Systemic and cognitive perspectives* (pp. 85–107). New York: Guilford Press.

Goldenberg, I., & Goldenberg, H. (1991). *Family therapy: An overview* (3rd ed.). Pacific Grove, CA: Brooks/Cole.

Goldenberg, I., & Goldenberg, H. (2003). *Family therapy: An overview* (6th ed.). Pacific Grove, CA: Brooks/Cole.

Gordon, S. B., & Davidson, N. (1981). Behavioral parenting training. In A. S. Gurman & D. P. Kniskern (Eds.), *Handbook of family therapy* (pp. 517–577). New York: Brunner/Mazel.

Huber, C. H., & Baruth, L. G. (1989). *Rational–emotive family therapy: A systems perspective.* New York: Springer.

Jacobson, N. S. (1991). Behavioral marital therapy. In A. S. Gurman & D. P. Kniskern (Eds.), *Handbook of family therapy* (pp. 556–591). New York: Brunner/Mazel.

Jacobson, N. S., & Addis, M. E. (1993). Research on couples and couples therapy: What do we know? Where are we going? *Journal of Consulting and Clinical Psychology, 61*(1), 85–93.

Jacobson, N. S., & Margolin, G. (1979). *Marital therapy: Strategies based on social learning and behavior exchange principles.* New York: Brunner/Mazel.

Leslie, L. A. (1988). Cognitive-behavioral and systems models of family therapy: How compatible are they? In N. Epstein, S. E. Schlesinger, & W. Dryden (Eds.), *Cognitive-behavioral therapy with families* (pp. 49–83). New York: Brunner/Mazel.

Liberman, R. P. (1970). Behavioral approaches to couple and family therapy. *American Journal of Orthopsychiatry, 40*, 106–118.

Madanes, C. (1981). *Strategic family therapy,* San Francisco: Jossey-Bass.

Margolin, G., Christensen, A., & Weiss, R. L. (1975). Contracts, cognition and change: A behavioral approach to marriage therapy. *Counseling Psychologist, 5*, 15–25.

Margolin, G., & Weiss, R. L. (1978). Comparative evaluation of therapeutic components associated with behavioral marital treatments. *Journal of Consulting and Clinical Psychology, 46*, 1476–1486.

McCubbin, H. I., Patterson, J. M., & Wilson, L. R. (1985). FILE: Family Inventory of Life Events and Changes. In D. H. Olson, H. I. McCubbin, H. Barnes, A. Larsen,

M. Muxen, & M. Wilson (Eds.), *Family inventories* (rev. ed., pp. 272–275). St. Paul: Family Social Science, University of Minnesota.

Minuchin, S. (1974). *Families and family therapy*, Cambridge, MA: Harvard University Press.

Minuchin, S. (1998). *Workshop: Family therapy for the new millennium.* New York: Minuchin Center for Family Therapy.

Munson, C. E. (1993). Cognitive family therapy. In D. K. Granvold (Ed.), *Cognitive and behavioral treatment: Methods and applications* (pp. 202–221). Pacific Grove, CA: Brooks/Cole.

Nichols, M., & Schwartz, R. (1998). *Family therapy: Concepts and methods* (4th ed.). Boston: Allyn & Bacon.

Nichols, M., & Schwartz, R. (2001). *Family therapy: Concepts and methods* (5th ed.). Boston: Allyn & Bacon.

Northey, W. M., Jr. (2002). Characteristics and clinical practices of marriage and family therapists: A national survey. *Journal of Marital and Family Therapy, 28*(4), 487–494.

Patterson, G. R. (1971). *Families: Applications of social learning to life.* Champaign, IL: Research Press.

Patterson, G. R. (1982). *Coercive family processes: A social learning approach* (Vol. 3). Eugene, OR: Castalia.

Patterson, G. R. (1985). Beyond technology: The next stage in developing an empirical base for parent training. In L. L'Abate (Ed.), *Handbook of family psychology and therapy* (Vol. 2, pp. 26–39). Homewood, IL: Dorsey Press.

Patterson, G. R., & Hops, H. (1972). Coercion, a game for two: Intervention techniques for marital conflict. In R. E. Ulrich & P. Mountjoy (Eds.), *The experimental analysis of social behavior* (pp. 424–440). New York: Appleton-Century-Crofts.

Patterson, G. R., McNeal, S., Hawkins, N., & Phelps, R. (1967). Reprogramming the social environment. *Journal of Child Psychology and Psychiatry, 8,* 181–195.

Russell, T., & Morrill, C. M. (1989). Adding a systematic touch to rational–emotive therapy for families. *Journal of Mental Health Counseling, 11*(2), 184–192.

Sanders, M. R., & Dadds, M. R. (1993). *Behavioral family intervention,* Needham Heights, MA: Allyn & Bacon.

Satir, V. M. (1967). *Conjoint family therapy.* Palo Alto, CA: Science & Behavior Books.

Schindler, L., & Vollmer, M. (1984). Cognitive perspectives in behavioral marital therapy: Some proposals for bridging theory, research and practice. In K. Hahlweg & N. S. Jacobson (Eds.), *Marital interaction: Analysis and modification* (pp. 146–162). New York: Guilford Press.

Schwebel, A. I., & Fine, M. A. (1992). Cognitive-behavioral family therapy. *Journal of Family Psychotherapy, 3,* 73–91.

Schwebel, A. I., & Fine, M. A. (1994). *Understanding and helping families: A cognitive-behavioral approach.* Hillsdale, NJ: Erlbaum.

Sexton, T., Weeks, G., & Robbins, M. (Eds.). (2003). *Handbook of family therapy: The science and practice of working with families and couples.* New York: Brunner-Routledge.

Stuart, R. B. (1969). Operant-interpersonal treatment of marital discord. *Journal of Consulting and Clinical Psychology, 33*, 675–682.

Stuart, R. B. (1976). Operant interpersonal treatment for marital discord. In D. H. L. Olsen (Ed.), *Treating relationships* (pp. 675–682). Lake Mills, IA: Graphic Press.

Teichman, Y. (1992). Family treatment with an acting-out adolescent. In A. Freeman & F. M. Dattilio (Eds.), *Comprehensive casebook of cognitive therapy* (pp. 331–346), New York: Plenum Press.

Thibaut, J. W., & Kelly, H. H. (1959). *The social psychology of groups*. New York: Wiley.

Vincent-Roehling, P. V., & Robin, A. L. (1986). Development and validation of the Family Beliefs Inventory: A measure of unrealistic beliefs among parents and adolescents. *Journal of Clinical and Consulting Psychology, 54*, 693–697.

Watts, R. E. (2001). Integrating cognitive and systemic perspectives: An interview with Frank M. Dattilio. *The Family Journal, 9*(4), 422–476.

Weiss, R. L. (1984). Cognitive and strategic interventions in behavioral marital therapy. In K. Hahlweg & N. S. Jacobson (Eds.), *Marital interaction: Analysis and modification* (pp. 337–355). New York: Guilford Press.

White, M., & Epston, D. (1990). *Narrative means to therapeutic ends*. New York: Norton.

Wright, J. H., & Beck, A. T. (1993). Family cognitive therapy with inpatients: Part II. In J. H. Wright, M. E. Thase, A. T. Beck, & J. W. Ludgate (Eds.), *Cognitive therapy with inpatients: Developing a cognitive milieu* (pp. 176–190). New York: Guilford Press.

Index

Abandoned Child mode
  in borderline personality disorder,
    276, 278
  definition, 276
  and DSM-IV criteria, 278
  image of therapist in, 296
  and reparenting approach, 280, 281
  treatment of, 287, 288
  dangers, 288
Abused children, personality disorder,
  325
Addictions, 206–227
  automatic thoughts, 212, 213
  Beck's contribution, 10, 13
  behavioral rituals, 215, 216
  cognitive therapy empirical findings,
    217–219
  combined treatments, 223, 224
  cravings and urges, 213, 214
  high-risk stimuli, 209, 210
  lapses, 216, 217
  maladaptive beliefs, 210–212, 214,
    215
  myopic decision making, 128–130
  stages-of-change model, 221, 222
  therapeutic alliance importance, 219–
    221
Additive effects, medication, 342, 354
Adolescent personality disorder, 319–
  337
  arguments for and against, 324, 325
  assessment and diagnosis, 328–332
  and DSM-IV criteria, 320–322
  therapy process, 334, 335
  treatment conceptualization, 332, 333
  treatment costs, 333
Affect regulation
  borderline personality disorder, 284
  and looming vulnerability style, 78

schema therapy stage, 280–286
"Affect without recollection" 144, 145
Agoraphobia, 98, 108
Alcohol abuse, 206–227
  behavioral rituals, 215, 216
  combined treatments, 223, 224
  high-risk stimuli, 209, 210
  lapses, 216, 217
  maladaptive beliefs, 210–212, 214, 215
  myopic decision making, 128–130
  stages-of-change model, 221, 222
  therapeutic alliance importance, 219–221
Alprazolam
  combined treatment use, 348, 354
  discontinuation, 345
  memory effects, 344
Anger
  Beck's model, 9, 11
  limit setting, 292, 293
  and schema modes, 278
  and therapist–patient relationship, 292,
    293
Anger management, 286, 293, 294
Angry and Impulsive Child mode
  borderline personality disorder, 276, 278,
    292–295
  definition, 276
  image of therapist in, 296
  treatment, 292–295
  dangers, 295
Antidepressants
  in anxiety disorders, 348, 349, 354
  in bulimia nervosa, 349, 350
  cognitive reactivity differential effect, 34
  and cognitive therapy, 45–55, 346, 347
  early studies, 46–49
  outcome research interpretation, 352–
    354
  response rates, 48, 51, 52